POCKET CONSULT

# Obstetrics

## G.M. Stirrat
MA, MD, FRCOG
*Professor of Obstetrics and Gynaecology,
University of Bristol*

SECOND EDITION

Blackwell Scientific Publications

OXFORD LONDON EDINBURGH
BOSTON PALO ALTO MELBOURNE

© G.M. Stirrat 1981, 1986

Blackwell Scientific Publications
Editorial offices:
Osney Mead, Oxford, OX2 0EL
8 John Street, London, WC1N 2ES
23 Ainslie Place, Edinburgh,
 EH3 6AJ
52 Beacon Street, Boston
 Massachusetts 02108, USA
667 Lytton Avenue, Palo Alto
 California 94301, USA
107 Barry Street, Carlton
 Victoria 3053, Australia

All rights reserved. No part of this publication may be reproduced, stored in a retrieval system, or transmitted, in any form or by any means, electronic, mechanical, photocopying, recording or otherwise without the prior permission of the copyright owner

First published 1981
Second edition 1986

Photoset by Enset (Photosetting), Midsomer Norton, Bath, Avon

Printed in Great Britain
by the Alden Press, Oxford

DISTRIBUTORS

USA
 Year Book Medical Publishers
 35 East Wacker Drive
 Chicago, Illinois 60601

Canada
 The C.V. Mosby Company
 5240 Finch Avenue East,
 Scarborough, Ontario

Australia
 Blackwell Scientific
 Publications
 (Australia) Pty Ltd
 107 Barry Street
 Carlton, Victoria 3053

British Library
Cataloguing in Publication Data

Stirrat, Gordon, M.
Obstetrics.—2nd ed.—(Pocket consultant)
1. Obstetrics
I. Title
618.2   RG524
ISBN 0-632-01394-X

# Contents

Prefaces, iv

Acknowledgements, v

1.0 Introduction, 1

2.0 Physiological changes in pregnancy, 7

3.0 Fetal growth and development, 23

4.0 The placenta and amniotic fluid, 33

5.0 Antenatal care, 45

6.0 Congenital malformation, 61

7.0 Medical complications of pregnancy, 77

8.0 Rhesus iso-immunization, 119

9.0 Maternal and fetal infections, 127

10.0 Some practical problems, 145

11.0 Labour, 167

12.0 Obstetric emergencies, 225

13.0 Perinatal and infant mortality, 241

14.0 Maternal mortality, 249

15.0 The neonate, 255

16.0 The puerperium, 277

17.0 Prescribing during pregnancy and lactation, 287

Suggested further reading, 301

Abbreviations, 303

Conversion tables, 304

Useful addresses, 306

Index, 308

# Prefaces

### To first edition
This book is designed to be a mine of useful information for all who look after pregnant women. House officers, obstetricians (budding and otherwise), GPs, midwives and medical students will find within its pages facts which should help to make the physiology and pathology of pregnancy clearer to them and their patients.

This is not a text book, nor can it replace that most valuable of schoolmasters, experience. It must, by its very nature, be selective and it may seem dogmatic. The reader is encouraged to use the blank sheets provided for personal notes and additions. While every effort has been made to ensure that everything in the book is factually correct there remain 'ifs and buts' behind many of the statements. The range of normality is wide and our knowledge still only partial.

### To second edition
The material in this second edition represents a comprehensive updating of changes in knowledge, practice and fashion since the first edition was published as well as correction of any errors of omission or commission. Several subjects are covered in detail for the first time (e.g. ultrasound in pregnancy, AIDS, the management of the third stage and neonatal screening for cystic fibrosis) because they are currently matters of debate. Everything written in the first edition has been re-thought and the author hopes it will be even more useful for all who care for pregnant women.

The author is grateful for the helpful comments and criticisms he has received from readers of the first edition and has responded to them.

# Acknowledgements

In addition to those who gave invaluable assistance with the first edition I am deeply indebted to the following whose suggestions have helped me in preparing the second: Dr. Peter Fleming, Dr. David James, Mr. Walter Prendiville, and Dr. Trevor Thomas.

The work of a multitude of authors over many years has contributed to the body of knowledge incorporated in the book and I would particularly like to thank the following authors and publishers for permission to reproduce material:

Blood coagulation cascade (p. 16) adapted from Scientific Tables. p. 622 published by Documenta Geigy 1970. Centile values of Birthweight for Gestational Age in Scottish Infants (p. 26) by Mary Smalls and J. Forbes. Social Paediatric Research Unit, University of Glasgow 1984. Uterine fundal height (p. 31) Robinson *et al., Brit. J. Obstet. Gynaec.* **88,** 115, 1981.

Oestrogen/creatinine ratios (p. 42) derived from data provided by D.J. Goldie, Department of Clinical Chemistry, Southmead Hospital, Bristol. Antacid therapy (p. 210) and hypotensive regimes (p. 233) by T.A. Thomas, Department of Anaesthetics, Bristol Maternity Hospital. Action-line analysis adapted from Whitfield, *Amer. J. Obstet. and Gynaecol.* **108,** 1239, 1970. Biophysical profile scoring by Chamberlain and Manning, *Medicine* **1,** 1658, 1983. External cephalic version (p. 161) derived from Hofmeyr, *Brit. J. Obstet. Gynaecol.* **90,** 293, 1983. Characteristics of uterine activity by Steer *et al., Brit. J. Obstet. Gynaecol.* **91,** 220, 1984. Anticonvulsant regimes, (p. 231) Dr. I.G. Robertson St. Mary's Hospital, Manchester. Perinatal mortality in England and Wales 1981 (p. 245) from OPCS DH3 84/3 and 4. Maternal mortality (p. 251) from Confidential Enquiry into Maternal Mortality in England and Wales 1979–81, HMSO. Clinical assessment of gestational age in the newborn infant (p. 263) from Dubowitz *et al., J. Pediat.* **77,** 1, 1970 and Farr *et al., Develop. Med. Child Neurol.* **8,** 507, 1966. Neonatal diagnosis of cystic fibrosis (p. 274) by A.F. Heeley, regional Neonatal Screening Laboratory, Peterborough General Hospital. Procedures relating to AIDS and labour from Prof. C.N. Hudson.

# 1.0 Introduction

**1.1 Length of pregnancy, 3**

**1.2 Fertilization and implantation, 3**

**1.3 Expected date of delivery, 3**

**1.4 Parity and gravidity, 4**

## 1.0 Introduction

### 1.1 Length of pregnancy
Ovulation occurs 14 days before the onset of the next menses. Only in a regular 28 day cycle is this 14 days from the first day of the last menstrual period (LMP). Pregnancy begins with fertilization of the ovum which is difficult to time with certainty and it is therefore conventional to date **gestational age** from the first day of the LMP.

The mean length of pregnancy is 278±15 days whereas the time from ovulation to delivery is 265±12 days.

### 1.2 Fertilization and implantation
The ovum is fertilized in the outer third of the fallopian tube and the **stages of formation of the blastocyst** are as follows:

| | | |
|---|---|---|
| Stage 1 | 1 cell | 0–24 hours |
| Stage 2 | 2 cells | 24–36 hours |
| | 3–4 cells | 36–48 hours |
| | 5–8 cells | 48–72 hours |
| | 9–16 cells | 72–96 hours (arrives in uterus) |
| Stage 3 | Free blastocyst | 4–5 days |
| | 50–60 cells | about 96 hours |
| | 100–110 cells | about 108 hours |
| Stage 4 | Implantation | 6–9 days |
| Stage 5 | Avillous blastocyst | 10–12 days |
| | Lacunae in trophoblast contain maternal blood | 12 days |
| Stage 6 | Primitive chorionic villi | 13–15 days |

### 1.3 Expected date of delivery
To calculate the **expected date of delivery** (EDD) add 7 days and

# 1.0 Introduction

1.4 Parity and gravidity

9 months to the date of onset of the LMP. The **gestational age** can be calculated quickly by remembering that in each quarter of a year there are 13 weeks, e.g. if one wishes to calculate gestational age on 27th October when the LMP began on 13th June.

| | |
|---|---:|
| From 13 June to 13 September is | 13 weeks |
| and from 13 September to 27 October is | 6 weeks |
| therefore gestational age is | 19 weeks |

## 1.4 Parity and gravidity

The parity of a woman is the number of her previous pregnancies which have lasted more than 28 weeks. When written (e.g. Para 1+1) the second figure denotes pregnancies ending before 28 weeks. The term gravidity includes all pregnancies at whatever gestation they have ended as well as any current pregnancy. Thus, a woman who is Para 1+1 but who is not pregnant is Gravida 2; if she is pregnant she is Gravida 3. A multiple pregnancy is best counted as one in parity and gravidity.

# 2.0 Physiological changes in pregnancy

- **2.1 Cardiovascular dynamics, 7**
- **2.2 Respiratory function, 8**
- **2.3 Composition of blood, 9**
- **2.4 Blood coagulation in pregnancy, 15**
- **2.5 Renal function, 17**
- **2.6 Adrenal function, 18**
- **2.7 Thyroid function, 18**
- **2.8 Hypothalamo-pituitary function, 19**
- **2.9 Alimentary function, 20**
- **2.10 Carbohydrate metabolism in pregnancy, 20**
- **2.11 Weight gain during pregnancy, 21**

## 2.0 Physiological changes in pregnancy

### 2.1 Cardiovascular dynamics
**Plasma volume** increases progressively to its maximum at 34 weeks.
The mean total increase in
> primigravidae is about 1250 ml
> multigravidae is about 1500 ml

From 34 weeks the volume falls by 200–300 ml, and a further drop of 500–600 ml occurs at delivery. It has returned to non-pregnant levels by 6–8 weeks postpartum. **Cardiac output** rises by about 1.5 l/minute within the first 10 weeks of pregnancy and is maintained at this increased level. The sleeping **heart rate** is raised by about 15 beats/minute and the **stroke volume** from 64 to 71 ml from early pregnancy. In labour the heart rate accelerates at the onset of a contraction and begins to decelerate at its height. The **arterio-venous oxygen difference** of the blood is reduced because cardiac output is raised with a smaller rise in oxygen consumption. It is at its lowest in early pregnancy.

### Blood pressure
Specific levels cannot be given for pregnancy because the individual variation is so great. The **systolic blood pressure** (SBP) falls slightly in early pregnancy but rises again in late pregnancy. The **diastolic blood pressure** (DBP) is well below non-pregnant levels from early in pregnancy. It returns to those levels after 30–32 weeks gestation. The pulse pressure is therefore increased in the first and second trimesters. Blood pressure falls significantly during sleep. Uterine contractions in labour are associated with a rise in blood pressure. The sphygmomanometer overestimates SBP by about 7 mmHg and the DBP by about 12 mmHg in pregnancy.

### Other cardiovascular changes
**Peripheral resistance** is low at the beginning of pregnancy but gradually increases thereafter.

## 2.0 Physiological changes in pregnancy

2.2 Respiratory function

**Circulation time** changes very little.

**Venous pressure** is greatly increased in the femoral and other leg veins but not in the arms. This is due to compression of the inferior vena cava by uterus and fetus, and the pressure of blood returning from the uterus. About 300 ml of blood is expelled from the uterus during a contraction. Venous distensibility increases in pregnancy. The heart increases in size: it is pushed upwards and forwards and ECG changes may occur as listed below:

- T wave flattening or reversal in lead III
- depression of S-T segment in both chest and limb leads (possibly)
- lower voltage QRS complexes
- deep Q waves and occasional U waves.

Ectopic beats are common and occasional episodes of supraventricular tachycardia may occur.

### 2.2 Respiratory function

The lower ribs flare out; the subcostal angle increases from 68° in early pregnancy to 103° at term. The transverse diameter of the chest increases by 2 cm. The diaphragm is raised 4 cm and its excursion in breathing is greater.

The **respiratory rate** does not change.

The **tidal volume** (the volume of gas inspired and expired in each respiration) rises progressively in pregnancy by 0.1–0.2 l.

The **expiratory reserve volume** (the maximum amount of air expired from the resting end-expiratory positions) falls by about 15%.

The **residual volume** (the volume of gas remaining at the end of maximal expiration excluding that in dead space) falls by 20%. This fall, combined with the increased tidal volume, causes more efficient gas mixing.

**Vital capacity** (the maximum volume of gas which can be expired after maximum inspiration) does not change.

**Inspiratory capacity** (the maximum volume of gas which can be

## 2.0 Physiological changes in pregnancy

### 2.3 Composition of blood

inspired from the resting end expiratory position) rises by about 5%.

The **minute volume** (tidal volume×respiration rate) increases by 40%.

Airway resistance is reduced, possibly by an increase in airway cross-section.

Oxygen consumption rises by about 15% in late pregnancy (circa 32 ml/min). This increase is met by the increased oxygen carrying capacity of the blood. The increase in ventilation in pregnancy greatly exceeds the increase in oxygen consumption. The alveolar concentration of $CO_2$, therefore falls.

Alveolar $PCO_2$ falls slightly in the luteal phase of the cycle from about 37–39 mmHg (5.0–5.2 kPa) and this fall continues in pregnancy to about 31 mmHg (4.1 kPa) at 28 weeks gestation. This may be an effect of progesterone. The respiratory centres are more sensitive to changes in $PCO_2$ possibly due to oestrogen. For every 1 mmHg rise in $PCO_2$ in the non-pregnant ventilation increases by 1.5 l/min. In pregnancy the increase is 6.0 l/min. This may cause some dyspnoea and reduces maternal plasma bicarbonate and thus plasma sodium and osmolality. The fetus benefits by being able to get rid of $CO_2$ without itself having a high $PCO_2$.

### 2.3 Composition of blood

#### 2.3.1 Haematological indices (Table 2.1)
**Red cell mass** decreases initially by about 100 ml at 12 weeks gestation. It then increases gradually towards term when it is about 250 ml above the non-pregnant level if no iron supplements are given. The increase is up to 400 ml if iron is given. Some changes are still present 8 weeks postpartum but the red cell mass is normal by 4–6 months.

**Red cell fragility**: The erythrocytes are more spherical in pregnancy due to a fall in colloid osmotic pressure. They therefore are more susceptible to haemolysis by taking up water.

## 2.0 Physiological changes in pregnancy

### 2.3 Composition of blood

**Table 2.1.** Haematological indices in pregnancy.

|  | Non-pregnant A* | B† | 12 weeks A | B | 36 weeks A | B |
|---|---|---|---|---|---|---|
| White cell count ($\times 10^9$/l) | 5.6 | 6.3 | 6.9 | 8.1 | 10.2 | 10.0 |
| Red cell count ($\times 10^{12}$/l) | 4.7 | 4.6 | 4.0 | 4.1 | 3.9 | 4.1 |
| Haemoglobin concentration (g/dl) | 13.3 | 13.4 | 12.0 | 12.1 | 11.1 | 12.7 |
| Haematocrit (l/l) | 0.4 | 0.4 | 0.35 | 0.35 | 0.33 | 0.37 |
| Mean cell volume (fl) | 83.7 | 85.7 | 86.2 | 86.0 | 85.0 | 88.8 |
| Mean cell haemoglobin (pg) | 28.4 | 29.0 | 30.1 | 29.4 | 28.7 | 30.8 |
| Mean cell haemoglobin concentration (g/dl) | 33.8 | 33.6 | 34.2 | 34.1 | 33.5 | 34.5 |

*A No haematinics
†B Iron and folic acid supplements given

**Erythrocyte deformibility index** increases from about 0.85 before pregnancy to 0.97 by 12 weeks. It is at its highest (1.16) by 32 weeks declining gradually towards a term value of 1.0.

**Leucocytes:** The increase in white cell count is due almost entirely to a change in neutrophils which are at their maximum at 30 weeks. Despite conflicting reports it is likely that lymphocyte concentrations and the proportion in each subset are unchanged.

**Platelets:** The normal platelet count is 150–400 $\times 10^9$/l. Counts in normal pregnancy vary from patient to patient but do not change significantly as a result of the pregnancy.

**Plasma viscosity,** which is a balance between rising fibrinogen and falling total protein levels, is at its highest by 12 weeks then falls slowly. It is still above non-pregnant levels at term.

**Whole blood viscosity** is unchanged in the first half of pregnancy because the rise in plasma viscosity is matched by the fall in haematocrit. It is at its lowest between 24 and 36 weeks then rises along with the haematocrit.

Cigarette smoking increases blood viscosity.

**Blood sedimentation rate** (BSR) or erythrocyte sedimentation

## 2.0 Physiological changes in pregnancy

2.3 Composition of blood

rate (ESR) rises from the non-pregnant level of 20 mm in the first hour, to between 44 and 114 mm (mean 78) during pregnancy. The rise is due to increased globulin and fibrinogen levels.

### Erythropoiesis

The normal daily diet contains 10–15 mg of iron of which 5 to 10% is absorbed. Only 65% of it is used for haemoglobin. The iron requirements in the second and third trimesters of pregnancy are about 2.7 mg/day to compensate for fetal needs and blood loss at delivery. Lactation adds another 0.8 mg/day to the requirements. The average serum iron concentration in late pregnancy is 35% below the non-pregnant level of 11–27 $\mu$mol/l. This can be modified but not prevented by iron supplements. The iron binding capacity doubles in pregnancy from 50 $\mu$mol/l to about 100 $\mu$mol/l.

Folic acid is obtained from fresh green vegetables, liver and kidneys. The normal **serum folate** is 14–48 nmol/l but it falls progressively towards term to below 8 nmol/l.

**Red cell folate** makes up 95% of blood folate. The normal level is > 360 nmol/l but this falls gradually in pregnancy. Levels of < 180 nmol/l are often associated with megaloblastic anaemia. Diagnosis needs to be confirmed by bone marrow examination. Red cell folate levels can be maintained in pregnancy by 100 $\mu$g supplementary folic acid daily (see page 000).

**Vitamin $B_{12}$** levels fall from 400 $\mu$mol/l in early pregnancy to 325 $\mu$mol/l at term. They may be at their lowest between 16–20 weeks gestation. True deficiency of Vitamin $B_{12}$ is rare in pregnancy.

### Serum electrolytes

**Sodium** falls in early pregnancy from 140 to 137 mmol/l and remains relatively constant thereafter.

**Potassium** falls similarly from 4.3 to 4.0 mmol/l by 28 weeks but may rise in late pregnancy to near non-pregnant levels. **Calcium** falls from 2.5 to 2.3 mmol/l at term in line with the decrease in

## 2.0 Physiological changes in pregnancy

### 2.3 Composition of blood

albumin. **Magnesium** gradually falls from 0.8 to 0.7 mmol/l to term. **Copper** increases from a non-pregnant level of 1.14 mg/l to 2.39 mg/l at term. Most of this is contained in caeruloplasmin. **Serum osmolality** falls quickly within the first 8 weeks by 10 m osmol/kg $H_2O$ to 280 m osmol/kg $H_2O$ at which level it remains throughout the remainder of the pregnancy.

### Non-protein nitrogen (Table 2.2)

The concentration of urea falls in early pregnancy by up to 25% compared to non-pregnant levels. Levels above 5.0 mmol/l are abnormal in pregnancy.

The range of **uric acid** levels is wide before, during, and after pregnancy. Levels tend to remain low until about 24 weeks then gradually rise to above pre-pregnancy levels by term. Any changes which may occur in relation to pre-eclampsia must be interpreted in this light.

**Creatinine** levels are reduced in normal pregnancy due to increased renal clearance.

**Table 2.2.** Non protein nitrogen levels in pregnancy.

| Gestational age (weeks) | Serum urea (mol/l) | Serum uric acid (mmol/l) | Serum creatinine ($\mu$m/l) |
|---|---|---|---|
| 12 | 3.5 | 0.17 | 60 |
| 24–26 | 3.3 | 0.20 | 45 |
| 38–40 | 3.1 | 0.27 | 40 |
| Non-pregnant | 4.3 | 0.25 | 70 |

### Serum proteins

The **total protein concentration** falls in the first trimester and reaches a plateau around mid-pregnancy lying about 10 g/l below the non-pregnancy level.

**Albumin** concentration falls quickly in the first trimester and continues to fall more slowly until late pregnancy. The overall fall is about 10 g/l. Pre-eclampsia leads to an even greater fall.

## 2.0 Physiological changes in pregnancy

### 2.3 Composition of blood

**Alpha 1-globulin** rises progressively by about 1 g/l. It is not affected by pre-eclampsia.
**Alpha 2-globulin** rises by about 1 g/l.
**Beta-globulin** rises progressively by up to 3 g/l. There is no further effect from pre-eclampsia.
**Gamma-globulin** falls by up to 1 g/l.
**Pregnancy-associated and pregnancy-specific proteins**—(See Chapter 4).

Most of these serum protein changes can be mimicked in non-pregnant women by giving ethinyl oestradiol 0.5 mg for 20 days.

**Colloid osmotic pressure** falls rapidly from 37 cm $H_2O$ to 31 cm $H_2O$ by 26 weeks. A slower fall to 30.5 cm $H_2O$ continues to term. These changes exactly follow the fall in albumin.

### Serum lipids
These rise from about 6 to 10 g/l.
The **triglycerides** rise progressively from $<$ 1 g/l to between 2 and 3 g/l at term.
**Cholesterol** falls in the first trimester from 2.0 to 1.8 g/l and then increases in a linear fashion to 2.7 g/l at 36 weeks. Pre-eclampsia causes a greater rise.
**Phospholipids** rise from 2.5 g/l to between 3.5 and 4 g/l. Cephalin levels treble, lecithin and sphingomyelin almost double but lysolecithin falls.
**Prostaglandins** (PG) are biologically active lipids synthesized in almost every tissue in the body from long-chain unsaturated fatty acids such as linoleic and arachidonic acids. They belong to the biochemical family of endoperoxides. At least 13 different prostaglandins (or prostanoids) have been identified. In parturition the most important of these are $PGF_2\alpha$ and $PGE_2$ both of which derive from arachidonic acid and cause the myometrium to contract. The most important sites of synthesis in parturition (roughly in order of importance) are decidua, fetal membranes, myometrium, cervix and placenta. Oestrogen promotes and

## 2.0 Physiological changes in pregnancy

### 2.3 Composition of blood

progesterone inhibits PG synthesis by making lyosomal membranes more labile or more stable respectively. The oestrogen/progesterone ratio is therefore an important factor in inhibiting or promoting uterine contractility.

Other important endoperoxides include prostacyclin ($PGI_2$) and thromboxane ($TXA_2$). Prostacyclin is a very potent vasodilator and inhibitor of platelet aggregation. The main site of production is vascular endothelium and synthesis is increased in maternal blood vessels during pregnancy. This contributes to the drop in peripheral resistance which normally occurs in pregnancy. The placenta also synthesizes $PGI_2$. $TXA_2$ is a potent vasoconstrictor and platelet aggregator but the effect of $PGI_2$ predominates in normal pregnancy.

**Serum enzymes**
The levels of the following are *unchanged* in pregnancy:
- Lactate dehydrogenase (LDH)
- Isocitrate dehydrogenase (ICDH)
- $\alpha$-hydroxybutyrate dehydrogenase (HBDH)
- Aspartate aminotransferase (glutamate-oxaloacetate transaminase—GOT)
- Alanine aminotransferase (glutamate-pyruvate transaminase—GPT)

High levels of GOT and GPT occur in the presence of a hydatidiform mole.

Creatine kinase is reduced in the first half of pregnancy only. (N.B. This may mask abnormalities when testing for carriers of Duchenne muscular dystrophy.)

Lipase may be reduced markedly.

Cholinesterase is unchanged but pseudocholinesterase activity may be depressed by up to 30% in late pregnancy. This can occasionally prolong succinyl-choline activity, for example at caesarean section.

Alkaline phosphatase is a large family of iso-enzymes, the activity of which rises markedly in pregnancy. This is due to a

## 2.0 Physiological changes in pregnancy

2.4 Blood coagulation in pregnancy

heat stable fraction (HSAP) which appears during the first trimester and increases until, in the third trimester, it forms 40 to 70% of the total serum alkaline phosphatase activity. It derives from the trophoblast and has been used as a monitor of placental function.

Acid phosphatase activity in the peripheral circulation is unchanged but the placental activity falls in late pregnancy.

Leucine aminopeptidase activity (the enzyme which splits angiotensin) quadruples between early and late pregnancy.

Cystine aminopeptidase (oxytocinase) activity increases tenfold between early and late pregnancy. Multiple pregnancy produces even greater rises in these two enzymes.

Deoxycytidylate deaminase (DCD) levels do not change in normal pregnancy but may rise in pre-eclampsia.

Relaxin (a polypeptide mainly synthesized in the corpus luteum) is detectable in plasma by 7–10 weeks and reaches its maximum between 38 and 42 weeks. Its main functions are cervical ripening and softening the ligaments of the pelvic girdle.

### 2.4 Blood coagulation in pregnancy (Fig. 1)

Plasma **fibrinogen** rises from about 2.4 g/l before pregnancy to 3.2 g/l by 12 weeks. It reaches a maximum of 3.7–3.8 g/l by 36 weeks then gradually falls to around 3.5 g/l by term. Clotting time and bleeding time are unchanged. Placental separation activates clotting.

**Fibrinolytic system**

Fibrin is broken down gradually by plasmin which, in some circumstances, will also break down fibrinogen and other proteins in the coagulation system. Plasmin is formed from plasminogen by a complex of plasminogen activators. Despite elevated fibrinogen and plasminogen levels, fibrinolytic activity decreases in plasma during pregnancy. This is probably due to low levels of fibrinolytic activators and impaired release of them from vessel walls. Inhibition of plasminogen activation does not

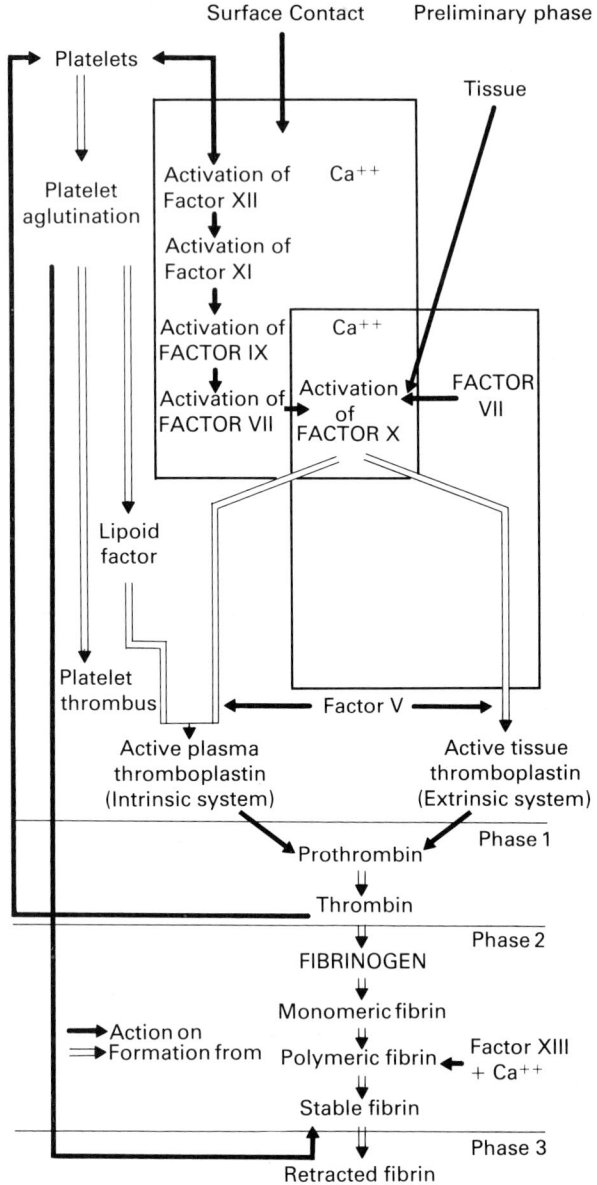

**Fig. 1.** Blood coagulation. *Note*: factors with raised levels in pregnancy are shown in capitals.

## 2.0 Physiological changes in pregnancy

2.5 Renal function

change in the circulation but the placenta contains high levels of fibrinolytic inhibitors.

The plasmin inhibitors, antiplasmin and $\alpha_2$ macroglobulin, increase substantially during pregnancy. Fibrinolytic activity returns to normal within 15 minutes of delivery of the placenta.

### 2.5 Renal function

The renal tracts begin to dilate by 10 weeks of pregnancy and the right ureter and renal pelvis are more severely affected. This is partly, but not solely, due to mechanical pressure. The involvement of progesterone is now questioned.

**Renal plasma flow** (RPF) is raised throughout pregnancy by 200–250 ml/min.

**Glomerular filtration rate** (GFR) rises from about 100 ml/min to about 170 ml/min.

**Creatinine clearance** rises to between 150 and 200 ml/min at the end of the second trimester but may fall to non-pregnant levels during the last trimester. Urea and uric acid clearances are also raised. The passage of normal urine volumes in the face of low plasma osmolality (down to 10 mosmols/kg) and a raised extracellular fluid volume is unique to pregnancy.

Renal clearance of amino acids is increased markedly and further affected by, for example, pre-eclampsia.

**Renin** is an enzyme produced in the kidney acting on an $\alpha$-2 globulin substrate to form the inactive decapeptide angiotensin I. This is converted by another enzyme to angiotensin II. Plasma renin concentration rises markedly in the first trimester and falls thereafter. Only 10% is active; the rest comes from the myometrium and chorion. Plasma renin activity (PRA) still rises two to four-fold within the first trimester and remains constant thereafter. Renin substrate increases particularly in the second half of pregnancy in response to oestrogen. Plasma angiotensin II is markedly elevated in normal pregnancy though the range of values is wide.

## 2.0 Physiological changes in pregnancy

2.6 Adrenal function

### 2.6 Adrenal function

Elevated **aldosterone** levels are necessary to conserve sodium which would otherwise be lost due to an increased GFR and the sodium-losing/potassium-sparing action of progesterone. The rise in plasma aldosterone occurs within days of fertilization, governed by an increase in angiotensin II.

**Desoxycorticosterone** levels are high towards the end of pregnancy. They are not suppressed by a high salt intake and do not rise during ACTH administration.

**Plasma cortisol** levels, both bound and free, are elevated throughout pregnancy, being highest in early morning and lowest around midnight.

**Catecholamines** do not change significantly during pregnancy.

### 2.7 Thyroid function

Renal clearance of **iodine** doubles in the first trimester and remains stable thereafter. It is normal by six weeks postpartum. The result is a low **plasma inorganic iodine** (PII).

Free **tri-iodothyronine** ($T_3$) and **thyroxine** ($T_4$) circulate in reverse equilibrium with protein bound hormone although $T_3$ is only weakly protein-bound. $T_3$ is three times more active than $T_4$. Since the level of thyroid binding proteins (globulin, pre-albumin and albumin) more than double in pregnancy (due to an oestrogen effect on the liver) the proportion of free $T_4$ falls and the **protein bound iodine** (PBI) rises from 4.0–8.0 $\mu g/100$ ml to 7.5–13.5 $\mu g/100$ ml. This is corrected by an increased $T_4$ production. Both free $T_3$ (0.75–1.5 $\mu g/100$ ml) and $T_4$ (2–4 $\mu g/100$ ml) are, therefore, normal in pregnancy. Only 0.5% of $T_3$ and 0.05% of $T_4$ are present free in serum. Thus the nett hormonal turnover is increased in pregnancy but because hormonal requirements depend on body size, the daily turnover rate is normal. The **basal metabolic rate** (BMR) is increased by up to 30% by the third trimester due to the needs of the uterus and fetus (60%) and increased maternal respiratory, cardiac and renal work (40%).

## 2.0 Physiological changes in pregnancy

2.8 Hypothalamo-pituitary function

The **$T_3$ resin uptake test** ($T_3R$) and the **free thyroxine index** ($FT_4I = PBI \times T_3R$) are useful tests of thyroid function in pregnancy because the $T_3R$ is low despite a high PBI (c.f. thyrotoxicosis with high $T_3R$ and PBI).

**Thyroid stimulating hormone** (TSH) is probably unchanged by pregnancy but chorionic thyrotrophin and long-acting thyroid stimulator (LATS) can affect thyroid function in normal pregnancy. LATS is an IgG acting on the thyroid microsomes.

**Hydatidiform mole** may result in a marked increase in thyroid activity due to molar thyrotrophin. The thyroid also secretes thyrocalcitonin which inhibits bone resorption and therefore lowers serum calcium. Information on pregnancy changes is inadequate.

### 2.8 Hypothalamo-pituitary function

The pituitary gland enlarges in pregnancy. Serum follicle stimulating hormone (FSH) falls when human chorionic gonadotrophin (hCG) begins to rise and remains low throughout the pregnancy. The effect of pregnancy on luteinizing hormone is not known. The levels of thyroid stimulating hormone (TSH) and growth hormone do not change. Adreno-corticotrophic hormone (ACTH) levels are depressed.

The number of prolactin-secreting cells increases in pregnancy and serum prolactin levels double by term from the non-pregnant level of 600 nmol/l.

Oxytocin is a monopeptide synthesized by neurons in the supra-optic and paraventricular nuclei of the hypothalamus. Levels in the peripheral blood are very low, the mean level at term being about 20 pg/ml. It is released in a neuro-endocrine reflex in response to tactile stimulation of the reproductive tract e.g. stretching of the cervix increases myometrial contractility (Ferguson reflex); nipple stimulation facilitates milk let down during lactation. Despite the oxytocin surges which occur in labour, its function is not clear and its role in the initiation of parturition is doubted.

## 2.0 Physiological changes in pregnancy

2.9 Alimentary function
___

Vasopressin levels are also very low in pregnancy (< 2 pg/ml throughout).

### 2.9 Alimentary function
Pregnant women have an early surge in appetite which decreases as pregnancy progresses. The daily food intake increases by about 200 Kcal by the beginning of the second trimester and remains stable thereafter. Secretion of saliva is not usually increased in pregnancy. There is disagreement as to whether tooth caries increases in pregnancy or not. Gingival oedema occurs as part of the general changes in connective tissue in pregnancy. Heartburn may occur due to reflux oesophagitis. The whole gastro-intestinal tract suffers from reduction in muscle tone and motility. For example the stomach emptying time is doubled during pregnancy. Acid and pepsin secretion are reduced.

In the large intestine water reabsorption increases which, together with motor sluggishness, may lead to constipation.

The **liver** is rarely palpable in pregnancy unless it is diseased or the patient is in congestive cardiac failure. Blood flow through the liver increases by 60–70% during pregnancy.

**Bilirubin** levels tend to remain normal but up to 15% of normally pregnant women will have levels > 17 $\mu$mol/l. Bromsulphthalein (BSP) is cleared more slowly in pregnancy. The standard 45 and 60 minute levels are higher but still within normal limits. The BSP excretion rate from liver to bile falls by up to 60% (75% in multiple pregnancies). These changes can be mimicked by oestrogens.

**Cephalin flocculation** and **thymol turbidity** remain normal although they may be raised in late pregnancy.

The gall bladder is affected by the general smooth muscle atony. Gall stones may be more common in pregnancy.

### 2.10 Carbohydrate metabolism in pregnancy
A fall in fasting blood sugar levels of about 0.5 mmol occurs in

## 2.0 Physiological changes in pregnancy

2.11 Weight gain during pregnancy

the first trimester of pregnancy. Only a very small fall occurs thereafter. There is also a delay in time taken to reach peak plasma glucose levels in response to a 50 g oral glucose load. In pregnancy the peak is reached about 45 minutes after the flucose is taken and the curve of glucose response is shifted to the right. The glucose tolerance test (GTT) is discussed in greater detail on page 000.

Insulin resistance also occurs during pregnancy; and although there is an increase in basal and post-prandial insulin values of 150–300% compared to the non-pregnant state, there is no causal relationship between higher insulin and lower fasting glucose levels.

**Glycosuria** Glucose is filtered at the glomerulus and reabsorbed in the proximal tubule. Pregnancy is associated with reduced reabsorption and because glomerular filtration is increased to 150–200 ml/min, glucose can spill into the urine at blood levels of 5–6.7 mmol/l. Glycosuria is therefore not an effective screening test for diabetes in pregnancy.

## 2.11 Weight gain in pregnancy

The components of weight gain in pregnancy are given in Table 2.3, and the rate of maternal weight gain are shown in Table 2.4.

**Table 2.3.** Components of weight gain (in grams).

|  | \multicolumn{4}{c}{Gestational age (weeks)} |  |  |  |
|---|---|---|---|---|
|  | 10 | 20 | 30 | 40 |
| Total maternal weight gain | 650 | 4000 | 8500 | 12500 |
| Fetus | 5 | 300 | 1500 | 3400 |
| Placenta | 20 | 170 | 430 | 650 |
| Amniotic Fluid | 30 | 350 | 750 | 800 |
| Total | 55 | 820 | 2680 | 4850 |
| Products of conception as a proportion of total maternal weight gain | 8% | 20% | 32% | 40% |

## 2.0 Physiological changes in pregnancy

2.11 Weight gain during pregnancy

**Table 2.4.** Rate of maternal weight gain.

| | |
|---|---|
| To 16 weeks gestation | 0.36 kg/wk |
| 17–26 weeks | 0.45 kg/wk |
| 27 weeks–term | 0.36–0.41 kg/wk |

**Notes on weight gain**
- The range of weight gain is wide.
- No single figure can be regarded as 'normal'.
- The optimum is 12.5 kg for the whole of pregnancy and 9 kg for the second half.
- Mothers who gain little or no weight tend to have smaller babies than those who gain more weight.
- One week after delivery the average woman is 4.4 kg above pre-pregnant weight, but this extra weight is usually lost gradually.
- Weight gain in second or subsequent pregnancies is about 1 kg less than during a first pregnancy but this relates to maternal age rather than directly to parity.
- Socio-economic status has no influence on weight gain, except in situations of severe malnutrition.

# 3.0 Fetal growth and development

3.0 Fetal growth and development, 25
3.1 Average measurements of normal fetuses, 25
3.2 Birth weight, 25
3.3 Assessment of gestational age, 28
3.4 Low birth weight, 31

## 3.0 Fetal growth and development

All the cells in a term fetus arise from only 42 divisions of the fertilized ovum. Only 5 further divisions are required to attain adult size. The pattern of growth shows little variability in the first half of pregnancy when genetic control is dominant. The influence of other factors gives rise to greater variability in the second half of pregnancy.

### 3.1 Average measurements of normal fetuses (Table 3.1)

**Table 3.1.**

| Menstrual age (wks) | Foot length (mm) | Knee–heel length (mm) | Crown–rump length (mm) | Bi-parietal diameter (mm) | Fetal weight (g) |
| --- | --- | --- | --- | --- | --- |
| 10 | 6  | 8  | 33 | —  | —  |
| 11 | 7  | 11 | 47 | —  | —  |
| 12 | 8  | 13 | 58 | 18 | 14 |
| 13 | 10 | 17 | 72 | 23 | 18 |
| 14 | 14 | 24 | 80 | 26 | 36 |
| 15 | 18 | 31 | —  | 31 | 66 |
| 16 | 21 | 36 | —  | 35 | 97 |
| 17 | 23 | 40 | —  | 37 | 122 |
| 18 | 25 | 43 | —  | 40 | 150 |
| 19 | 30 | 51 | —  | 45 | 234 |
| 20 | 33 | 56 | —  | 48 | 294 |
| 21 | 35 | 60 | —  | 50 | 338 |
| 22 | 39 | 66 | —  | 53 | 434 |
| 23 | 42 | 72 | —  | 55 | 517 |
| 24 | 45 | 77 | —  | 58 | 606 |
| 25 | 48 | 82 | —  | 60 | 702 |
| 26 | 51 | 87 | —  | 61 | 805 |

### 3.2 Birth weight

Birth weight varies directly with maternal height and weight. Tall, heavy mothers will have babies up to 500 g heavier than short, light mothers. Mothers who gain no weight during pregnancy have babies weighing 300–400 g less than those who

## 3.0 Fetal growth and development

### 3.2 Birth weight

gain 20 kg or more. Average birth weight falls as socioeconomic and nutritional status deteriorate. The average difference between a baby from social classes I & II (professional and managerial) and IV & V (semi-skilled and unskilled manual workers) is 150 g but much of this difference depends on maternal size.

**Table 3.2.** Ethnic differences in average birth weight.

| European | 3400 g |
| South West & East Asian | 3200 g |
| Indonesian and African | 3100 g |
| Indian | 2900 g |

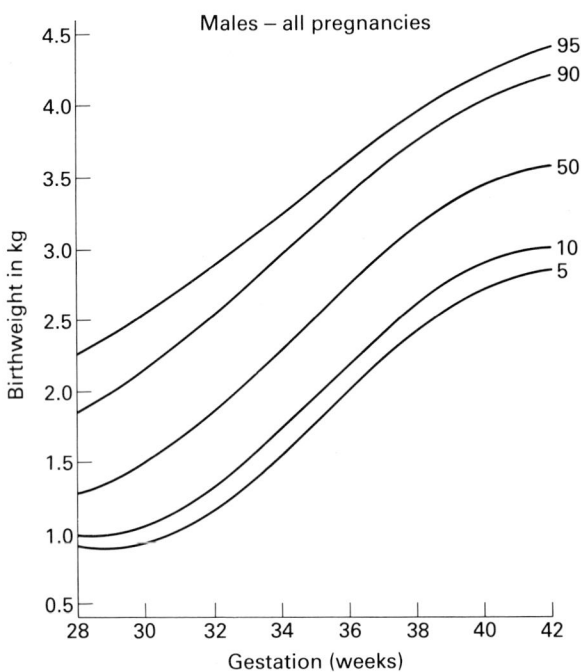

**Fig. 2a.** Percentile values for birthweights and gestational age at birth.

# 3.0 Fetal growth and development

## 3.2 Birth weight

In first pregnancies, males are on average 140 g heavier than females at term. In subsequent pregnancies this increases to 180 g. The difference is negligible up to 33 weeks gestation. Birth weight usually rises from first to second pregnancies with a smaller rise in the third pregnancy. This may be due to increased maternal weight.

Smoking in pregnancy reduces the mean birth weight by 100–200 g from 34 weeks gestation onwards. Babies are also shorter and have smaller head circumferences. The effect is on growth and not as a result of maternal nutritional deficiencies.

### Weight for gestation standards

The charts on pages 26 and 27 have been prepared to allow

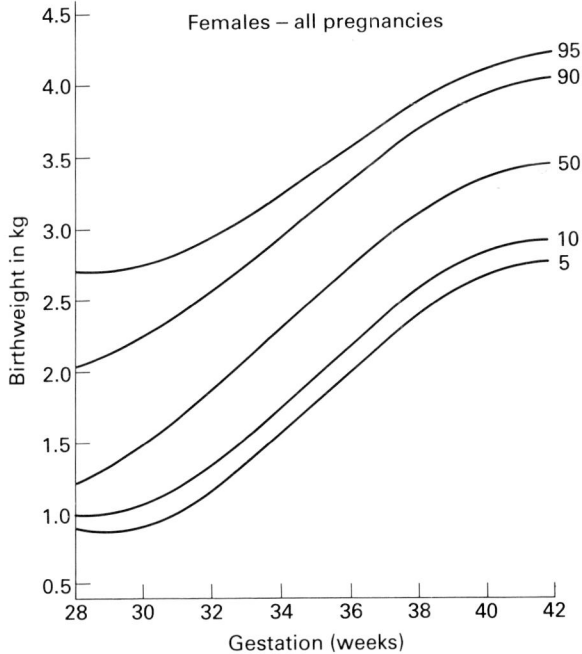

**Fig. 2b.** Percentile values for birthweights and gestational age at birth.

## 3.0 Fetal growth and development

3.3 Assessment of gestational age

---

simple comparison between babies from similar populations in terms of weight, sex, gestational age and parity.

### 3.3 Assessment of gestational age

#### Crown–rump length
This can be measured ultrasonically and provides an accurate estimate of gestational age up to 14 weeks (see chart on p. 00).

#### Cephalometry
The most widely used measure of fetal growth is the ultrasonic assessment of the bi-parietal diameter (BPD) at a velocity of 1600 m/s. When used to indicate fetal maturity it is most

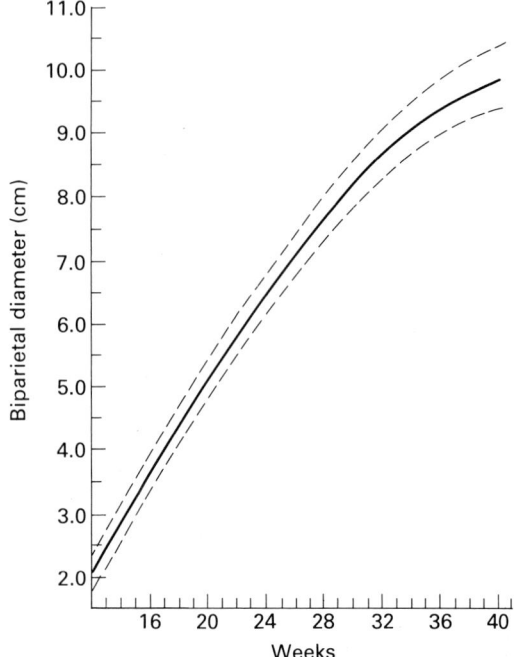

**Fig. 3.** Biparietal diameter ±2s.d.

## 3.0 Fetal growth and development

### 3.3 Assessment of gestational age

accurate before 24 weeks gestation but unreliable after 34 weeks (Fig. 3).

The mean growth of the BPD is 3.4 mm/week at 17 weeks, falling to 1.2 mm/week at 39 weeks.

Ultrasonic measurement of the ratio of the head circumference (at the level of the third ventricle) and the abdominal circumference (at the level of the umbilical vein) is a very useful measure of fetal growth. This ratio (head circumference/abdominal circumference) falls progressively reaching <1:1 at term. In intra-uterine growth retardation (IUGR) the ratio is high (e.g. 1.5:1) because of sparing of brain growth in this condition (Fig. 4). The safety of ultrasound is discussed on p. 000.

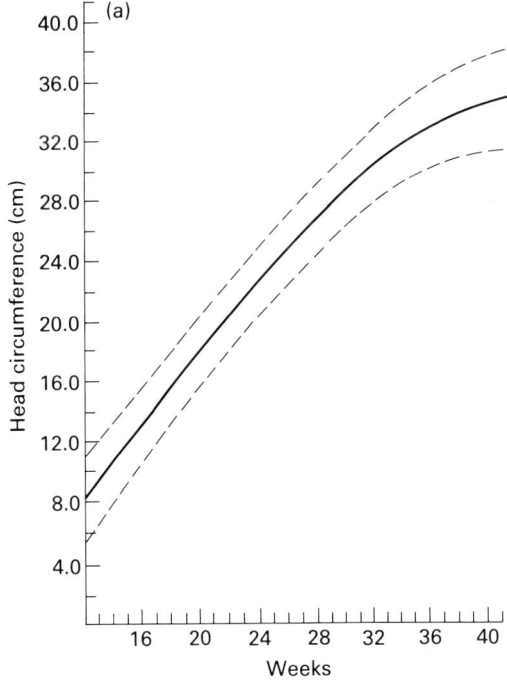

**Fig. 4.** (a) Head circumference ±2s.d.

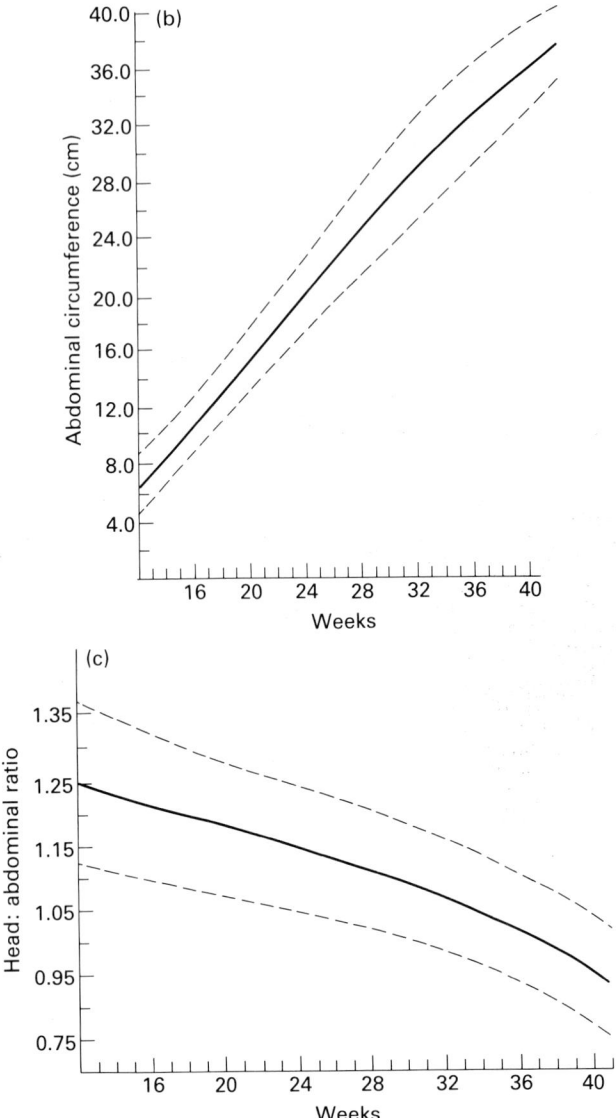

**Fig. 4.** (b) Abdominal circumference ±2s.d.
(c) Head abdominal ratio (head circumference: abdominal circumference) ±2s.d.

# 3.0 Fetal growth and development

## 3.4 Low birth weight

### Ossification centres
Radiology will reveal calcification of fetal epiphyses but their appearance is delayed in IUGR. Table 3.2 shows times of usual appearance.

**Table 3.2.**

| Ossification centres | Times of appearance |
|---|---|
| Os calcis | 24–26 weeks |
| Distal femoral epiphysis | 36 weeks |
| Proximal tibial epiphysis<br>Femoral head | 40 weeks |

### Height of uterine fundus
Clinical judgement of fundal height is not an accurate measure of gestational age. It is most helpful when measured in cm from the symphysis pubis (see Fig. 5).

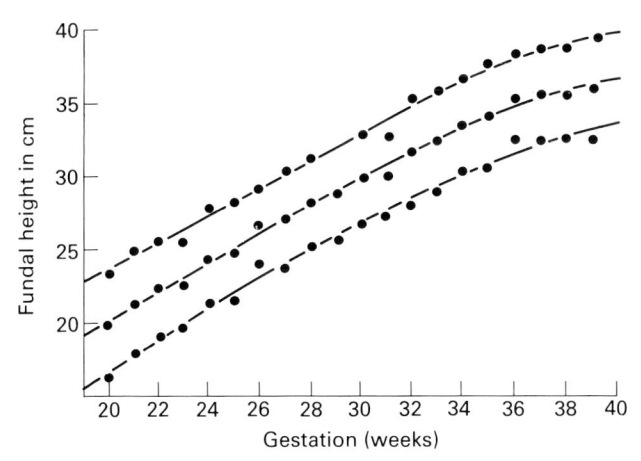

**Fig. 5.** Fungal height ±2s.d.

## 3.4 Low birth weight
The words prematurity and postmaturity have now been discarded to be replaced by the following definitions.

## 3.0 Fetal growth and development

### 3.4 Low birth rate

> Pre-term: born under 259 days (37 completed weeks) menstrual age.
>
> Term: born between 259 and 293 days (37–42 weeks completed weeks) menstrual age
>
> Post-term: born at or over 294 days (42 completed weeks) menstrual age.

Six to seven per cent of infants in the UK are less than 2.5 kg at birth. Of these 50% are born after 37 completed weeks and only 29% are delivered pre-term after spontaneous labour. Infants born weighing less than the 10th centile for their gestational age and sex are 'small-for-dates', or 'light-for-dates'. A more rigorous definition uses the 5th centile of birth weight for gestational age. The problems of low birth weight are discussed on pages 000 and 000.

# 4.0 The placenta and amniotic fluid

4.0 The placenta and amniotic fluid, 35

4.1 Feto-placental synthetic function, 35

4.2 Amniotic fluid, 37

4.3 Placental synthetic function as a test fetal well-being, 40

## 4.0 The placenta and amniotic fluid

## 4.0 The placenta and amniotic fluid
The contribution made by the placenta and amniotic fluid to the total weight gain of the mother as pregnancy advances is shown on page 21. However placental weight is a poor indicator of its functional adequacy because it does not usually work at its maximum capacity.

## 4.1 Feto-placental synthetic function

### Oestrogens
The 3 main oestrogens produced in pregnancy are **oestrone** ($E_1$), **oestradiol** $17\beta$ ($E_2$), and **oestriol** ($E_3$). The ultimate site of their production is the trophoblast. Both the fetus and the placenta contribute to $E_3$ synthesis. Essential enzymes lacking in one are present in the other. Oestrogens stimulate growth of the uterus and breasts and probably have important effects on fetal development. They promote PG synthesis.

$E_1$ and $E_2$ are less dependent on the fetus for synthesis. Fetal precursors contribute to 90% of $E_3$ but only 60% of $E_1$ and $E_2$.

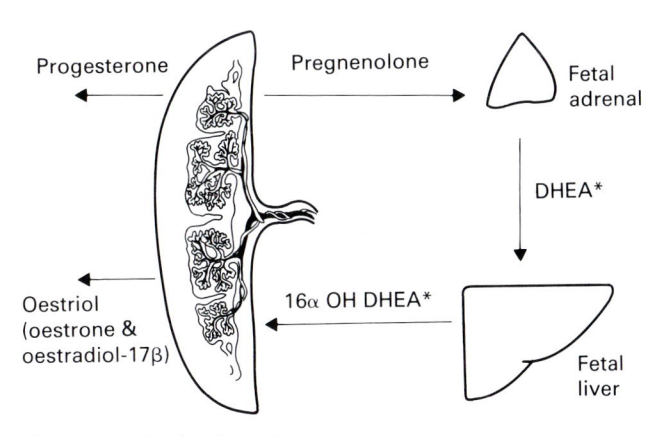

*Dehydroepiandrosterone

**Fig. 6.** The feto-placental unit.

## 4.0 The placenta and amniotic fluid

### 4.1 Feto-placental synthetic function

The daily production rates of oestrogens at term are:
- $E_1$ 12 mg/24 hrs
- $E_2$ 15 mg/24 hrs
- $E_3$ 19 mg/24 hrs

Oestrogens are excreted as conjugates in urine. Conjugated $E_3$ makes up 80–90% of oestrogens in pregnancy urine.

### Progesterone
Progesterone is initially produced by the corpus luteum but this source is unimportant by 70 days from the LMP as the syncytiotrophoblast takes over.

**Table 4.1.** Levels of progesterone.

|  | Daily output | Levels in maternal blood |
|---|---|---|
| Early pregnancy | 250–300 mg/24 hrs | 20 $\mu$g/l |
| Late pregnancy | 300–400 mg/24 hrs | 150–200 $\mu$g/l |

90% is bound in maternal plasma—mostly to albumin
10–15% is excreted in urine as pregnanediol

Among the main functions of progesterone in pregnancy are that:
- it is catabolic
- it promotes sodium loss to balance the sodium sparing effect of aldosterone
- it provides an important substrate pool for the fetal adrenal to produce gluco- and mineralo- corticoids
- it inhibits PG synthesis.

### Placental proteins
The placenta produces a wide range of proteins, some of them in large quantities, many of which do not have any counterpart in the adult. The more important of these specific proteins are shown in Table 4.2. The true function of most of them is unknown.

## 4.0 The placenta and amniotic fluid

### 4.2 Amniotic fluid

The production of the placental proteins depends on the mass of trophoblast and blood flow in the intervillous space. When measured on a linear scale their levels in maternal serum rise slowly in early pregnancy, rapidly in the mid-trimester, plateauing from 36 weeks onwards. This mirrors the pattern of fetal growth. A more accurate picture of relative production rates is given by logarithmic transformation of the data. This shows early pregnancy to be the time of greatest increase. The exception is hCG which shows a large peak at 60 days of gestation. This suggests that the first trimester peak may be due to a variant coming from a different and unknown site.

### 4.2 Amniotic fluid

Until the fetal skin becomes keratinized in mid-pregnancy, fluids can pass freely between the fetal extracellular fluid (ECF) and amniotic fluid (AF) compartments the composition of which is therefore very similar. In the second half of pregnancy AF has the composition and osmolality of dilute fetal urine. In the first half of pregnancy AF is yellow (from pale to deep) due to its bilirubin content. By 36 weeks gestation AF is colourless. Thereafter white floccules of lipid (vernix) and desquamated epithelial cells may appear. The presence of even small amounts of blood can produce a deep red colour. Meconium causes a distinctive green coloration initially which gradually darkens.

### Amniotic fluid volume

Table 4.3 shows the correlation between menstrual age and amniotic fluid amounts.

**Table 4.3.**

| Menstrual age (wks) | 10 : 12 : 14 : 16 : 18 : 20 : 30 : 40 |
|---|---|
| Amniotic fluid (ml) | 30 : 50 : 100 : 175 : 250 : 350 : 750 : 800 |

**Table 4.2.** The major specific proteins produced by the placenta.

| Protein | Molecular weight (daltons) | Chemistry | Effects (this does not assume function) | Site of production | Levels in pregnancy |
|---|---|---|---|---|---|
| Human chorionic gonadotrophin (hCG) | $50 \times 10^3$ | Glycoprotein with $\alpha$ and $\beta$ subunits $\beta$ subunit shared with LH | Can maintain corpus luteum (but peak level occurs after CL has faded). May stimulate fetal adrenals | Cytotrophoblast stored by syncytiotrophoblast | Peak levels at about 60 days of pregnancy |
| Human placental lactogen (hPL) | $22 \times 10^3$ | Single chain protein | Breast development? Causes insulin resistance | As for hCG or produced by syncytiotrophoblast | Up to 20 $\mu$g/ml; 1.3 g produced daily at term (10–20% of all proteins produced by placenta. See figure on p. 00 |
| Human chorionic thyrotrophin (hCT) | $45 \times 10^3$ | Glycoprotein with 2 subunits | Thyrotrophic | Trophoblast | — |
| Pregnancy-specific $\beta_1$-glycoprotein (SP$_1$) | $90 \times 10^3$ (90%) $20 \times 10^4$ (10%) | Glycoprotein | Suppresses mixed lymphocyte reactions but *in vivo* role unknown by trophoblast | Syncytiotrophoblast for maternal liver with absorption contains 30 mg | 140–200 ($\pm$40–55) mg/l at 38 weeks gestation. Average term placenta |

| Placental protein —5 (PP$_5$) | $36 \times 10^3$ | Glycoprotein | Protease inhibitor | Syncytiotrophoblast | Average term placenta contains 1.5 mg 45 $\mu$g/l at 36 weeks to term |
|---|---|---|---|---|---|
| Pregnancy-associated plasma protein A (PAPP-A) | $75 \times 10^4$ | $\alpha_2$-globulin | Inhibition of fibrinolysis | Syncytiotrophoblast | Actual levels unknown; peak late in third trimester |
| Pregnancy-associated plasma protein B (PAPP-B) | $1 \times 10^6$ | $\beta_1$-globulin | Unknown | Syncytiotrophoblast | Actual levels unknown; peak in third trimester |
| Heat-stable alkaline phosphatase (HSAP) | — | Heat-stable at 65°C | Hydrolyses orthophosphoric acid | Cytotrophoblast | 20 weeks—25 iu/l 38 weeks—80 iu/l |
| Cystine aminopeptidase (oxytocinase) (CAP) | — |  | Splits oxytocin and vasopressin |  | 20 weeks—1.5 iu/l 38 weeks—5 iu/l |

## 4.0 The placenta and amniotic fluid

4.3 Placental synthetic function as a test of fetal well-being

**Alpha-feto protein**
(AFP) is an alpha-globulin of similar molecular weight to albumin. It is synthesized by the yolk sac and the fetal liver. It passes from fetal serum into amniotic fluid and maternal serum. Its concentration in fetal serum at 16–18 weeks gestation is about 30,000 times that of maternal serum and 150 times that of amniotic fluid. It reaches its maximum level in maternal serum at about 30 weeks of pregnancy. For a variety of complex reasons, levels of AFP in amniotic fluid do not correlate with those in maternal serum. Thus, in the diagnosis of neural tube defect, for instance, they are independent diagnostic aids (see page 71). A normal range of maternal serum AFP levels between 15 and 22 weeks gestation is shown on page 72.

### 4.3 Placental synthetic functions as a test of fetal well-being

Assays of hormones or other products as tests of placental function and, by inference, fetal well-being are being relied on less and less. This is not only due to fashion but also because the measurement of placental products does not reflect its vital transport function on which fetal growth and well-being depends.

Among the other factors which affect their clinical relevance are:
- the variable maternal component (e.g. renal function and maternal size).
- clearance rates differ among individuals.
- biological and technical variations in serial levels which can explain large falls in levels but which have no pathological significance.
- maternal liver disease (e.g. intrahepatic cholestasis), or antibiotic therapy reduce oestrogen concentrations by influencing clearances through the liver.
- the fetal risk is often already obvious before placental function tests become consistently abnormal.

## 4.0 The placenta and amniotic fluid

### 4.3 Placental synthetic function as a test of fetal well-being

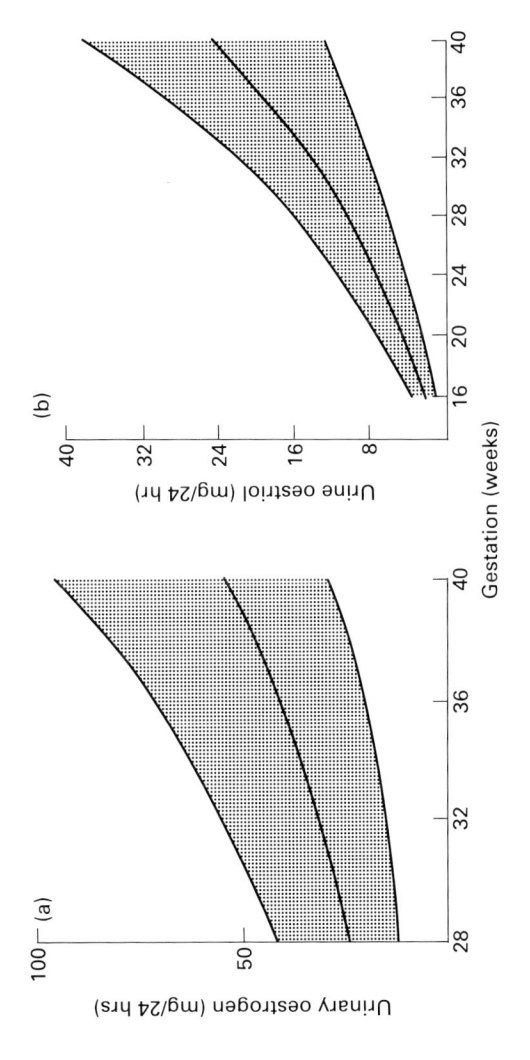

**Fig. 7.** (a) Urinary total oestrogen values in pregnant women (mean ±2s.d.) (b) Normal range of urinary oestriol levels in pregnancy (mean and the 10th and 90th percentiles).

## 4.0 The placenta and amniotic fluid

### 4.3 Placental synthetic function as a test of fetal well-being

Because published ranges do not take into account difference in assays and populations, each laboratory must define its own limits for normal and abnormal subjects, but the charts below provide a guide to generally accepted normal ranges (see Fig. 7).

### Commonly used tests of placental function

#### Urinary oestrogens
Total conjugated oestrogens or conjugated oestriol ($E_3$) may be used. The patient is instructed to empty her bladder on rising on the day of collection. This specimen is discarded. She then collects every specimen of urine passed during the following 24 hours including the first one on the following morning (see Fig. 7).

#### Oestrogen/creatinine ratio
The ratio of oestrogen to creatinine in an early morning urine sample has been found to be as useful as 24 hour urinary

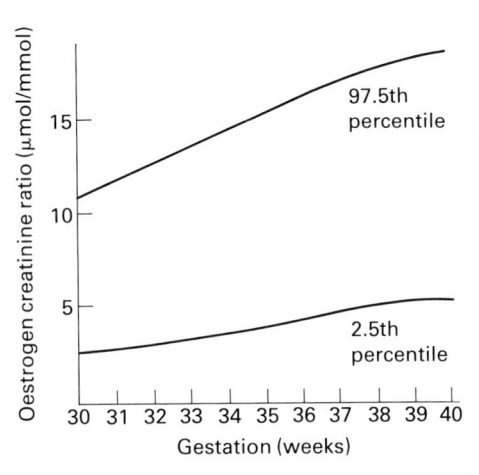

**Fig. 8.** Normal range of oestrogen-creatinine ratios in pregnancy.

## 4.0 The placenta and amniotic fluid

4.3 Placental synthetic function as a test of fetal well-being

---

oestrogen measurement. Figure 8 shows the 97.5 and 2.5 centiles from 30 weeks. Low levels of oestrogen are more likely to signify a deterioration in welfare of the fetus if they are the start, or form part of a continuing trend. Persistent very low urinary or plasma oestrogen levels may be associated with maternal corticosteroid therapy or a placental sulphatase deficiency. Apart from the association of the latter with prolonged pregnancy and possible poor uterine action, neither is of any significance to the fetus.

### Human Placental Lactogen (hPL)

Levels of plasma hPL repeatedly below 4 $\mu$g/ml after 30 weeks gestation suggest some deterioration in placental function.

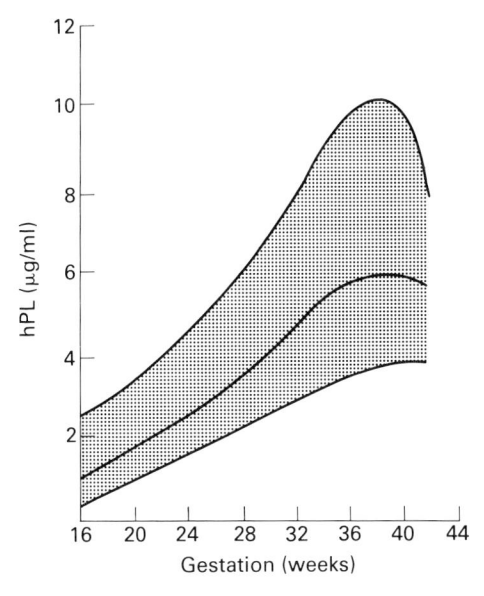

**Fig. 8.** Normal range of plasma hPL levels in pregnancy (mean ±2s.d.)

# 5.0 Antenatal care

5.0 Antenatal care, 47
5.1 Early diagnosis of pregnancy, 47
5.2 Recommended criteria for hospital confinement, 48
5.3 Booking criteria for GP unit confinement, 48
5.4 Provision of antenatal care, 49
5.5 Diet in pregnancy, 59

## 5.0 Antenatal care

The aim of antenatal care is to assess the risk of harm to mother and baby, and apply the appropriate level of surveillance to minimize or eradicate its effects.

### 5.1 Early diagnosis of pregnancy

**Symptoms**

Amenorrhoea, nausea, frequency of micturition, tingling sensation in areola of breasts.

**Signs**

'Active' breasts (i.e. enlargement of Montgomery's tubercles), slight pigmentation, venous engorgement; bluish coloration of vaginal skin and cervix, uterus (including cervix) soft with increasing enlargement.

**Tests**

Immunological pregnancy tests become positive about two weeks after first missed period, especially in early morning specimen of urine. The test reagents are an anti-hCG antibody and hCG bound to latex or erythrocytes. Pregnancy urine contains hCG which neutralizes the anti-hCG antibody when they are mixed. On addition of the latex or erythrocyte suspension no change occurs because all the antibody has been 'used up'. In non-pregnant urine the unneutralized antibody causes flocculation of the latex or sedimentation of the erythrocytes. Therefore no reaction is a positive test. False positives may occur especially in the presence of proteinuria.

False negative tests are commoner than is supposed, and the test usually becomes negative at 16–18 weeks when hCG levels are falling. Tests may remain positive for up to 48 hours after abortion has occurred or become inevitable.

Oral pregnancy tests using oestrogen/progestogen tablets are absolutely contra-indicated because they may cause virilization of some female infants.

## 5.0 Antenatal care

5.2 Recommended criteria for hospital confinement

A gestation sac may be seen by careful ultrasound as early as six weeks from the LMP.

### 5.2 Recommended criteria for specialist unit confinement
- nulliparae under 20 or over 30 years of age
- all women 35 years of age or over
- from the fifth pregnancy onwards
- gross obesity
- poor social conditions
- previous pre-term delivery (i.e. before 37 completed weeks)
- height 1.54 m (5 ft) or less
- previous stillbirth, neonatal death or severe congenitally abnormal infant
- previous low birth weight infant ($<$ 2.5 kg)
- previous caesarean section, myomectomy or hysterotomy
- previous placental abruption or third-stage abnormality (e.g. PPH, retained placenta)
- previous third degree tear, cervical or pelvic floor repair
- medical disorders (e.g. cardiac disease, diabetes, hypertension, anaemia, thyroid disease, psychiatric disease)
- multiple pregnancy
- rhesus negative with antibodies
- elevated serum AFP (without fetal NTD)
- malpresentations (persisting after 34 weeks gestation).

### 5.3 Booking criteria for GP unit confinement
The practice of booking women with a low risk of pregnancy pathology to be delivered by their own midwife and general practitioner in a GP Obstetric Unit is to be commended. The problem lies in adequately assessing risk. The following are broad criteria for such bookings in units isolated from maternity hospitals:
- nulliparae between ages of 20 and 30 over 1.54 mg (5 ft) in height

# 5.0 Antenatal care

5.4 Provision of antenatal care

- second, third or fourth pregnancy under 35 years of age
- no medical, psychological or obstetric contra-indications
- no rhesus or other antibodies

Regrettably some maternal and perinatal mortality and morbidity arises because of inappropriate booking. In general however the results are excellent. Criteria for booking when the GP and consultant units are integrated may not need to be so strict, but agreement as to what is appropriate should be reached locally. Obstetricians are happy to advise on any case in which significant doubt exists as to suitability for GP unit confinement. Deviation of any patient from normality during pregnancy (particularly in labour) requires prompt referral to the consultant unit.

The option of home confinement is still open in the UK but only about 1.4% of all women delivered each year do so at home and many of these do so accidentally. Among the criteria for suitability are a mother at very low risk of pregnancy pathology, good home circumstances (with e.g. a bathroom on the same level as the bedroom), a midwife and GP willing and able to cope with home delivery, and an obstetric flying squad available should the need arise. Nulliparous women are by definition not suitable for home confinement because labour problems cannot be predicted adequately. Some women who are totally unsuitable for home confinement insist on it. Specialist units can provide valuable moral and practical support to the unfortunate GP caught in this predicament both in convincing the woman that she should book into the hospital and assisting him if things go wrong with the pregnancy or labour in the home.

## 5.4 Provision of antenatal care

### Antenatal booking clinic procedures

### History
- Administrative details: Age, first day of LMP and menstrual cycle, marital status.

## 5.0 Antenatal care

### 5.4 Provision of antenatal care

- Medical and surgical history: including urinary infections, viral infections, (e.g. rubella contact), sexually transmitted diseases, hypertension (particularly on the pill) and blood transfusions. Ask about recent drug therapy.
- Obstetric history: dates of previous delivery or abortions; pregnancy complications; pre-term or post-term labours; induction of labour and indications; duration of labour; modes of delivery; birthweight and well-being of children; puerperium; mode of infant feeding.
- Family history: e.g. multiple pregnancy; diabetes; hypertension; pre-eclampsia; congenital anomalies; tuberculosis.
- Social history: housing problems; number of cigarettes smoked daily; alcohol ingestion.

**Examination**

**Preliminary**
Weight; height; urinalysis—glucose, protein and ketones; midstream urine sample (MSU) for culture; blood pressure.

**General**
Teeth, gums, lymphadenopathy, thyroid enlargement; respiratory system; heart—a soft systolic murmur and splitting of the second sound at the aortic and pulmonary areas are usually physiological; breasts—exclude masses and check nipples for inversion etc. (advise accordingly); abdomen—the clinical assessment of uterine size is not an accurate method of assessing gestational age but the height of the fundus (in cm above the symphisis pubis) correlates fairly well with gestational age (see page 00); legs—oedema, varicose veins; pelvic examination; a cervical smear for cytology should be carried out if none has been done within the previous five years; check cervical competence; exclude ovarian cysts; this is not the best time to assess pelvic dimensions.

## 5.0 Antenatal care

5.4 Provision of antenatal care

### Routine blood tests
- Full blood count and film. Exclude haemoglobinopathy and sickle cell trait disease in susceptible women (see page 00).
- ABO and rhesus blood group. Check for antibodies.
- Rubella antibody status. If negative, immunize in puerperium. Tests for syphilis (see page 51).

Alpha-feto protein—(see page 40). Serum can be taken to screen for neural tube defects (NTD) between 16–22 weeks (optimum 16–18 weeks).

- Australia antigen ($HB_s$ Ag). There is a potential but unquantified risk of hepatitis from contact with blood from $HB_s$ Ag-positive individuals (Chapter 9.2). The risk must be very small for unsuspected $HB_s$ AG-positive mothers have been delivered for many years without undue problems. However, blood samples and request cards in such patients should be clearly marked 'hepatitis risk' and be handled separately. There is no way to avoid blood contamination at delivery. The small risk is reduced even further if the patient carries antibody to the Australia antigen.

### Ultrasound in antenatal care
As many as 70% of mothers in the UK have a routine ultrasound scan during the antenatal period and a further 15% have a scan at some other time. The safety and effectiveness of the procedure are, therefore, important matters.

### Safety of ultrasound
In considering the safety of ultrasound the following must be considered:
- Diagnostic imaging uses 1 microsecond pulse of ultrasound followed by a 1 millisecond gap for detection of the returning sound wave. Thus for an average examination lasting 15 minutes the fetus is exposed to sound for only 1 second.
- Experiments testing for deleterious effects use continuous

## 5.0 Antenatal care

### 5.4 Provision of antenatal care

wave ultrasound or very long pulses over a prolonged period.

- Ultrasound of much higher intensity than is used in diagnostic equipment can produce effects in cells by, e.g. heating, the production of bubbles (cavitation), or eddies (microstreaming).
- There is, to date, no experimental evidence to show that any of these effects occur to any significant degree in human tissues under diagnostic imaging ultrasound conditions.
- The balance of evidence is against ultrasound causing chromosome breaks even at much higher intensity and for longer periods than are used diagnostically.
- No clinical study has shown any association between antenatal use of diagnostic ultrasound and congenital abnormalities, intra-uterine growth retardation, childhood cancer or damage to maternal or fetal germ cells.

Careful scrutiny of the evidence by the American Institute for Ultrasound in Medicine (1983), European Federation for Ultrasound in Medicine & Biology (1984), British Medical Ultrasound Society (1984), and the Royal College of Obstetricians & Gynaecologists (1984) (see suggested further reading) has led them to conclude that there is still no evidence of adverse bioeffects from diagnostic ultrasound on mammalian tissues. The lack of well designed, long-term, prospective studies is noted and the search for possible hazards should continue.

**Use of diagnostic ultrasound**
An ultrasound scan can be helpful diagnostically in many clinical situations during pregnancy. Among those suggested in reports from the NIH in the USA and the RCOG in the UK are:
- assessment of bleeding and/or pain in early pregnancy
- differential diagnosis of troublesome vomiting
- ascertainment of gestational age when it is otherwise uncertain
- exclusion of multiple pregnancy in mothers who have been

# 5.0 Antenatal care

## 5.4 Provision of antenatal care

given fertility drugs or in whom the uterus is large for gestational age

- examination of the fetus when the risk of congenital anomaly is high and before such diagnostic procedures as amniocentesis or chorious biopsy
- to check fetal size and liquor volume when the uterus is either large or small for gestational age
- monitoring fetal growth in high risk pregnancies
- assessing placental site, and identifying the source of antepartum haemorrhage
- determination of fetal presentation if it is unclear by palpation.

The performance of a routine scan at 16–18 weeks' gestation sometimes followed by another at 32–36 weeks' is an increasingly common practice in Europe and the USA.

Among the aims of the early routine scan are:

- **Accurate assessment of gestational age** is one of the greatest benefits because menstrual history may be unreliable in up to 45% of women. It allows more exact interpretation of other tests (e.g. serum AFP); better identification of IUGR; more confident timing of any intervention; and hopefully, elimination of inappropriate induction for supposed post maturity.

- **Diagnosis of multiple pregnancy**. Although there is as yet no good evidence of an improvement in outcome as a result, early diagnosis and closer observations of these high risk pregnancies are fundamentally sound clinical practices (see page 162).

- **Placental localization**. This allows identification of a group of women at high risk of complications due to placenta praevia (see page 151). But, since only 1 in 10 of 'low lying' placentae at early scan remain as placenta praevia later in pregnancy, too great a weight placed on early information can cause unnecessary anxiety to some women.

- **Detection of serious fetal anomalies**. Craniospinal, urinary

# 5.0 Antenatal care

## 5.4 Provision of antenatal care

tract and gut anomalies and anterior abdominal wall defects can be detected by expert use of ultrasound. If a maternal serum AFP screening programme is practised the early scan should probably be at 16 weeks gestation. Otherwise routine scanning at 18 weeks allows more detailed intracerebral and cardiac scanning to be carried out. The sensitivity (i.e. false negative rate) and specificity (i.e. false positive rate) of routine early scanning for fetal anomalies has still not been fully assessed. It must not be assumed that termination of pregnancy is the only appropriate response when a fetal anomaly is detected. Some may be amenable to ante-natal manipulation (e.g. distended bladder due to posterior urethral valves) and others have a high chance of successful correction after delivery (e.g. exomphalos, duodenal atresia).

The main aim of a routine scan at 32–36 weeks gestation is to screen for IUGR and detect unsuspected but correctable fetal anomalies (e.g. diaphragmatic hernia). The value of this policy, given the additional work-load involved, has yet to be determined.

**Conclusions**
- There is as yet no convincing evidence that ultrasound is anything but safe for mother, baby and operator.
- The skill of the operator is of prime importance. Misleading information will lead to wrong management decisions.
- A routine scan at 16–18 weeks gestation is a helpful adjunct to clinical practice. Information from the scan should be freely communicated to the mother and her partner.
- Ultrasound equipment should be sited conveniently for the mother.

**Other tests**
**Chest X-ray** is advisable in women from communities in which tuberculosis is endemic (e.g. Asian immigrants) or if there is a recent personal or family history.

## 5.0 Antenatal care

### 5.4 Provision of antenatal care

**Genetic counselling** should be arranged for mothers at special risk of congenital anomaly (Chapter 6).

### Health education and advice
**Diet**: See page 59.
**Breastfeeding**: Advice on care of nipples.
**Dental care**: Free throughout pregnancy and for one year afterwards.
**Smoking**: advise strongly against it.
**Coitus**: May be best avoided until 14 weeks and from 36 weeks onwards. The lateral position is preferable later in pregnancy because penetration is less and the risk of supine hypotension not so great.
**Rest**: The ideal is over eight hours sleep at night throughout and two hours rest in the afternoon in late pregnancy.
**Travel**: Seat-belt wearing is controversial in pregnancy. In the last trimester the pregnant woman should avoid driving if possible and sit in the back seat as a passenger. Long unbroken car journeys carry a potentially increased risk of deep vein thrombosis. Air travel is medically safe but is not permissible by normal scheduled services from 34 weeks of pregnancy.
**Vaccination**: Vaccines using live attenuated viruses are contraindicated in pregnancy (Chapter 16).

### Maternity benefits
Full details of conditions of maternity benefits available are provided in leaflet NI.17A issued by the DHSS. Up-to-date rates are to be found in leaflet NI.196. These are available in antenatal and child health clinics and social security offices. A maternity grant is available to almost all mothers (see NI.17A) and is paid as a lump sum. It can be claimed at any time from 26 weeks of pregnancy until up to 3 months after the birth. A weekly maternity allowance is payable if the mother has in her own right paid (or been credited with) National Insurance contributions under a variety of rather complicated conditions (See

## 5.0 Antenatal care

5.4 Provision of antenatal care

NI.17A). The current basic requirements are that contributions must have been paid on earnings of at least 25 times the lower earnings limit in any one tax year and in the relevant tax year. Claims for the allowance should be made as soon as possible from 26 weeks of pregnancy because late claims may lead to some loss of benefit. If the claim is made before confinement, payment is for 18 weeks commencing at 28 weeks. If the claim is made after delivery, payment is made only for the week of, and 6 weeks following, confinement. Both benefits are claimed on form BM4 available through antenatal or child health clinics or social security offices.

Other free benefits for expectant mothers include:
- milk and vitamins
- dental care
- glasses
- prescriptions.

Fares to the Hospital can be claimed by low income families through supplementary benefits. The medical social work departments are only too willing to help if there are any special difficulties.

### Continuing antenatal care

Patterns of care are presently under scrutiny. The traditional scheme of visits every 4 weeks until 28, every 2 weeks from 28 to 36, and weekly thereafter, has not been proved necessary in women at low risk of developing complications. It has been suggested that, in the absence of complications the patient should be seen by a midwife and/or doctor at:
- 12 weeks—to arrange booking and confirm dates
- 16 weeks—baseline weight and BP; screening tests (e.g. ultrasound, AFP)
- 26 weeks—to check fetal growth
- 36 weeks—to check presentation
- 40 weeks—assessment near delivery.

Any additional visits should have a clearly specified objective.

## 5.0 Antenatal care

5.4 Provision of antenatal care

**Routine examinations and investigations**

**Every antenatal visit**
Weight; urinalysis; blood pressure; exclude oedema; measure fundal height.

**Each visit in third trimester**
Fetal lie and presentation; presence of fetal heart; record patient awareness of fetal movement (see chapter 10).

**At 26 and 36 weeks (as a minimum)**
Full blood count; Rh-D antibodies in Rh negative women and other antibodies if already detected at the first visit.

**At 36 weeks**
Pelvic assessment in primigravidae (see page 190–1). If care is being shared by hospital and GP a cooperation card should be completed at each visit. Some clinics will have optimum schedules different from the above depending on local needs. If abnormal features develop closer attention is required.

### 5.5 Diet in pregnancy
The recommended daily dietary intake during pregnancy and lactation is shown in Table 5.1.

**Suggested diet in pregnancy**
**Milk.** One pint daily *or* ½ pint milk+2 plain yoghurts or 40 g cheese.
**Cereal.** Wholewheat bread, wholegrain breakfast cereals.
**Meat, fish, cheese or eggs.** Two good servings daily.
**Fats.** Fried foods should be eaten in moderation using oils rather than animal fats. Use soft margarine or butter according to taste.
**Vegetables.** Potatoes, green vegetables, roots or pulses at least once a day (can be taken as soups). Fresh vegetables or salad daily.

**Table 5.1.** Recommended daily dietary intake during pregnancy and lactation.

| | Energy* kcal | Mega-joules | Protein (g) | Calcium (mg) | Iron (mg) | Folate (µg) | Vitamin A (µg) | Thiamine (mg) | Ribo-flavin (mg) | Nicotinic acid (mg) | Vitamin D (µg) |
|---|---|---|---|---|---|---|---|---|---|---|---|
| Pregnancy | 2400 | 10.0 | 60 | 1200 | 13 | 500 | 750 | 1.0 | 1.6 | 18 | 10 |
| Lactation | 2750 | 11.5 | 69 | 1200 | 15 | 400 | 1200 | 1.1 | 1.8 | 21 | 10 |

*1 megajoule = 240 kcal

## 5.0 Antenatal care

### 5.5 Diet in pregnancy

**Fruit.** At least once a day. Include citrus fruit, tomato or blackcurrants 3–4 times weekly.

**Alcohol.** In moderation if at all (see p.114): none if overweight.

**Supplements.** Iron (100 mg) and Folic Acid (300 $\mu$g) daily. Other vitamin supplements are not routinely necessary. Iodized salt is recommended if iodine is deficient locally.

**Fluid.** Sweetened drinks are best avoided but it is a good idea to drink plenty of fluids.

# 6.0 Congenital malformations

6.0 Congenital malformations, 63

6.1 Chromosome disorders, 63

6.2 Single gene disorders, 66

6.3 Neural tube defects, 70

6.4 Congenital heart lesions, 73

6.5 Other conditions, 73

6.6 Irradiation, 74

6.7 Rubella, 74

6.8 Diagnostic amniocentesis, 75

6.9 Chorionic villus sampling, 76

$\quad\quad$ B   N.
$\quad$ AB.  AA.

AB   AB.   AA   AA?
AB   AB   N.   B.


$\quad\quad$ B $\quad\quad$ N.
$\quad\quad$ ||  $\quad\quad$ ||


|| $\quad$ || $\quad$ || $\quad$ ||

## 6.0 Congenital malformations

## 6.0 Congenital malformations
Major congenital malformations constitute:
- 2.0–2.5% of all deliveries
- 1.6% of live births
- 32% of all stillbirths
- 20% of perinatal deaths
- 33% of neonatal deaths
- 28% of infant deaths.

Perinatal mortality (defined on page 243) due to malformations is around 2.0–2.5/1000 births. Thirty per cent of all children born alive with major malformations die within 5 years. The incidence is more than doubled in multiple pregnancy, especially in monozygotic twins.

## 6.1 Chromosomal disorders
Ninety-five per cent of gametes with chromosome abnormalities are not viable. The defects are usually:
- abnormality in number of chromosomes (aneuploidy) usually by mutation
- translocation of fragment between chromosomes—often inherited.

A balanced translocation exists when the genome contains the correct amount of genetic matter, they usually have no outward manifestation. If one parent has a balanced translocation the outlook for any conceptus is:
- 1 in 4 will have the same balanced translocation
- 1 in 4 will have normal chromosomes
- 1 in 2 will have an unbalanced translocation.

Unbalanced translocations always declare themselves and occur when the genome contains extra genetic matter. Loss of a substantial part of a chromosome (deletion) is nearly always lethal. Deletion of part of the short arm of chromosome 5 produces the rare 'cri-du-chat' syndrome. Some cells can be chromosomally normal while others are not. This is called mosaicism.

63

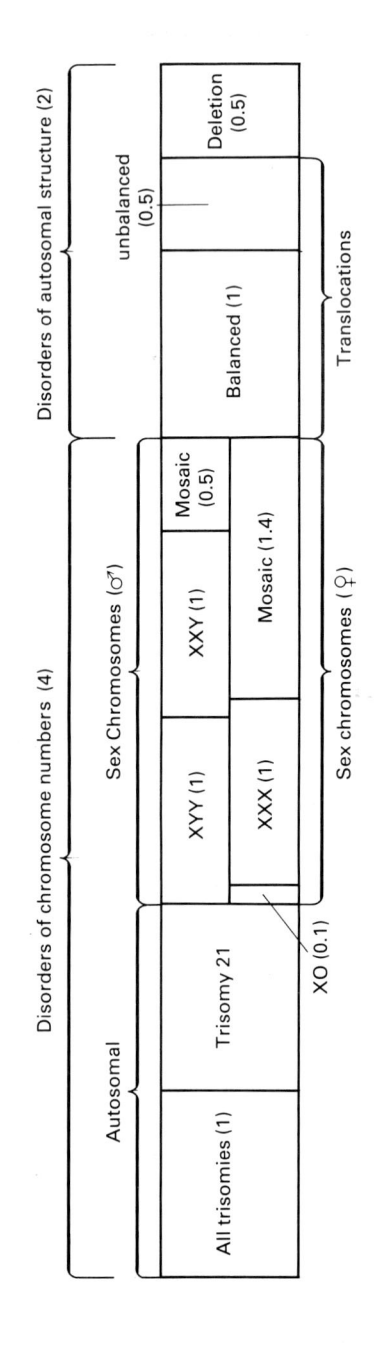

**Fig. 10.** Chromosomal disorders (approx. incidence/1000 live births).

# 6.0 Congenital malformations

## 6.1 Chromosome disorders

### Chromosomal disorders
See Fig. 10

### Downs syndrome
The overall incidence is about 9 per 10,000 total births. Up to 50% of all affected conceptuses miscarry early and only one-third survive to viability.

### Genetic abnormalities in Downs syndrome

| | |
|---|---|
| Trisomy 21 | 95% (maternal age related) |
| Translocation 14:21 | 2% |
| Other translocations | 2% |
| Mosaicism | 1% |

### Maternal age related risk of trisomy 21
The age-related risks are shown in Table 6.1.

**Table 6.1.**

| Maternal age | Approximate risk of affected child per 1000 live births |
|---|---|
| 20 | 1 in 2000 |
| 25 | 1 in 2000 |
| 30 | 1 in 900 |
| 35 | 1 in 365 |
| 36 | 1 in 290 |
| 37 | 1 in 225 |
| 38 | 1 in 180 |
| 39 | 1 in 140 |
| 40 | 1 in 110 |
| 41 | 1 in 85 |
| 42 | 1 in 70 |
| 43 | 1 in 50 |
| 44 | 1 in 40 |
| 45 | 1 in 30 |
| 46 | 1 in 25 |
| 47 | 1 in 20 |
| 48 | 1 in 15 |
| 49 | 1 in 12 |

## 6.0 Congenital malformations

6.2 Single gene disorders

The risk of future children being affected by Downs syndrome due to Trisomy 21 if one child is already affected is between 1 in 70 and 1 in 100. The risk of translocation 14:21 recurring is about 1 in 10 if the mother has a balanced translocation, and 1 in 50 if the father has it.

The standard method of antenatal diagnosis is by analysis of chromosomes in fetal cells from amniotic fluid at 16–18 weeks but chorionic villus sampling at about 8 weeks is becoming possible (page 76). Antenatal diagnosis should be offered to all pregnant women from the age of 38 onwards and be available for those who want it from the age of 35. A serum AFP level at or below 0.5 MOM (see p. 72) at 14 to 20 weeks may predict an increased risk of fetal trisomy 21. It may, therefore, be appropriate to offer such mothers an ammocenterin.

Other trisomies are rare and infants do not usually survive long.

### Sex chromosome disorders
See Fig. 10. Individuals with these anomalies are often sterile.

### 6.2 Single gene disorders
See Table 6.2 on pp. 68–9.

In **autosomal dominant** conditions the gene need only be inherited from one parent to be evident. Such conditions are usually relatively mild (e.g. polydactyly), arise after reproductive years (e.g. Huntington's chorea) or have various degrees of manifestation. If a gene is present but its effects can only be seen in 80% of individuals carrying it, it is said to have a penetrance of 80%. Fifty per cent of children of affected individuals will inherit the gene. Molecular genetic techniques are beginning to offer hope of early pregnancy diagnosis.

In **autosomal recessive** conditions the gene must be inherited from both parents to be evident. The effects are usually severe. Fifty per cent of children of affected individuals will be carriers.

## 6.0 Congenital malformations

### 6.2 Single gene disorders

In conditions in which the biochemical defect has been elucidated (e.g. Tay-Sachs) detection of carriers is possible.

**X-linked disorders** can be recessive or dominant. Table 6.3 does not include the X-linked glucose-6-phosphate dehydrogenase (G6PD) deficiency. It is very common globally but not in northern European populations.

There are considerable racial differences in the frequency of genetic disease as is shown in Table 6.3.

**Table 6.3.**

| Disease | Race | Frequency/100,000 births |
|---|---|---|
| **Cystic fibrosis** | N. Europeans | 40–50 |
|  | Negroes, Orientals | 1.0 |
| **Tay-Sachs disease** | Ashkenazi Jews | up to 40 |
|  | Sephardi Jews/Gentiles | < 0.5 |
| **Thalassaemia** | Mediterranean peoples, Orientals | up to 2000 |
|  | N. Europeans | insignificant |
| **Sickle-cell anaemia** | Negroes | up to 2000 |
|  | N. Europeans | insignificant |

### PKU

Phenylketonuria (PKU) cannot be detected antenatally but neonatal screening is routinely carried out. The incidence in the UK is about 1/10,000 births (higher in the NW than SE). A mother with PKU has about an 8% chance of giving birth to a child with PKU. She must receive a phenylalanine-free diet from before conception, otherwise the risk of spontaneous abortion, infant death or severe mental retardation is high, even if the child has not inherited the disorder.

### Cystic fibrosis

Cystic fibrosis (CF) is the commonest inherited metabolic disease in Western populations with an incidence of about 1 in

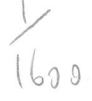

**Table 6.2.** Incidence of the commoner single gene disorders in Europe per 1000 live births.

|  | Autosomal dominant |  | Autosomal recessive |  | X-linked recessive/1000 males |  |
|---|---|---|---|---|---|---|
| Neuromuscular | Huntington's chorea | 0.5 | Neurogenic muscle atrophies | 0.01 | Duchenne's muscular dystrophy | 0.2 |
|  | Neurofibromatosis | 0.4 | Tay-Sachs disease | 0.004 | Mucopolysaccharidosis 2 (Hunter's) | 0.01 |
|  | Myotonic dystrophy | 0.2 | Severe mental retardation | 0.5 | Mental retardation | 0.1 |
|  | Tuberous sclerosis | 0.01 |  |  |  |  |
| Skeletal/skin | Diaphyseal aclasis | 0.5 |  |  | Ichthyosis | 0.1 |
|  | Thanatophoric dwarfism | 0.08 |  |  |  |  |
|  | Osteogenesis imperfecta | 0.04 |  |  |  |  |
|  | Marfan's syndrome | 0.04 |  |  |  |  |
|  | Achondroplasia | 0.02 |  |  |  |  |
|  | Ehler Danlos syndrome | 0.01 |  |  |  |  |
|  | Osteopetrosis tarda | 0.01 |  |  |  |  |
| Vascular | Monogenic hypercholesterolaemia | 2.0 |  |  |  |  |
| Haematological | Congenital spherocytosis | 0.2 | Sickle cell anaemia | 0.1 | Haemophilia factor VIII deficiency | 0.1 |
|  |  |  | $\alpha$ and $\beta$ Thalassaemia-variable depending on community |  | factor IX deficiency | 0.01 |

| | | | | |
|---|---|---|---|---|
| Visual | Dominant forms of blindness | 0.1 | Recessive forms of blindness | 0.1 | Colour blindness (red/green) | 80 |
| | Retinoblastoma | 0.03 | | | Childhood blindness | 0.02 |
| Auditory | Childhood deafness | 0.1 | Congenital deafness | 0.2 | | |
| | Otosclerosis | 0.01 | | | | |
| Facial | Cleft lip and/or palate | 0.01 | | | | |
| Dental | Dentinogenesis imperfecta | 0.1 | | | | |
| | Amelogenesis imperfecta | 0.02 | | | | |
| Intestinal | Multiple polyposis coli | 0.1 | | | | |
| Renal/Adrenal | Polycystic disease | 0.8 | Adrenal hyperplasia | 0.1 | | |
| Metabolic | Acute intermittent porphyria | 0.01 | Cystic fibrosis | 0.5 | | |
| | Variegate porphyria | 0.01 | Classical phenylketonuria | 0.1 | | |
| | | | Alpha-1 anti-trypsin deficiency | 0.3–0.8 | | |
| | | | Galactosaemia | 0.02 | | |
| | | | Galactokinase deficiency | 0.01 | | |
| | | | Cystinuria | 0.06 | | |
| | | | Cystinosis | 0.01 | | |
| | | | Mucopolysaccharidosis I | 0.02 | | |
| | | | Mucopolysaccharidosis II | 0.01 | | |

## 6.0 Congenital malformations

6.3 Neural tube defects

1600 births in the UK. The carrier frequency in the population is about 1 in 22. Early pregnancy diagnosis is not routinely possible as yet. The most promising method currently being investigated relies on the presence in second-trimester amniotic fluid of 2 major alkaline phosphatase iso-enzymes in constant proportions. One, derived from fetal intestinal mucosa, is inhibited by phenylalanine, the other by homoarginine. In pregnancies in which the fetus has CF, the concentration of the phenylalanine inhibitable form in amniotic fluid is very low.
For neonatal diagnosis see p. 274.
Parents with CF are now living longer and a small but increasing number of pregnancies are being reported in women with CF. Data are sparse but the risk of pre-term delivery, maternal and perinatal mortality seems to be increased. Pregnancy should be avoided in women with severe respiratory impairment.

### Alpha and beta thalassaemia

These thalassaemias (see p. 79) are amenable to antenatal diagnosis by chorionic villus sampling (p. 76) or by fetoscopy and fetal blood sampling for women at high risk. The risk of miscarriage from fetoscopy is $\leq 10\%$.

### 6.3 Neural tube defects (NTD)

Anencephaly and spina bifida comprise 95% of NTD's and encephalocele the other 5%. In the UK the incidence increases from the South and East to the North and West and is higher in

**Table 6.4.** Incidence of NTD in England and Wales 1974–83 (per 10,000 total births).

|      | Anencephaly | Spina bifida |
|------|-------------|--------------|
| 1974 | 13          | 18           |
| 1977 | 10          | 15           |
| 1980 | 5           | 11           |
| 1983 | 2           | 7            |

## 6.0 Congenital malformations

### 6.3 Neural tube defects

lower Socio-economic groups. It has dropped steadily in the UK over the past 20 years (Table 6.4). This is not entirely accounted for by antenatal screening programmes resulting in termination of affected pregnancies.

**Recurrence rate of NTDs**
See Table 6.5.

**Table 6.5.**

| Number of affected children | Recurrence rate |
| --- | --- |
| 1 | ten-fold |
| 2 | twenty-fold |
| 3 | forty-fold |

With an open NTD the neural tube is completely exposed or only covered by thin membrane; it comprises 80% of NTDs and includes anencephaly. Of the babies born with open spina bifida:
- 30% survive to 5 years of age
- 85% of these will be severely handicapped
- 10% will be moderately handicapped
- 5% will not be handicapped.

A closed NTD is completely covered by skin or thick opaque membrane.

**Screening for open NTDs**
The aim is to identify a population of women at high enough risk to justify diagnostic procedures. Policies for and against screening should be determined by the incidence of the condition within each district or region. At present, screening (Fig. 11) relies on the levels of alpha feto-protein (AFP) in maternal serum, but concentrations vary with gestational age. There is no particular level which discriminates totally between mothers at high and low risk. A 'cut-off' level set low enough to include

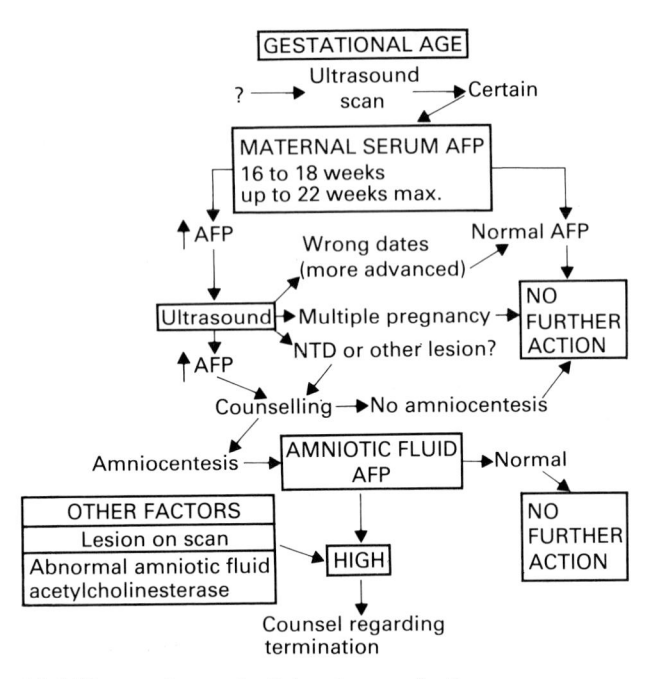

**Fig. 11.** AFP screening: potential sequence of action.

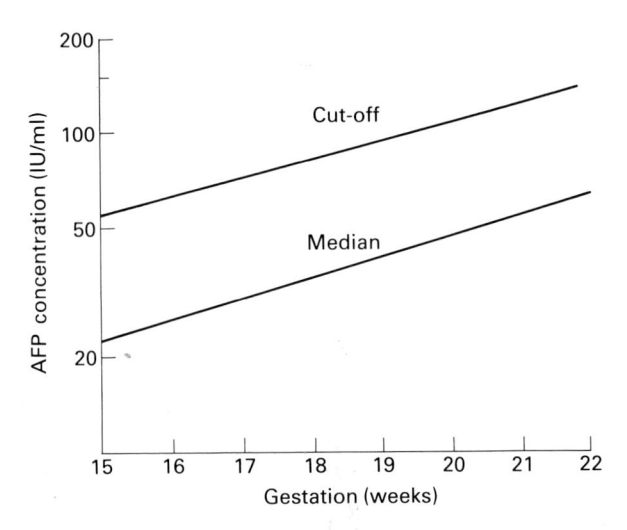

**Fig. 12.** Maternal serum AFP: median and cut-off levels.

# 6.0 Congenital malformations

## 6.4 Congenital heart lesions

nearly all affected pregnancies would include a large proportion of normal ones. A high cut-off to exclude normal pregnancies would miss most open NTDs. A cut-off level (Fig. 12) around 2.5 multiples of the normal median (MoM) at 16–18 weeks gestation will detect 90% of anencephaly, 80% of open spina bifida, but will include 3% of unaffected singleton pregnancies. Each laboratory must work out the 'cut-off' levels suited to their circumstances. Corrections should be made for maternal weight. The larger the woman, the greater the circulating blood volume. The AFP is therefore at a lower concentration per ml of maternal blood. One possible sequence of action is outlined below.

Relying on serum and amniotic fluid testing alone the false positive diagnosis rate could be 2 per 1000 unaffected viable pregnancies. Modern ultrasound techniques can reduce these errors significantly and may indeed totally supplant AFP measurement as an effective screening procedure.

**Prevention of NTD**

It is possible that the risk of recurrence of NTD may be reduced if the mother takes multivitamin tablets (vitamin A, vitamin D, thiamin, riboflavin, pyridoxine, nicotinamide, ascorbic acid, folic acid, ferrous sulphate and calcium phosphate). The dose is one tablet three times daily from at least one month before conception to about eight weeks of pregnancy.

## 6.4 Congenital heart lesions

The overall incidence has increased from 10 per 10,000 births in 1974 to 16 per 10,000 in 1983. The reason is unknown. Lesions cannot be routinely diagnosed antenatally but the rapid improvements in ultrasound resolution means that some major defects can be detected from about 18 weeks. Incidence and recurrence rate of some malformations are given in Table 6.7.

## 6.0 Congenital malformations

6.6 Irradiation

**Table 6.7.**

| Malformation | Incidence | Recurrence Rate |
|---|---|---|
| Patent ductus arteriosus<br>Ventricular septal defect | 1 in 1000 births | 1 : 30 |
| Atrial septal defect<br>Pulmonary stenosis<br>Coarctation of aorta<br>Transportation of great vessels<br>Fallot's tetralogy | 1 in 2000 births | 1 : 40 |

## 6.5 Other conditions

### Cleft palate and/or cleft lip
Risks are listed in Table 6.8.

### Pyloric stenosis
The incidence is approximately 3 in 1000 live births in the UK but there are large regional variations. It may be becoming more

**Table 6.8.**

| Birth frequency | Subsequent risk | |
|---|---|---|
| 1 in 1000 | To sibs and children | 1 in 25 |
| | To nephews and nieces | 1 in 140 |
| | To first cousins | 1 in 400 |
| | If parents and one child, or two sibs already affected | 1 in 12 |

**Table 6.9.**

| Relationship | Risk |
|---|---|
| Male sibs and male children | 1 in 20 |
| Female sibs and male children | 1 in 40 |
| Male sibs and female children | 1 in 8 |
| Female sibs and female children | 1 in 20 |

## 6.0 Congenital malformations

### 6.8 Diagnostic amniocentosis

common. The sex ratio is 5 male:1 female. Risks are given in Table 6.9.

### 6.6 Irradiation

Although the increased risk of any congenital abnormality or later malignancy being due to X-rays during pregnancy is negligible in practice, this form of investigation should be avoided if at all possible. A standard intravenous pyelogram may expose the pelvis to a dose of 100–300 mrad. Termination of pregnancy has been recommended if the fetus is exposed to 25 rads or more in the first eight weeks of pregnancy. If such heavy irradiation occurs after about 12 weeks gestation the maximum risk of developing leukaemia or other malignancies is about 1 in 500.

### 6.7 Rubella

This is considered fully in Chapter 9.

### 6.8 Diagnostic amniocentesis

This is best carried out by a small experienced team between 16 and 18 weeks gestation. The liquor volume is by then adequate, and there is still enough time for chromosome culture and analysis which takes 2–3 weeks.

The additional risk of miscarriage is 1.0–1.5%; other risks are more controversial.

Ultrasound scanning is mandatory at the time of the test to localize the placenta and locate the liquor pool. It is also helpful in confirming gestational age, and detecting multiple pregnancy or intrauterine death.

The procedure is as follows:
- A 20 gauge lumbar puncture needle (with stilette) should be used.
- Infiltrate down to the rectus sheath with local anaesthetic.
- No more than 16–18 ml of amniotic fluid should be removed.
- If the first puncture fails, scan again to relocate the liquor pool

## 6.0 Congenital malformations

### 6.9 Chorionic villus sampling

and try again. If the uterus has contracted wait for 15–20 minutes to allow the uterus to relax.

- If the second attempt fails also wait a few days and then repeat.
- A sequestrene blood sample should be taken before, and 20 minutes after, the test to check for feto-maternal transfusion (using the Kleihauer test).
- All antibody-negative Rh-D-negative women (and those in whom the Rh group is unknown) should be given anti-D immunoglobulin 100 $\mu$g. More can be given if a significant feto-maternal transfusion occurs (see p. 121).

### 6.9 Chorionic villus sampling

Chromosome analysis and culture are now becoming possible by chorionic villus sampling at around 8 weeks gestation. It is not an easy procedure and cannot yet be considered to be a routine practice. The transcervical route is preferred using a plastic or silver cannula under ultrasound guidance. Analysable samples are currently being obtained in over 90% of attempts. Any patient undergoing the analysis must be warned that later amniocentesis may be necessary.

The abortion rate after the procedure is 3–5% with a background spontaneous abortion rate of 3% at this gestation. Chorionic villus sampling should only be carried out in centres close to cytogenetic laboratories.

### Advantages
- It can be carried out earlier in pregnancy than amniocentesis.
- DNA analysis and gene probing are possible.
- Initial results can be ready in about 48 hrs (full cultures still take 2–3 weeks).

# 7.0 Pregnancy and associated diseases

7.1 **Haematological disorders,** 77

7.2 **Hypertensive disorders,** 82

7.3 **Diabetes mellitus,** 90

7.4 **Cardiac disease in pregnancy,** 97

7.5 **Thyroid disorders,** 102

7.6 **Systemic lupus erythematosus,** 104

7.7 **Myasthenia gravis,** 104

7.8 **Epilepsy,** 105

7.9 **Pituitary tumours,** 107

7.10 **Respiratory disease,** 107

7.11 **Diseases of the liver and alimentary tract,** 108

7.12 **Psychiatric disorders,** 111

7.13 **Malignancy,** 115

# 7.0 Pregnancy and associated diseases

## 7.1 Haematological disorders
For normal haematological indices see page 10.

**Abnormal indices** are as follows:

$$\begin{aligned}
\text{Hb} &< 10.5 \text{ g/dl} \\
\text{PCV} &< 0.33 \text{ l/l } (33\%) \\
\text{MCV} &< 78 \text{ fl} \\
\text{MCH}^1 &< 27 \text{ pg} \\
\text{MCHC}^2 &< 28 \text{ g/dl} \\
\text{Serum Iron} &< 11 \ \mu\text{mol/l} \\
\text{Binding capacity (TIBC)} &> 100 \ \mu\text{mol/l} \\
\text{Saturation (Fe/TIBC)} &< 30\% \\
\text{Serum ferritin} &< 15 \ \mu\text{g/l} \\
\text{Platelets}^3 &< 150 \times 10^9/\text{l}
\end{aligned}$$

[1] MCH is the average Hb content of one red cell
[2] MCHC is the average percentage Hb concentration per unit volume of red cells.
[3] Risk of bleeding increases only with counts $< 100 \times 10^9/\text{l}$

## Causes of falling haemoglobin in pregnancy
See Table 7.1.

## Prophylaxis of anaemia in pregnancy
The amount of iron required for pregnancy cannot be fully coped with by diet. If supplements are not given iron stores will become depleted and serum ferritin will be low (approximately 6 $\mu$g/l) by 28 weeks. Routine prophylactic therapy is recommended throughout pregnancy, and certainly from 28 weeks onwards. 100 mg elemental iron and 300 $\mu$g folic acid per day are all that is necessary. Gastro-intestinal intolerance occurs to some iron preparations and may be helped by changing to chelated or delayed release preparations.

## Use of parenteral iron in pregnancy
Parenteral iron is best given as a total dose intravenous infusion

Table 7.1. Causes of falling haemoglobin in pregnancy

| Cause | Features | Management |
|---|---|---|
| 'Physiological' | Due to haemodilution Hb > 10 g/dl | Continue routine haematinics (Fe 100 mg, folic acid 300 µg daily) |
| Iron deficiency | Blood film hypochromic and microcytic. MCH ↓ TIBC ↑ Se ferritin < 15 µg/l Se Fe may be as low as 30 µg/dl with < 16% TIBC saturation. No stainable Fe in marrow | Responds to oral Fe as quickly as to parenteral (see below for severe anaemia). Increase dietary sources (liver, meat, fish, eggs and spinach) |
| Folate deficiency | Blood film normochromic, macrocytic. Hypersegmented (more than 4 lobes) and giant polymorphs. Howell-Jolly nuclear inclusion bodies in RBC. Nucleated RBC present (25% of cases show up in puerperium) | Check Se folate and $B_{12}$ (Red cell folate low in both folate and $B_{12}$ deficiency). Treatment is 5–15 mg folic acid daily. Increase dietary sources (as for Fe) |
| Vitamin $B_{12}$ deficiency | Megaloblastic—as for folate deficiency. Higher incidence in strict vegetarians | A daily folate supplement of 300 µg daily will not mask $B_{12}$ deficiency. Treatment is 1000 µg vitamin $B_{12}$ weekly |
| Infection | Inhibits erythropoiesis; therefore causes a normochromic normocytic anaemia. TIBC ↓ marrow Fe ↑ | Treat infection (urinary infection is a frequent cause). Do not use parenteral iron during infection |
| Haemoglobinopathies | see p. 79 | |
| Miscellaneous | Haemolytic and aplastic anaemias    see p. 82<br>Chronic myeloid leukaemia<br>Hodgkin's lymphoma | |

## 7.0 Pregnancy and associated diseases

### 7.1 Haematological disorders

(TDI) of the iron-dextran compound. The rise in Hb is no better than with oral Fe but one does not need to rely on patient compliance in taking tablets. The maximum response takes 6 weeks.

- use parenteral iron sparingly and avoid if there is any significant allergic history
- side-effects tend to occur more frequently in pregnancy
- check Se Fe and TIBC beforehand and stop oral Fe
- the usual TDI dose is 1000–1750 mg calculated on an expected rise of 0.7 g Hb/100 ml for each 100 mg elemental iron plus 500 mg to replenish iron stores
- give an oral antihistamine (e.g. perphenazine 25 mg) half an hour before starting the infusion
- the infusion rate should be no more than 10 drops per minute (dpm) for the first 15 minutes.

### The management of severe anaemia in pregnancy
If Hb < 6.0 g/dl consider exchange transfusion or plasmaphaeresis. If Hb is between 6.0 and 8.0 g/dl transfuse slowly with 3–5 units of packed cells. Use intravenous frusemide 20 mg to prevent circulatory overload.

### Haemoglobinopathies

### Thalassaemias
These are the inherited defects in the rate of synthesis of one or more globin chains. The resulting imbalance in globin chain production leads to ineffective erythropoiesis, haemolysis and a variable degree of anaemia. The defects are uncommon among people from Northern Europe and the western hemisphere, and commoner in tropical or subtropical areas of Africa, Asia and Europe.

$\alpha$-thalassaemia occurs when structural DNA genes are deleted from the genome affecting the $\alpha$-Hb chains. The fetus can be affected because HbF contain $\alpha$ chains. If both linked

# 7.0 Pregnancy and associated diseases

## 7.1 Haematological disorders

pairs of $\alpha$-genes are missing, hydrops fetalis and stillbirth will result. Deletion of one of the linked pairs of $\alpha$-genes will lead to neonatal hypochromic anaemia. Heterozygotes will have mild anaemia, microcytosis and abnormal red cells. $\beta$-thalassaemia is due to a variety of abnormalities in messenger RNA. In $\beta^\circ$ thalassaemia no $\beta$-chains are produced, and in $\beta^+$ disease reduced amounts are produced. Heterozygotes are asymptomatic, but patients with homozygous $\beta^\circ$ and severe $\beta^+$ variants have severe thalassaemia major, from which up to 100,000 children die worldwide each year. There are no intrauterine effects because HbF is not affected. Infants become susceptible from about 3 months of age. This also applies to sickle-cell disease.

### Sickle-cell disease
Sickle-cell diseases are due to structural alterations in one of the globin chains. There are more than 80 $\alpha$-chain and 180 $\beta$-chain variants. The most important are the $\beta$-chain variants Hb S and Hb C. They may occur in conjunction with thalassaemia gene disorders.

Sickle-cell trait (Hb A/S or Hb A/C) is not a serious problem, but there is an increased risk of pyelonephritis in these patients. Hb S/S has its highest incidence and is most troublesome in tropical Africa, where heterozygote frequency is 20–40%. It also present among North American blacks (heterozygote frequency 9%), in the Middle East, India and the Mediterranean littoral. Hb S/C disease is unpredictable in pregnancy. It affects West Indian negro populations particularly severely.

Homozygosity predisposes to abortion, pre-term labour, stillbirth and sickling crises. HbSS, HbSC and HbS-$\beta$ thalassaemia have a fetal mortality of up to 50%.

**Sickling crises.** Hb A and Hb S function similarly when well oxygenated but Hb S polymerizes when deoxygenated. The red cells become sickle shaped and occlude vessels causing widespread vascular damage, severe pain, and haemolytic anaemia.

# 7.0 Pregnancy and associated diseases

## 7.1 Haematological disorders

To prevent crises give folate supplements and oral bicarbonate (to alkalize the urine), and carry out blood transfusions (3–4 units) at six week intervals.

The best treatment of crises is by exchange transfusion as follows:
- ask patient to empty bladder
- give oral frusemide 40 mg
- wait until bladder fills; ask patient to empty it again
- commence exchange transfusion removing 2.5 l of blood and replacing it with 3.0 l of carefully cross-matched blood.

### Antenatal screening for haemoglobinopathies
Routine Hb electrophoresis at the antenatal clinic is indicated when the indigenous or immigrant population makes the risk of haemoglobinopathy high. If routine screening is not necessary a sickling test (e.g. Sickledex) should be carried out on all black patients.

### Antenatal diagnosis
If a woman is found to be a heterozygous carrier for thalassaemia or sickle cell disease then her husband should be tested. If he too is heterozygous then antenatal diagnosis can be offered. The most effective method still depends on obtaining a sample of fetal blood by fetoscopy (see p. 70) at 16 to 18 weeks gestation. Newer methods involve the analysis of DNA using complex molecular biological techniques in fetal fibroblasts obtained at amniocentesis, or better still, chorionic villi which can be obtained at about 8 weeks (see p. 70). The ultimate aim is to understand how the globin genes are regulated and to discover if the defective genes which cause the problem can be replaced.

### Idiopathic thrombocytopaenic purpura (ITP)
Neonatal thrombocytopaenia occurs in 50% of ITP cases but is self-limiting. It may occur even though the mother has had a

## 7.0 Pregnancy and associated diseases

### 7.2 Hypertensive disorders

splenectomy in the past. Splenectomy is not advisable during pregnancy and treatment of maternal thrombocytopaenia ($< 100 \times 10^9$/l) is by prednisolone (up to 15 mg q.d.s.). Caesarean section is indicated only for obstetric reasons. Vaginal delivery should be attempted if at all possible avoiding laceration and episiotomy. Platelet transfusion may be given but the platelets are destroyed quickly.

### Haemolytic Anaemia
Glucose-6-phosphate dehydrogenase deficiency (G-6-PD) is the commonest cause, though rare in the UK. The gene is sex-linked recessive so male infants are affected. It occurs most commonly along the Mediterranean littoral, in Africa and the Far East. In these areas it is not an uncommon cause of neonatal jaundice. Jaundice is induced by oxidative drugs, particularly salicylates, sulphonamides and vitamin K analogues.

### Aplastic anaemia
Is rare and maternal prognosis is poor. The anaemia affects red cells, granulocytes and platelets. Infection and haemorrhage are therefore particularly hazardous.

**Chronic myeloid leukaemia and Hodgkin's lymphoma** are not affected adversely by pregnancy but treatment may be complicated because cytotoxic drugs may affect the fetus severely. Previously diagnosed and fully treated Hodgkin's disease (HD) is not a contra-indication to pregnancy, but it may be best to wait for at least a year after the end of therapy. If HD is diagnosed in early pregnancy termination may be indicated. Localized disease discovered in late pregnancy can await delivery for full work-up and therapy. Advanced disease should be investigated and treated fully whenever it is discovered.

### 7.2 Hypertensive disorders
Hypertension (H/T) is not a disease, it is a sign. Its correct management during pregnancy depends on identification of the

## 7.0 Pregnancy and associated diseases

### 7.2 Hypertensive disorders

underlying cause (whenever possible), the stage of pregnancy at which it is recorded, and assessment of the degree of risk to mother and fetus.

**BP measurement**. The criteria to be fulfilled are:
- patient relaxed
- upper arm level with heart
- patient sitting on examination couch or in bed
- take diastolic BP on muffling of Korotkoff sounds (phase IV) rather than their disappearance (phase V).

BP readings of 140/90 and over, or an increase of SBP > 30 mmHg and DBP of > 20 mmHg over the earliest recorded pregnancy reading are abnormal because the risk of fetal mortality and morbidity begins to rise concomitantly.

### Causes of hypertension in pregnancy
See Table 7.2.

**Table 7.2.** Classification of hypertension in pregnancy.

| Feature | Likely diagnosis |
| --- | --- |
| Abnormal BP, arising in the second half of pregnancy (usually in primigravidae) and returning to normal postpartum | Pregnancy-induced (gestational) H/T |
| Abnormal BP before pregnancy or noted in the first half of pregnancy | Pre-existing H/T |
| Exacerbation in second half of pregnancy of previously noted hypertension | Pre-existing H/T with superimposed pregnancy-induced H/T |

### (a) Pregnancy induced (gestational) hypertension
The hypertension itself may be:
**mild** a sustained BP > 140/90 but < 160/110 with the woman resting in bed; or
**severe** a sustained BP ≥ 160/110 while resting in bed.

# 7.0 Pregnancy and associated diseases

## 7.2 Hypertensive disorders

**Pre-eclampsia**
Is a condition peculiar to pregnancy of unknown aetiology usually characterized by hypertension, renal impairment, and fluid retention and often accompanied by proteinuria and increased intravascular coagulation. In mild pre-eclampsia mild H/T arises in the second half of pregnancy with some alteration in renal function but without proteinuria. It occurs in about 10% of pregnancies. In severe pre-eclampsia a BP $\geq$ 160/110 mmHg in the second half of pregnancy is accompanied by proteinuria of $\geq$ 0.5 g/l in the absence of urinary tract infection.

*Predisposing factors*
- **Primigravidity.** The incidence of proteinuric pre-eclampsia in a first pregnancy is about 6 percent. It affects about 2 percent of second pregnancies rising to 12 percent if the first pregnancy were affected and falling to 0.7 percent if the first was a singleton, normotensive pregnancy. Pregnancy by a new partner increases the risk to that of a first pregnancy. Hypertension of apparently acute onset in multiparous women is more likely to be due to latent pre-existing hypertension. The protection offered by an early miscarriage is now disputed.
- **Genetic.** Pre-eclampsia is more likely among women whose mother or sisters developed it also or in whom there is a strong family history of hypertension, other cardiovascular disorders or auto-immune disease. There is no significant racial preponderance.
- **Medical.** Pre-existing hypertension (see below) predisposes to pre-eclampsia as does diabetes mellitus. Women with a history of migraine, Raynaud's phenomenon or who became hypertensive while taking 'the pill' seem to be more prone to it.
- **Socio-economic.** The incidence increases as socio-economic status deteriorates. This may partly be due to diet, or be associated with failure to attend for antenatal care. The incidence is lower in women who smoke but the fetal outlook is poor in smokers who develop pre-eclampsia.

## 7.0 Pregnancy and associated diseases

### 7.2 Hypertensive disorders

- **Obstetric.** Multiple pregnancy and hydatidiform mole can be associated with very early and severe pre-eclampsia. It also tends to occur when hydrops fetalis (rhesus and non-rhesus) is present.

### (b) pre-existing hypertension
Among the causes are:
- Essential H/T—cause unknown.
- Renal H/T due to chronic pyelonephritis, glomerulonephritis, renal artery stenosis, nephropathy secondary to diabetes or analgesics, polycystic disease.
- Adrenal H/T—phaeochromocytoma, Cushing's syndrome, primary aldosteronism (Conn's syndrome), acromegaly, myxoedema, diabetes mellitus.
- Connective tissue disorders—systemic lupus, polyarteritis nodosa, scleroderma.
- Coarctation of aorta.
- Drug—oral contraceptives, corticosteroids, monoamine oxidase inhibitors (etc.).

### Guidelines to the management of mild H/T
The patient should be seen at least every two weeks until about 32 weeks gestation and weekly thereafter. Bed rest is usually effective in reducing mild H/T. The use of sedatives or tranquillizers is of no additional value and anti-hypertensive therapy is not indicated in this group (see below). Uncomplicated mild H/T is suitable for careful supervision at home by community midwives.

**Admission to hospital** is indicated when:
- SPB is $\geq$ 160 and/or DBP $\geq$ 100 mmHg.

(N.B. blood pressures of the above order cannot be ignored merely because readings taken 5 to 10 minutes later are significantly lower. The tendency to develop hypertension has been demonstrated and that suggests the possibility of increased risk.)

# 7.0 Pregnancy and associated diseases

## 7.2 Hypertensive disorders

- proteinuria is detected in a clean (i.e. mid-stream) urine sample in the absence of a urinary infection
- the patient is symptomatic with e.g. visual disturbances, unusual headache, epigastric pain, vomiting or twitching
- there is clinical evidence of intrauterine growth retardation
- excessive weight gain (> 1 kg/week) accompanies a lesser degree of hypertension than above
- tests of fetal welfare have deteriorated (see page 153).
- a previous bad obstetric history suggests that closer surveillance would be worthwhile.

### Management of severe H/T

The maternal risk of cerebro-vascular accident, and left ventricular or renal failure begins to increase significantly when the BP is of the order of 170/110 mmHg after 24 hrs rest in bed, or without bed rest if there are two successive readings of $\geq$ 180/120 mmHg. In such circumstances the choice has to be made between delivery and anti-hypertensive therapy.

Among the factors influencing the decision are:
- gestational age—oral therapy is seldom justified from 34 weeks onwards
- availability of intensive neonatal care facilities
- symptoms and signs of severe pre-eclampsia (see above).

Anti-hypertensive therapy neither influences the progression of underlying pre-eclampsia nor significantly improves fetal outcome. It helps to protect the mother and enables many pregnancies to continue that otherwise would be ended because of maternal risk.

### Fulminating pre-eclampsia and eclampsia

This is discussed on page 231.

### Oral anti-hypertensive drugs for use in pregnancy

#### $\alpha$-methyldopa

Is the most thoroughly investigated hypotensive agent used in

## 7.0 Pregnancy and associated diseases

### 7.2 Hypertensive disorders

pregnancy, its use has been shown to be relatively safe. Its action is central, decreasing the sympathetic outflow from the brain.

**Dose**: Initially 500 mg, then 250 mg 6 hourly rising to a maximum of 750 mg 6 hourly.

**Side-effects**: Drowsiness (which usually passes within 24–48 hrs) and faintness on standing. It is contra-indicated in patients with a history of depressive illness. If necessary it can successfully be combined with oral hydralazine (see below).

### Hydralazine

Is a non-specific vasodilator. It is used extensively parenterally in hypertensive emergencies (see page 000). It is used orally in conjunction with, for example, $\alpha$-methyl dopa or labetalol.

**Dose**: Initially 25 mg 6–8 hourly rising to a maximum of 75 mg 6 hourly.

**Side-effects**: It may mimic impending eclampsia (headache, tremor, nausea) but this is rare after oral use. The vasodilated skin is hot and looks flushed. Only more prolonged treatment than occurs in pregnancy is liable to produce a systemic lupus-like illness.

### Beta-adrenergic blocking agents

Reduce sympathetic stimulation of the heart and may suppress the renin–angiotensin system. Their use is contra-indicated with a history of asthma. **Propranolol** is not recommended in pregnancy.

Among the alternatives which have been used successfully in the management of hypertension in pregnancy are:

- **oxprenolol**—80 mg twice daily up to a maximum of 480 mg per day.
- **atenolol**—50 mg once or twice daily. Side-effects: bradycardia, bronchospasm, peripheral vasoconstriction.
- **labetalol**—it has combined alpha- and beta-adrenergic receptor blocking effects, the latter predominating. It can be

# 7.0 Pregnancy and associated diseases

## 7.2 Hypertensive disorders

used intravenously to control hypertensive crises (see p. 233). The oral dose is 100 mg 8 hourly rising to a maximum of 200 mg 8 hourly. Side effects: postural hypotension, tiredness, headache

### Nifedipine
Is a calcium channel blocker and vasodilator the use of which is now being reported in pregnancy. Further studies are necessary. It can be used as an adjunct to beta-blocking agents.
**Dose**: 5–10 mg twice daily (maximum 40 mg twice daily).
**Side effects**: flushing, headache and ankle-swelling.
**Angiotensin—converting enzyme inhibitors** such as captopril are not recommended in pregnancy.

### Diuretics
Should only be used for the treatment of heart failure and severe oliguria. Peripheral oedema does no harm and all satisfactory trials of diuretics have failed to show any benefit.
They are contra-indicated in pre-eclampsia because they:
- obscure the interpretation of plasma uric acid and urea levels (see below)
- further reduce circulating blood volume
- may cause thrombocytopaenia in the infants.

### Sedatives and tranquillizers
Neither have a beneficial effect and merely cause a false sense of security in medical staff. Fetal heart rate responses are affected and this may be crucial if antenatal fetal heart rate monitoring (see page 155) is being used as an indicator of fetal well-being.

### Antenatal monitoring of pregnancy hypertension

### Examination (over and above routine)
- palpation of the femoral pulses (to exclude coarctation of aorta)

## 7.0 Pregnancy and associated diseases

### 7.2 Hypertensive disorders

- exclude kidney enlargement
- check optic fundi for silver wiring, arterio-venous nipping, exudates and haemorrhages.

**Laboratory investigations**

*(a) Once only*
Urinary catecholamines and vanillyl mandelic acid (VMA—a catecholamine metabolite) are raised in the presence of a phaeochromocytoma. Although this tumour is very rare the consequences of failure to diagnose it can be catastrophic to mother and baby. It is therefore still justifiable to exclude it in all cases of which DBP is persistently > 90 mmHg (particularly if it is episodic). Test results are invalid if the patient is taking $\alpha$-methyl dopa.

*(b) Serial*
**Urine microscopy and culture.** Bacterial counts of $10^5/mm^3$ are significant (repeat if $10^4-10^5/mm^3$).

**Serum uric acid** increases are an early, sensitive indicator of the onset of pre-eclampsia. Levels > 350 $\mu$mol/l are abnormal in pregnancy, but gradually increasing levels are most significant.

**Serum urea and creatinine.** Rising levels are significant but not such sensitive indicators of pre-eclampsia as uric acid. The upper normal limits in pregnancy are 5 mmol/l for serum urea and 100 $\mu$mol/l for creatinine, but trends are even more important than specific levels.

**Creatinine clearance**—see page 17.

**Platelet count** gradually falls if disseminated intravascular coagulation is occurring.

**Coagulation factors.** Fibrin degradation products (FDPs) are of little diagnostic or prognostic value. Coagulation studies are not routinely necessary.

**Tests of fetal growth and well-being** are vital and are discussed fully on pages 28 and 153.

## 7.0 Pregnancy and associated diseases

7.3 Diabetes mellitus

**Optimum time for delivery**
Pre-eclampsia is the commonest cause of intrauterine growth retardation. The optimum time for delivery depends on the availability of intensive neonatal care facilities. If these are not adequate locally the woman should be transferred antenatally to the nearest hospital with appropriate facilities. Transfer of a very sick neonate is hazardous and not to be recommended if it can be avoided.

The most common grounds for delivery are:
- progressive fetal compromise, i.e. when the baby is obviously safer delivered
- unacceptable risk to maternal health e.g. uncontrollable BP, impending renal failure or heart failure, increasing jaundice or intravascular coagulation or eclampsia (see page 231).

The mode of delivery (caesarean section or vaginal) depends on the seriousness of the situation, the gestational age and the degree of fetal/maternal compromise.

**Long-term outlook**
Severely pre-eclamptic/eclamptic primigravidae are not at increased risk of developing chronic hypertension (given that there is no pre-existing hypertension). Later chronic H/T is, on the other hand, very prevalent among severely pre-eclamptic multiparous women because it is their latest hypertension which predisposes them to pre-eclampsia in the first place.

## 7.3 Diabetes mellitus

**Definitions**
Symptoms and signs (polydipsia, polyuria, weight loss and glycosuria) plus a random venous plasma glucose concentration $\geq$ 11.0 mmol/l or a fasting concentration $\geq$ 8.0 mmol/l. In the absence of symptoms a fasting value $> 8.0$ mmol/l and/or a concentration $> 11$ mmol/l 2 hrs after a 75 g glucose load are diagnostic.

## 7.0 Pregnancy and associated diseases

7.3 Diabetes mellitus

**Impaired glucose tolerance** (IGT) is present if the fasting level is < 8.0 mmol/l but is between 8.0 and 10.9 mmol/l, 2 hrs after a 75 g glucose load.

### Antenatal screening
Carbohydrate intolerance must be suspected in all women with:
- glycosuria on routine testing
- a history of diabetes in first degree relatives
- a previous baby weighing > 90th centile for gestational age, and sex (see p. 26)
- previous unexplained stillbirth
- diabetes in previous pregnancy
- obesity (> 85 kg or > 20% above ideal weight)
- polyhydramnios.

Blood should be taken for glucose estimation before (fasting) and 2 hrs after a 50 g glucose load. An oral GTT is indicated if the fasting plasma glucose concentration is > 5 mmol/l and/or the 2 hr level is > 7 mmol/l.

Unfortunately about 30% of gestational diabetics do not show any of the above features in their history; not all women with IGT or even diabetes have persistent glycosuria; and glycosuria can be found in up to 50% of all pregnant women at some time. Routine antenatal screening has therefore been recommended. To do this blood is taken at booking and 28–32 weeks for random blood glucose measurement. A glucose tolerance test (GTT) is indicated if concentrations are $\geq$ 6.4 mmol/l within 2 hrs of the last meal or $\geq$ 5.8 mmol/l more than 2 hrs after it.

### The oral glucose tolerance test
Despite being unphysiological the GTT will reveal impaired carbohydrate homeostasis better than any other available test. It should be carried out under the following standard conditions:
- 12 hours of fasting and 30 minutes sitting quietly beforehand
- patient remains seated and does not smoke during the test

# 7.0 Pregnancy and associated diseases

## 7.3 Diabetes mellitus

- after the fasting blood specimen is taken 75 g of glucose in 200–250 ml of water (or equivalent volume of 'Lucozade') is drunk within 5 minutes
- zero time is the beginning of the drink and samples are withdrawn at 30 minute intervals for at least two hours.

The criteria of normality for a GTT depend on the type of blood sample taken and the method for estimating the blood glucose. Plasma glucose is about 10% higher than whole blood, and capillary levels are different from venous. In addition enzymatic methods (e.g. the glucose oxidase method) give lower levels than chemical estimations.

Using the glucose oxidase method on venous plasma after a 75 g glucose load the criteria for normality should roughly be as follows:

- fasting plasma glucose $<$ 5.8 mmol/l
- 1 hour level $<$ 12.5 mmol/l
- 2 hour level $<$ 9.5 mmol/l
- 3 hour level $<$ 7.5 mmol/l.

However, each hospital has its own normal ranges for the GTT and these should be ascertained and used.

### Risks associated with diabetes in pregnancy

Retinopathy, nephropathy and neuropathy may be adversely affected by pregnancy. There is an increased risk of obstetric complications such as polyhydramnios, pre-term labour, pre-eclampsia, urinary tract infection, monilial vaginitis and other infections. The risk of congenital malformations is greater and perinatal morbidity and mortality are increased. Sudden unexpected intrauterine death may occur, usually after 36 weeks. Delivery may be complicated because of excess fetal growth (macrosomia). For the neonate there are increased risks from birth trauma, respiratory distress (increased six-fold), hypoglycaemia, hypocalcaemia and jaundice. The incidence of all problems is greatly increased by poor control of the diabetes

# 7.0 Pregnancy and associated diseases

## 7.3 Diabetes mellitus

(especially if maternal keto-acidosis develops) and by inadequate antenatal obstetric supervision.

## Management of diabetes in pregnancy

### 1. Pre-pregnancy
Women with established diabetes should be seen *before* pregnancy in order to:
- provide general counselling particularly about the importance of tight control
- plan for pregnancy
- review diet
- examine optic fundi
- establish good blood glucose control.

### 2. Antenatally (pre-existing diabetes)

*General aspects*
- encourage early booking and establish a plan for the pregnancy
- care should be jointly between obstetrician and physician
- see 2–4 weekly (depending on control).

*Diabetic control*
- ask dietitian to provide appropriate high fibre diet
- oral hypoglycaemia agents cause fetal hyperinsulinaemia and are therefore contra-indicated
- blood glucose profiles should be carried out 2–3 times weekly (more if control difficult) at home using filter paper strips and a reflectance meter. The timing is before and 2 hours after breakfast, lunch and supper, and last thing at night (and sometimes at 3–4 a.m.). Pre-prandial levels of < 5.0 mmol/l and 2 hour levels of < 7.0 mmol/l are ideal
- regular urinalysis for glycosuria—this is of limited value in

# 7.0 Pregnancy and associated diseases

## 7.3 Diabetes mellitus

assessing control but keeps a check on loss of dietary carbohydrate
- glycosylated haemoglobin estimates are also of limited value for control but can provide retrospective assessment at the end of each trimester and a check on the validity of the home glucose monitoring.

### Insulin treatment
A regime using a combination of soluble and intermediate-acting insulins morning and evening is preferable. Use of the new human insulins or highly purified porcine insulin reduces the risk of insulin antibodies (which can cross the placenta). If control is difficult, meal times or calorie distribution can be adjusted. A third dose of soluble insulin is sometimes necessary in late evening or, occasionally, before the midday meal.

### Maternal health
- check optic fundi early in pregnancy and 3 monthly in severe cases
- monitor blood pressure carefully
- carry out baseline assessment of renal function (urea, electrolytes, urate and creatinine clearance) at booking and thereafter as indicated.

### Monitoring fetal welfare
- offer alpha-fetoprotein screening at 16–18 weeks (N.B.—the levels of AFP are on average 10% lower in diabetic compared with normal pregnancy)
- carry out baseline ultrasound scan for gestational age and gross normality at 16–18 weeks
- assess fetal growth by BPD and AC measurements monthly
- kick chart from 26 weeks—(see p. 153)
- biophysical profiles (see p. 156) can be carried out weekly (or more frequently if indicated) from 26 weeks

## 7.0 Pregnancy and associated diseases

### 7.3 Diabetes mellitus

- if pre-term delivery is contemplated carry out amniotic fluid phospholipid analysis.

*Indications for admission to hospital*
- good glucose control not possible as out-patient
- hypertension or proteinuria
- excessive weight gain
- deterioration of renal function, pyelonephritis
- concern over fetal growth or well-being.

### 3. Gestational diabetes
When impaired glucose tolerance is diagnosed for the first time during pregnancy the patient should be admitted for pre-prandial glucose estimations on her normal diet. If concentrations are $\geq$ 5.8 mmol/l treatment is indicated. If diet does not control it then insulin should be started. Management is then as above.

### 4. Delivery
When diabetes is well controlled and pregnancy uncomplicated, vaginal delivery between 38–40 weeks should be anticipated. Caesarean section is only indicated for obstetric reasons. The obstetrician and physician in charge, and the paediatrician should be kept informed at all times.

*Programme for vaginal delivery*
If prostaglandin pessaries are being used as part of induction of labour give normal diet and usual regime of insulin until labour is established then proceed as below.

When patient is in established spontaneous or induced labour:
- give nothing by mouth
- set up i.v. infusion of 500 ml 5% dextrose with 10 mmol potassium chloride at rate of 100 ml hourly

## 7.0 Pregnancy and associated diseases

7.3 Diabetes mellitus

- provide continuous infusion of soluble insulin in normal saline (by pump into the tubing of the i.v. line) at 1–2 units/hr (see below)
- if a Syntocinon infusion is required use normal saline
- check blood glucose hourly and serum potassium 4–8 hourly
- alter rate of insulin infusion to maintain blood glucose at 5–8 mmol/l and dextrose infusion to keep serum potassium at normal levels
- monitor fetal heart using continuous CTG (by scalp clip when possible).

*Programme for elective caesarean section*
- give normal diet and insulin dose on evening before
- nil by mouth from midnight
  On day of delivery:

*08.00* check blood glucose and electrolytes; give pre-medication.

*08.30* set up i.v. glucose infusion (5%) with 10 mmol potassium chloride/500 ml, at a rate of 100 ml hourly; give insulin infusion as above.

*09.00* caesarean section. Monitor infusions throughout as for vaginal delivery.

**After delivery**: insulin sensitivity increases immediately after delivery of the placenta.

Maintain i.v. infusions of dextrose, potassium and insulin carefully monitoring the rates of infusion until the woman can eat and drink normally. The infusion can then be stopped and the usual diet recommenced.

The insulin dosage usually needs to be reduced by ⅓–½.

Monitor diabetic control with blood and urine glucose measurements and alter insulin dosages as indicated.

**Points to note**
- Hyperglycaemia should be avoided during labour because it produces neonatal hypoglycaemia.

## 7.0 Pregnancy and associated diseases

7.4 Cardiac disease in pregnancy

- Treatment of pre-term labour with beta-sympathomimetic agents causes marked hyperglycaemia. They should, therefore, either be avoided or covered by insulin infusions of up to 32 units/hr.

### Post-natal care
The baby should remain with the mother and only be transferred to a special care unit if specifically indicated. Hypoglycaemia is quite common in the baby and requires treatment if plasma glucose falls below 1.1 mmol/l or if signs and symptoms develop. Breast-feeding has little effect on diabetic control and should be encouraged. The perinatal mortality for diabetic pregnancies should now be approaching that of other pregnancies once congenital malformations are excluded.

### 7.4 Cardiac disease in pregnancy
The prevalence of **rheumatic heart disease** (RHD) varies from community to community but its incidence has fallen dramatically over the past 25 years. The relative contribution of **congenital heart defects** (CHD) has increased (6–8 per 1000 live births).

A classification based on symptoms is no longer recommended. Pregnancy has no permanent deleterious effects on RHD.

Pre-conception counselling is important for women with known heart disease in order to:

- provide general counselling and optimize treatment
- plan for pregnancy e.g. in some women cardiac surgery may be indicated beforehand
- advise accordingly those women suffering from a condition with which increased maternal mortality is associated e.g. Marfan's syndrome, inoperable cyanotic heart disease, primary pulmonary hypertension, Eisenmenger's syndrome. Pregnancy may be best avoided in these conditions.

## 7.0 Pregnancy and associated diseases

### 7.4 Cardiac disease in pregnancy

**Routine antenatal management**

Termination of pregnancy is not medically indicated (except, perhaps, for above conditions).

- arrange regular antenatal visits to obstetrician and cardiologist
- ensure adequate rest
- ban smoking
- prevent anaemia
- treat respiratory infection promptly
- cover dental work with antibiotics
- be watchful for incipient pulmonary congestion and arrhythmias
- admit patients with RHD and uncorrected CHD between 36 and 39 weeks gestation depending on nature and severity of the disease.

**Management of labour**

Induction of labour should only be for good obstetric reasons. Prostaglandin pessaries (see p. 000) are preferred. When a patient starts labour with good cardiac reserve the risk of heart failure is low.

- aim for vaginal delivery at term
- cover labour with antibiotics e.g. crystalline penicillin or ampicillin and gentamicin
- provide adequate analgesia—epidural anaesthesia is safe in experienced hands as long as hypotension is avoided
- shorten the second stage by use of 'lift-out' forceps or vacuum extractor (without raising legs into lithotomy position if possible)
- ergometrine is best avoided
- do not attempt caesarean section in the presence of heart failure
- have oxygen and relevant drugs *immediately* available.

**Cardiac failure**

This can occur in young, previously asymptomatic women at

## 7.0 Pregnancy and associated diseases

7.4 Cardiac disease in pregnancy

any stage of pregnancy. The risk increases as pregnancy advances and the early post-partum period is the most hazardous.

The clinical features of cardiac failure are pulmonary congestion, frank pulmonary oedema and right heart failure.

### 1. Pulmonary congestion
**Signs:**
- dyspnoea
- persistent moist sounds at lung bases
- haemoptysis (serious)
- vascular congestion on X-ray.

**Management:**
- bed rest in hospital
- digitalize (guided by degree of tachycardia)
- diuretics and potassium supplements
- salt restriction
- vigorous treatment of any intercurrent infection.

### 2 and 3 Acute pulmonary oedema and right heart failure

Both are MEDICAL EMERGENCIES which are particularly liable to occur a few minutes or hours after delivery. The management is:
- nurse in semi-recumbent position
- give oxygen
- keep airways clear
- morphine 10–20 mg s.c. or i.v.
- aminophylline 250 mg i.v.
- frusemide 40 mg i.v.
- digoxin (if not previously digitalized)
- if there is no improvement proceed to endotracheal intubation and assisted respiration
- if the patient is in labour, the fetus must take second place until the situation is under control.

## 7.0 Pregnancy and associated diseases

7.4 Cardiac disease in pregnancy

### Infective endocarditis
This is mostly due to *Streptococcus viridans*. It occurs rarely in pure mitral stenosis. Blood cultures may be negative or only become positive on repeated testing. Treat energetically on suspicion in women with mitral incompetence without awaiting results of blood culture.

Antibiotic prophylaxis is required for dental work (3 days) and labour (7 days) as follows:

- either crystalline penicillin 0.5 mega units i.m. then penicillin V 250 mg orally twice daily *or*
- erythromycin 300 mg i.m. then 250 mg orally six hourly (Use if patient allergic to penicillin) *or*
- cephaloridine 2 g i.m. then cephalexin 250 mg six hourly *or*
- ampicillin 250 mg i.m. six hourly, gentamicin 40 mg i.m. six hourly for 24 hours to cover labour.

### Management of arrhythmias
**Atrial fibrillation** is a MEDICAL EMERGENCY and should be managed as follows:
- bed rest in hospital
- digitalize
- anticoagulate (possibly)
- if the ventricular rate does not fall consider use of beta adrenergic blocking agents
- consider electroconversion to re-establish sinus rhythm.

**Atrial tachycardia** can precipitate heart failure rapidly: try carotid sinus pressure and if that fails DC shock therapy.

### Cardiac surgery and pregnancy
Anticoagulant therapy (see page 148) must be maintained and carefully controlled in women who have had previous cardiac surgery. Consider closed mitral valvotomy during pregnancy:
- in pure severe mitral stenosis *and*
- if pulmonary congestion develops (particularly if profuse haemoptysis is occurring) *and*
- if there is no prompt response to medical therapy.

## 7.0 Pregnancy and associated diseases

7.4 Cardiac disease in pregnancy

**Congenital heart disease** (CHD)
See Table 7.3. Most patients with acyanotic CHD tolerate pregnancy well (except aortic stenosis and coarctation of the aorta). Patients with uncorrected cyanotic CHD, primary pulmonary hypertension and pulmonary hypertension as part of Eisenmenger's syndrome do badly.

**Table 7.3.** Congenital heart lesions and pregnancy.

| Type of lesion | Response during pregnancy when lesion is: Uncorrected | Corrected |
|---|---|---|
| Patent ductus arteriosus | Many develop heart failure or duct may become infected. Can be closed during pregnancy | Uncomplicated |
| Atrial septal defect | Heart failure → closure surgically. Atrial tachydysrhythmias may occur | Usually uncomplicated even after closure |
| Ventricular septal defect | Size of defect and pulmonary vascular resistance determine prognosis. With high pulmonary vascular resistance a bidirectional shunt may develop, and this is dangerous | Uncomplicated |
| Fallot's tetralogy | Prognosis poor if $Po_2 < 80\%$ of normal and haematocrit $> 60\%$ | Pregnancy possible but not advisable |
| Coarctation of aorta | Occasional risk of aortic rupture or dissection | Uneventful |
| Eisenmenger's syndrome | High fetal and maternal risk. Maternal death often due to syncope | Not correctable |
| Aortic stenosis | Slight to moderate → uneventful pregnancy. In severe cases LV failure and maternal syncope may occur | — |
| Pulmonary stenosis | Pregnancy usually well tolerated if there is no pulmonary hypertension | — |

## 7.0 Pregnancy and associated diseases

7.5 Thyroid disorders

### 7.5 Thyroid disorders
For normal thyroid function in pregnancy—see page 000.

**Hyperthyroidism**
The clinical features are as follows:
- goitre
- weight loss
- raised sleeping pulse rate
- exophthalmos
- lid retraction
- peri-orbital swelling.

Investigations show a raised $T_4$ and Free $T_4$ Index ($FT_4I$). In addition the $T_3$ resin uptake ($T_3RU$) is low for pregnancy. Radioactive iodine tests must be avoided.

**Treatment** is with carbimazole 15 mg or propylthiouracil 150 mg (PTU) eight hourly and thyroxine 0.1 to 0.2 mg daily. When control is achieved, (which can take 4–6 weeks) the antithyroid drugs can be gradually reduced to carbimazole $\leq 20$ mg daily, PTU $\leq 200$ mg daily. Propranolol 20 mg eight hourly may be used if necessary to control the serious peripheral effect of thyrotoxicosis. Control is assessed on clinical grounds and by serial $FT_4I$, serum $T_3$ and TSH levels. Combined treatment should be continued throughout the puerperium. Breast feeding is safe if the daily dose of carbimazole $\leq 15$ mg or of propylthiouracil $\leq 50$ mg.

**Subtotal thyroidectomy** may be indicated in the following situations:
- Large goitre is causing obstruction
- Failure to control symptoms with reasonable doses of drugs
- Toxic reactions to drugs

Babies born to thyrotoxic mothers should be screened for hyperthyroidism.

**Hypothyroidism**
The commonest causes are auto-immune thyroiditis and partial

## 7.0 Pregnancy and associated diseases

### 7.5 Thyroid disorders

thyroidectomy. The clinical features are as follows:
- excess weight gain
- cold intolerance
- undue fatigue
- dry skin
- slow pulse
- delayed relaxation of ankle jerk.

Investigations show a raised TSH ($\geq 10\,\mu$U/ml) with a low $T_3$ and $FT_4I$.

**Treatment** is with thyroxine 2 micrograms/kg body weight. The $T_4$, $T_3RU$, $FT_4I$ and TSH levels should be measured every 1 or 2 months. The dose can be reduced after delivery. Breast feeding is not contra-indicated. If the mother has previously had thyrotoxicosis check for neonatal thyrotoxicosis and if she has had autoimmune thyroiditis check the baby for hypothyroidism.

*Post-partum thyroiditis* is a relatively common and generally unrecognised condition which is said to occur after 5–9% of pregnancies. It presents with fatigue, palpitations, or other features of mild thyrotoxicosis, at between 2 and 4 months post-partum. It is often confused with 'post-partum blues'. A painless goitre occurs in up to 75% of cases. There is a common association with HLA DR 3, 4, and 5. 20–25% of affected women have a first degree relative with auto-immune thyroid disease.

T3 and T4 levels are raised, radioactive iodine uptake is low and antimicrosomal antibodies (AMAs) are usually present.

*Treatment.* Thyrotoxic phase —beta-blockers for palpitations
Hypothyroid phase —nothing if asymptomatic
or thyroxine for 4 to 6 months

It is usually a self-limiting condition but in a small minority of cases hypothyroidism may persist.

In some women with a family history of auto-immune thyroid disease AMAs are present in the first trimester (they may become negative later) and about 60% of them will develop post-partum hypothyroidism. AMAs should therefore be looked for in women with such a family history.

## 7.0 Pregnancy and associated diseases

7.6 Systemic lupus erythematosus

### 7.6 Systemic lupus erythematosus (SLE)
SLE is a multisystem disease of unknown aetiology that tends to occur in women of reproductive age. The best diagnostic test are anti-nuclear factor and anti-DNA antibodies.

Pregnancy has no specific effects on SLE although there may be flare-up during the puerperium. Women with SLE in pregnancy have an increased risk of:
- first trimester miscarriage and later intra-uterine death
- hypertension and pre-eclampsia, pre-term delivery (planned and spontaneous)
- neonatal SLE (e.g. transient congenital heart block)

#### Management during pregnancy
Close antenatal supervision is necessary. Carry out serial measurements of blood pressure, renal function and fetal growth.

The mainstay of treatment is corticosteroids but azathioprine may be needed in some circumstances.

The timing of delivery depends on the severity of the condition. Deteriorating renal function may be an indication for early delivery. If the fetus has congenital heart block then Caesarean section is warranted because of reduced ability of the fetus to respond to stress.

#### The lupus anticoagulant (LA)
A circulating anti-cardiolipin antibody has recently been described that is associated with a high prevalence of maternal thrombosis and fetal loss. It is not specific to SLE and may be found in any women with a history of unexplained fetal loss at any gestational age. A causal relationship is not yet definitely established. Low-dose aspirin and corticosteroid therapy may be helpful but this has not yet been proven in controlled trials.

### 7.7 Myasthenia gravis
This is a rare condition with a peak incidence between 20 and 30

## 7.0 Pregnancy and associated diseases

### 7.8 Epilepsy

years of age. It produces weakness and rapid fatigue of voluntary muscles. 75% of patients have a thymoma (or thymic lymphoid hyperplasia). Pregnancy does not worsen the disease but exacerbations can occur in up to 30% of women (most frequently in the puerperium). Maternal mortality is increased but only if the condition goes unrecognized.

**Management**:
- avoid infections (they may cause exacerbation)
- avoid sedatives, tranquillizers, analgesics and narcotics
- avoid general anaesthesia (regional analgesia is preferred for labour)
- treatment is with pyridostigmine, or neostigmine and atropine
- corticosteroids or ACTH may also be effective
- thymectomy may sometimes be necessary
- labour may be shorter than normal
- pushing in the second stage can be tiring and low forceps delivery helpful
- give neostigmine 0.5 mg i.m. in labour.

Transient myasthenic sigmus and symptoms can occur in the neonate of affected mothers.

### 7.8 Epilepsy

Women with epilepsy should be seen before becoming pregnant so that their requirements for anticonvulsants can be checked. Counselling helps to allay their fears. The risk of an epileptic mother having an epileptic child is about 1 in 40. It is greatest among those with an EEG pattern showing $3H_z$ spikes and wave discharges. Pregnancy does not provoke epilepsy in mothers but the frequency of seizures may increase because anticonvulsants are cleared more quickly.

**The effect of anticonvulsants on the fetus**

The incidence of congenital malformations is increased two to three fold in infants of women on anticonvulsants. No one drug

## 7.0 Pregnancy and associated diseases

### 7.8 Epilepsy

can be said to be free of problems. Among the problems are:
- cleft lip and/or palate (increased ten fold)
- congenital heart defect (increased four fold)
- hypoplasia of terminal phalanges of fingers
- characteristic facial appearance of wide-spaced eyes; low posterior hair line; short neck; prominent brow; trigoncephaly
- retarded growth, delayed development and, occasionally mental retardation.

These problems may be associated with drug-induced folic acid deficiency.

Phenytoin (especially if combined with primodone or phenobarbitone) is associated with a 2 to 3 fold increase in such malformations as cleft palate, and cardiac anomalies, and retarded growth, delayed development and, rarely, mental retardation. It is not certain that these are drug effects. They may be related to genetic or other environmental factors, anoxia secondary to fits, or drug-induced folic acid deficiency. Valproate may lead to NTD and carbamazepine may cause IUGR and microcephaly.

### Routine management of epilepsy in pregnancy
- regular (monthly) supervision by neurologist and obstetrician
- continue anticonvulsants in adequate dosage—the risks from seizures is greater than that of congenital anomalies
- folic acid 5 mg orally eight hourly throughout pregnancy
- vitamin K 10 mg orally daily from 32 weeks gestation
- vitamin K 1 mg i.m. to all neonates of treated mothers
- breast-feeding is not contra-indicated.

### Management of status epilepticus
- maintain airway and give oxygen
- diazepam 10 mg i.v. as a bolus injection then 40 mg in 500 ml dextrose/saline at 100 ml/hr reducing as seizures come under control.

## 7.9 Pituitary tumours

Women who were previously considered infertile because of secreting adenomas are now becoming pregnant due to the use of dopamine agonists (e.g. bromocryptine). The tumour may increase in size during pregnancy, therefore the sella turcica should be re-examined radiologically at 28 weeks and particular note must be taken of visual disturbances or unusual headaches. If the tumour enlarges and causes pressure on the optic chiasma a neurosurgical opinion must be sought urgently, because of the danger to the patient's sight.

## 7.10 Respiratory diseases

### Bronchial asthma
Pregnancy has no consistent effect on asthma and cases should be managed medically in the normal manner. Sympathomimetic bronchodilators (e.g. salbutamol or orciprenaline) do not affect labour adversely. Disodium cromoglycate can be used safely in pregnancy. If steroids are used (or have been within the last year) cover labour (or anaesthesia) with hydrocortisone 100 mg i.m. six hourly during labour, tailing off over the next 48 hours. Inhaled steroids are effective and do not need parenteral cover during labour.

### Management of status asthmaticus
- steroids in high doses
- bronchodilators
- artificial ventilation, if necessary, in intensive care unit.

### Pulmonary tuberculosis
Treatment of pulmonary tuberculosis (TB) in pregnancy is with streptomycin 1.0 g daily with isoniazid 300 mg daily and either para-aminosalicylic acid (PAS) 16 g/day or ethambutol 15 mg/kg/day. This regime can be reduced to two drugs only, when the sensitivities of the tubercle bacilli are known. Rifampicin can be

# 7.0 Pregnancy and associated diseases

7.11 Diseases of the liver and alimentary tract

used after the first trimester and isoniazid should be continued. Treatment needs to continue for 1–2 years (9 months if rifampicin can be used). Labour is not usually a problem. If a patient has open tuberculosis and inhalational anaesthesia is used the anaesthetic machine must be sterilized carefully after use.

### Management of infants of mothers with tuberculosis
BCG vaccination is necessary. Give isoniazid 20 mg/kg/day until the Mantoux test is positive. It is only necessary to separate the infant from the mother if mother has open TB and until Mantoux conversion occurs. Breast-feeding is only contra-indicated if the patient has sputum-positive TB.

### Pneumonia
**Bacterial pneumonia** causes a high fever and systemic toxicity which may lead to pre-term labour or intra-uterine death. Treatment is with penicillin G, 1 megaunit six hourly. The fever can be lessened by tepid sponging.

**Viral pneumonia** carries a high maternal mortality and there is no specific treatment. Additional bacterial infections (often staphylococcus) must be treated vigorously with penicillin and cloxacillin. Intensive supportive care (e.g. tracheostomy, renal dialysis) may be necessary in severe cases.

## 7.11 Diseases of liver and alimentary tract

### Jaundice in pregnancy
The incidence is approximately 1 in 1500 pregnancies. It can be considered under the following headings:

### 1. Jaundice caused by pregnancy
Intrahepatic cholestasis constitutes 20% of all cases of jaundice but the incidence is higher in, for example, Scandinavia and Chile. The patient typically complains of generalized pruritus in

# 7.0 Pregnancy and associated diseases

## 7.11 Diseases of the liver and alimentary tract

the second half of pregnancy. Some patients never become jaundiced. The bilirubin is raised but is usually < 100 $\mu$mol/l (6 mg/100 ml). The transaminases are mildly elevated (usually < 250 iu/l).

There is an increased risk of pre-term labour, fetal distress and perinatal death. Jaundice clears up within 4 weeks of delivery and does not proceed to chronic liver disease. It tends to recur in subsequent pregnancies and may also occur in association with oestrogen-containing oral contraceptives. Cholestyramine will reduce itching but is very unpleasant to take. Parenteral vitamin K is required if jaundice causes prolongation of the prothrombin time.

**Jaundice complicating pre-eclampsia** is a rare but very serious complication usually associated with disseminated intravascular coagulation and severe systemic upset. The only treatment is delivery after which it resolves rapidly.

**Acute fatty degeneration of the liver** is a rare but very serious complication of pregnancy. The incidence is increased in association with poor maternal nutrition and intravenous tetracycline therapy. It presents with abdominal pain, vomiting and headache usually after 36 weeks gestation. Rapid progression may occur through severe jaundice, uraemia, and haematemesis, to coma and death. Both maternal and fetal mortality are high. The frequent profound hypoglycaemia should be treated energetically and delivery must be expedited.

### 2. Intercurrent jaundice in pregnancy

Viral hepatitis which constitutes 40% of all cases is due either to Hepatitis B (long incubation, serum hepatitis) or Hepatitis A (short incubation, infective hepatitis). Hepatitis B is associated with Australia Antigen now known as $HB_s$ Ag. In these cases the infants may be protected by gamma-globulin rich in antibodies to $HB_s$ Ag, but its effectiveness is by no means certain. All viral hepatitis can be managed conservatively.

**Cholelithiasis** forms 6% of all cases. Modern ultrasound or

# 7.0 Pregnancy and associated diseases

7.11 Diseases of the liver and alimentary tract

transhepatic cholangiography may be useful in confirming the diagnosis. Cholecystectomy can be carried out in pregnancy, preferably in the second trimester rather than the first or last.

Drug toxicity and haemolysis are other causes of intercurrent jaundice in pregnancy.

### 3. Pre-existing liver disease
Pregnancy is uncommon in the presence of cirrhosis due, for example to active chronic hepatitis, or primary biliary cirrhosis. The prognosis is good for mother and baby in familial non-haemolytic jaundice, e.g. Gilbert's and the Dubin Johnson syndromes. Pregnancy may increase jaundice in the latter.

### Acute pancreatitis
This is a rare condition in pregnancy. Serum amylase levels increase slightly in pregnancy but this should not cause confusion in diagnosis.

Treatment is conservative as in the non-pregnant patient using:
- naso-gastric aspiration
- intravenous fluids
- blood or plasma if patient shocked
- careful monitoring of blood glucose and calcium levels
- anti-cholinergic drugs.

The value of antibiotics is unclear.

### 'Heartburn'
The lower oesophageal sphincter relaxes under the influence of pregnancy hormones allowing reflux of acid gastric content. Sometimes a 'sliding' hiatus hernia may be present. Mild symptoms may respond to frequent small meals and avoiding lying flat or simple antacids can be prescribed. If no relief is obtained 'floating' antacids (e.g. sodium alginate/sodium bicarbonate) or metoclopranhide can be tried. Dilute hydrochloric acid has also proved successful.

## 7.0 Pregnancy and associated diseases

### 7.12 Psychiatric disorders

**Peptic ulceration**
Peptic ulcers tend to improve in pregnancy. Any perforation requires early diagnosis and surgery. The $H_2$ receptor antagonists cimetidine or ranitidine may be necessary in some cases but their long-term use cannot be routinely recommended.

**Coeliac disease**
This may present in pregnancy as a folate-deficiency anaemia due to malabsorption. If untreated it may be associated with an increased risk of abortion or intra-uterine growth retardation. It is successfully treated by a gluten-free diet and vitamin supplements.

**Ulcerative colitis**
Ulcerative colitis does not affect pregnancy adversely and pregnancy does not increase the chance of relapse of quiescent colitis. If the colitis arises *de novo* in pregnancy or the puerperium it carries a poor prognosis. Treatment can continue during pregnancy with rectal and systemic steroids and/or sulphasalazine. In women who have required an ileostomy and become pregnant the most serious risk is of intestinal obstruction. Most pregnancies proceed to normal vaginal delivery despite the ileostomy.

**Crohn's disease**
Women with Crohn's disease tend to be subfertile. There may be a small adverse effect on fetal outcome due to the disease and the risk of IUGR is increased. The condition itself is usually unaffected by pregnancy and it should be managed as normal. Deterioration is most likely in the puerperium.

### 7.12 Psychiatric disorders
Anxiety is a common natural reaction early in pregnancy which may recur as delivery approaches. It is not an illness.

## 7.0 Pregnancy and associated diseases

7.12 Psychiatric disorders

### During pregnancy
There is no increased risk of psychiatric illness in pregnant women compared with those who are not pregnant but it does occur as at any other time. Emotional disorders may present as severe anxiety, depression or hypomania. Occasionally, delusions and hallucinations may point to a schizophrenic illness. Psychological and practical support may be all that is needed in milder cases. In severe cases a psychiatrist should be consulted so that the potential benefits and risks of medication and/or electro-convulsive therapy (ECT) can be evaluated.

### After delivery
A psychiatric illness is said to be puerperal if it occurs within 12 months of delivery. The three main types of disturbance are:

### 1. Postpartum 'blues'
This is a transient mild disturbance characterized by weeping, irritability, variation in mood, a feeling of helplessness, sensitivity to criticism and poor sleep. It tends to develop around the third postpartum day and may last for hours or days. It can be recognized in at least half of all women delivered. Treatment should be by psychological support and reassurance rather than medication.

### 2. Depressive illness
This may start at any time after delivery and can last for a few weeks or many months. The peak incidence is about 3 months postpartum with a lesser peak at 12 months, and about 10% of women who deliver are affected. Tiredness, lethargy, irritability and anxiety may be more prominent than depressive mood change. The condition is often brought on by psychological and social stress, and there may be a previous psychiatric history. Treatment is by psychological and practical support combined where necessary with tricyclic antidepressant drugs.

# 7.0 Pregnancy and associated diseases

## 7.12 Psychiatric disorders

### 3. Puerperal psychosis
This can take the form of an affective disorder with depression or hypomania, or schizophrenia with delusions and hallucinations. It usually begins 2–4 days after delivery and occurs in about 2 live births per 1000. There is a risk of suicide and harm or neglect of the child. A psychiatrist should be consulted because treatment usually entails admission of the mother and her baby to a mental hospital. The depressive form may require treatment with anti-depressants and ECT; hypomania should respond to chlorpromazine or haloperidol. Chlorpromazine is also helpful in the schizophrenic form of the illness.

There is an increased risk of psychotic illness in the future at any time. It will recur after pregnancy in 1 woman out of 6 who have been affected once before, increasing to 1 in 3 if they have been affected twice before.

### Psychotropic drugs in pregnancy
Monoamine oxidase inhibitors are contra-indicated in pregnancy but withdrawal must be gradual. Chlorpromazine 25 mg 6-hourly or promethazine hydrochloride 25 mg 6-hourly should be used during and after withdrawal. If anaesthetic intervention is necessary within two weeks of withdrawal the anaesthetist must be informed.

### Drug abuse and pregnancy
The social outlook for the baby in all forms of drug abuse is very poor. Drug abusers are, almost by definition, poor antenatal clinic attenders and may present for the first time in labour. Arms should be examined for scars, tattoo marks and thrombophlebitis.

### Opiates
Intravenous abuse (main-lining) of heroin or methadone (Physeptone) with dirty syringes carries among its risks hepatitis, septicaemia, syphilis and rhesus sensitization.

## 7.0 Pregnancy and associated diseases

7.12 Psychiatric disorders
___

Unbooked 'main-liners' should be given pethidine or methadone during labour. Sudden withdrawal can cause fetal death so gradual weaning is necessary. The infant must not be given opiate antagonists (e.g. malorphine). Signs of withdrawal in the infant are: irritability; shrill cry; sneezing; diarrhoea; diuresis; muscle tremors; and convulsions. These may not develop until several weeks after delivery. Treatment is by chlorpromazine 2 mg/kg as often as needed.

### Barbiturates
It is very difficult to wean patients from these drugs and the outlook for the infant socially and physically is poor.

### Alcohol and pregnancy
Excessive chronic alcohol ingestation is usually defined as $\geq$ 80 g/day. That is equivalent to at least 8 large glasses of wine. It is increasingly being associated with a group of fetal problems now called the **fetal alcohol syndrome**. This is reported as being common in the USA (at least 1/1000 births) but far less common in the UK despite a high level of alcohol abuse in society.

The principal features of the fetal alcohol syndrome are:
- mental retardation
- growth retardation
- facies with short palpebral fissures
- hypoplastic nasal philtrum
- micrognathia.

Other congenital anomalies are also said to be more common.

The effects of moderate alcohol ingestion (up to 40 g/day) are much more difficult to assess because:
- an accurate drink history is difficult to obtain
- its effects are compounded by such other variables as smoking, social class, age and parity.

There may be some women in whom the fetus is particularly susceptible to damage from even moderate alcohol ingestion. It has been suggested, but not confirmed, that this relates to the

## 7.0 Pregnancy and associated diseases

7.13 Malignancy

production of acetaldehyde by the mother during alcohol metabolism. Because susceptibility cannot be predicted avoidance of all alcohol is a counsel of perfection. Women can, however, in general be reassured that occasional alcohol ingestion is most unlikely to cause any problems.

### 7.13 Malignancy
Malignant disease is estimated to complicate about 1 in 1000 pregnancies. Pregnancy does not usually affect the course of the disease adversely. The exception to this is malignant melanoma. The poor prognosis of pregnant women with cervical cancer is more likely to be due to the aggressiveness of the tumour in women in that age group than to the pregnancy itself. The diseases can affect the pregnancy and fetus by:
1   Transplacental transmission of tumour cells—this occurs only very rarely.
2   Maternal effects, e.g. increased risk of infection in leukaemia, or cachexia.
3   Increased maternal mortality.
4   The effects of therapy, e.g. anomalies and IUGR.
Termination of pregnancy is not of itself therapeutic but it may be inevitable in some cases, either before or as a consequence of treatment (e.g. chemo- or radiotherapy).

### Cervical cancer and CIN
Women at greatest risk of developing cervical cancer are least likely to attend postnatal clinics which is the traditional time for checking cervical cytology.

### Suggested policy
1   Perform a cervical smear at the booking antenatal clinic if the woman has never had one before or not within the last 5 years.
2   If the smear is abnormal carry out colposcopy—colposcopically directed biopsies can be taken safely in pregnancy.
Cervical intra-epithelial neoplasia (CIN) should be serially

## 7.0 Pregnancy and associated diseases

### 7.13 Malignany

observed for the remainder of pregnancy and dealt with definitively at the end of the puerperium. Invasive carcinoma of the cervix poses several clinical problems in pregnancy.

- If discovered under 24 weeks' gestation advise termination (by hysterotomy) followed by definitive treatment.
- Between 24 and 28 weeks' gestation it may be justifiable to await fetal viability before ending the pregnancy.
- Thereafter delivery should be effected as soon as the fetal lungs are mature.

Vaginal delivery is contraindicated. Whatever the management the prognosis is poor.

### Ovarian cancer

Ovarian tumours of all varieties are said to complicate 1 in 1000 pregnancies although only 1 in 20 are malignant. The frequency of tumour types is as in the non-pregnant woman.

Ultrasound is useful for detection of ovarian swellings.

### Management

Treat as in the non-pregnant woman. The prognosis seems to be better for ovarian cancer in pregnancy with a 5-year survival rate of up to 75 per cent compared to an overall 25 per cent. This reflects the nature of the tumours in this age group.

### Breast cancer

This is the commonest malignant tumour to affect women. About 2 per cent of women under 45 years of age who have the disease are pregnant at the time of diagnosis.

Lymph node involvement seems to be increased in pregnancy. Prognosis is, therefore, poorer.

Antenatal and post-natal examination of the breasts should be routine.

### Management

- In the first half of pregnancy treatment should be as for the

# 7.0 Pregnancy and associated diseases

## 7.13 Malignancy

non-pregnant woman. If chemotherapy is necessary, termination is advisable.
- In the second half of pregnancy delivery should be effected if the fetus is viable. Treatment can then begin.

It may be justifiable to delay treatment for a short time to await fetal viability in some cases.
- Breast-feeding is probably contra-indicated.

Further pregnancies can be embarked on if desired after a post-treatment interval of 2 years.

### Hodgkin's disease
This affects about 1 in 6000 pregnant women.

### Management
1  In the first half of pregnancy radiotherapy can be carried out with shielding of the uterus and ovaries.
2  In later pregnancy chemo- and radio-therapy can sometimes be delayed until after delivery.

### Acute leukaemia
This rarely complicates pregnancy despite being among the commoner malignancies affecting young women.

### Management
The balance of risk and benefit is clearly in favour of aggressive chemotherapy. Termination of pregnancy can be offered in early pregnancy once remission has been achieved. Delivery can be accomplished when fetal survival is assured and the mother is in complete remission. Modern management has produced a marked improvement in maternal and fetal prognosis.

### Melanoma
Pregnant women with this tumour have a poor prognosis. Metastatic spread seems to be more rapid in pregnancy. Management is as for the non-pregnant woman.

# 8.0 Rhesus iso-immunization

8.1 The Rh factor, 121
8.2 Prediction of severity and timing of intervention in Rhesus iso-immunization, 122
8.3 Intra-uterine transfusion, 124
8.4 Maternal plasmaphoresis, 125
8.5 Testing the baby at birth, 126
8.6 Indications for neonatal exchange transfusion, 126

## 8.0 Rhesus iso-immunization

### 8.1 The Rh factor
Each Rh gene is made up of three components from three allelomorphic pairs—C or $\bar{c}$, D or d, E or e. Each parent passes on either the first or second half of his/her full genotype e.g. a CDe/$\bar{c}$de parent hands on either CDe or $\bar{c}$de. All Rh negative people have 'd' in each half of the genotype. Where 'D' occurs in both halves of the genotype a parent is homozygous and can only pass on the Rh-D positive gene.

Clinically significant rhesus iso-immunization is usually against the D antigen. It also occurs, though less often and less seriously against the $\bar{c}$ antigen usually in Rh-D positive women, and occasionally against the E antigen. Similar problems may be encountered with the K antigen of the Kell blood group system.

### Sensitization
This usually occurs at parturition due to feto-maternal haemorrhage. Other causes of transplacental haemorrhage include:
- abortion (spontaneous or induced)
- abruptio placentae
- amniocentesis
- external cephalic version.

Anti-D antibodies develop in 1–2% of first pregnancies (in the absence of previous blood transfusion).

### Prevention
Anti-D immunoglobulin 100 $\mu$g can eliminate up to 4.0 ml of Rh positive blood from the maternal circulation.

Prevention of sensitization by anti-D immunoglobulin in Rh (D)-negative women

This programme is about 90% effective in preventing Rh iso-immunization. The continued occurrence of sensitization is due to:
- Failure to give anti-D immunoglobulin when indicated. This is

## 8.0 Rhesus iso-immunization

8.0 Rhesus iso-immunization

| 100 µg with 60 hours of: | 50 µg as soon as possible after: |
|---|---|
| • delivery occurring from 20 weeks gestation onwards when the infant is Rh(D)-positive<br>• a serious placental abruption | • spontaneous or induced abortion before 20 weeks gestation<br>• amniocentesis<br>• external cephalic version<br>• mild to moderate placental abruption |

Check maternal blood for feto-maternal transfusion (FMT) by Kleihauer test.

| • cover FMT > 4.0 ml by additional anti-D | • cover FMT > 2.0 ml by additional anti-D |
|---|---|

totally avoidable. Error can be minimized if *all* Rh(D)-negative women are given anti-D before the blood group of the baby is known.

- Lack of protection even when anti-D is given. Reference to the Kleihauer test and giving extra anti-D when necessary should reduce this to a minimum.
- Sensitization during a first pregnancy in the absence of complications.

It has recently been suggested that all Rh(D)-negative primigravidae should be given anti-D 100 µg at 28 and 34 weeks gestation. This can reduce the incidence of Rh sensitization in primigravidae by a factor of 8. The cost-effectiveness is still disputed.

### Detection
In unsensitized women check for antibodies at booking, then at 28, 32 and 36 weeks gestation.

### 8.2 Prediction of severity and timing of intervention in Rhesus iso-immunization
This depends on:

## 8.0 Rhesus iso-immunization

8.0 Rhesus iso-immunization

### 1. Obstetric History
The disease tends to be more severe in successive affected pregnancies particularly when a previous infant has required intra-uterine transfusion or has died of haemolytic disease.

### 2. Husband's genotype
Unfortunately about 75% of the fathers of affected children are homozygous.

### 3. Maternal antibody levels
Check levels at least monthly once antibodies are detected; measurement of serum antibody protein levels is of more predictive value than antibody titres.

### Significance of serum antibody protein levels

| Serum antibody protein levels | Interpretation |
| --- | --- |
| $< 2.5$ IU/ml | Mildly affected pregnancy<br>Amniocentesis not necessary<br>Deliver at term |
| $> 20$ IU/ml | Severe haemolytic disease likely |
| Rapid increase | Acute haemolysis in progress |

### 4. Amniotic fluid analysis
Maternal IgG crosses the placenta and will cause a fetal haemolytic anaemia. Amniotic fluid bilirubin concentration correlates with the severity of the haemolytic disease in the baby.

Spectrophotometry at an optical density (OD) of 450 nm shows a peak directly proportional to the quantity of bilirubin. The level is predicted by the actual OD at 450 nm and a projected

## 8.0 Rhesus iso-immunization

8.0 Rhesus iso-immunization

baseline reading. The difference between the actual OD and the projected baseline is the ΔOD the significance of which is interpreted in relation to gestational age (see below).

**Timing of amniocentesis**

| | |
|---|---|
| **First amniocentesis** | not before 20 weeks gestation |

- 10 weeks before earliest previous intra-uterine transfusion, intra-uterine death or delivery of fatally/severely affected infant
- otherwise at 28–29 weeks if serum antibody protein > 2.5 IU/ml or, less satisfactorily, if antibody titre ≥ 1:8

| | |
|---|---|
| **Second amniocentesis** | three to four weeks later |

**Additional amniocenteses** and/or reduced intervals between them are indicated if bilirubin levels are high or rising sharply

**Timing of intervention**

The manner and timing of intervention can be determined by charting the ΔOD on the action line analysis shown in Fig. 13. When the ΔOD at 450 nm is on or above the action line before 31–32 weeks (or the trend in levels would take it across the line before that time) intra-uterine transfusion is indicated. After 35–36 weeks a ΔOD which is beyond the line suggests that delivery is indicated. Action between these two gestational ages depends on fetal lung maturity determined by phospholipid analysis (see page 158). If the first ΔOD is below the horizontal broken line, the pregnancy can continue to term without further amniocentesis.

## 8.3 Intra-uterine transfusion (IUT)

The established method involves intraperitoneal transfusion under ultrasound guidance. Direct intravascular fetal blood

## 8.0 Rhesus iso-immunization

8.0 Rhesus iso-immunization

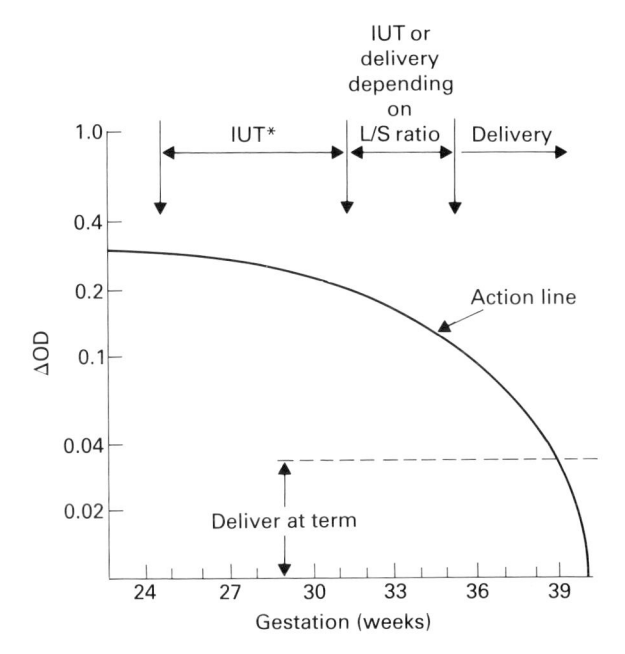

*IUT = intrauterine transfusion

**Fig. 13.** Action-line analysis.

transfusion by fetoscopy is increasingly successful in skilled hands. Transfusion into the hepatic part of the umbilical vein under ultrasound guidance has also been reported. IUT is not indicated before 22 weeks gestation. The transfusion can be repeated fortnightly. The expertise required for these techniques demands that they be concentrated in regional or supraregional centres.

### 8.4 Maternal plasmaphoresis

In very severely affected cases plasmaphoresis of maternal blood can be used as an adjunct or even alternative to IUT. Two to 4 units of plasma are removed 2 or 3 times each week from as early as 12 weeks gestation. The red cells are separated from all

## 8.0 Rhesus iso-immunization

8.0 Rhesus iso-immunization

blood withdrawn and returned to the mother, resuspended in plasma from healthy Rh-D negative donors or with plasma-protein fraction (PPF). It can be a psychological ordeal for the mother.

### 8.5 Testing the baby at birth
Cord blood is taken for:
- haemoglobin and blood film
- Coombs' test
- bilirubin levels.

### 8.6 Indications for neonatal exchange transfusion
These are:
- cord Hb $< 15.5$ g/dl
- pre-term infants with a positive Coombs' test regardless of Hb level
- positive Coombs' test with previously severely affected sibling
- very rapidly increasing jaundice with bilirubin $> 80$ $\mu$mol/l.

# 9.0 Maternal and fetal infections

9.1 Sexually transmitted diseases, 129

9.2 Rubella, 138

9.3 Cytomegalvirus, 140

9.4 Other viral infections, 141

9.5 Beta-haemolytic streptococcus, 141

9.6 Toxoplasmosis, 142

9.7 Malaria, 142

9.8 Listeriosis, 143

9.9 Urinary tract infections, 144

## 9.0 Maternal and fetal infections

### 9.1 Sexually transmitted diseases (STD)
- tend to be clinically less obvious during pregnancy
- infections with *Candida* and wart virus are more common in pregnancy
- a patient with one STD may also have others.

### Candidiasis
This is the commonest infection in pregnancy, due to *Candida albicans*

### Manifestations
- it may be asymptomatic or present as balanitis in the male
- pruritus
- 'cream-cheese' discharge in variable amounts
- adherent white film on vaginal skin
- marked erythema.

### Diagnosis
- microscopy of wet and stained smears for mycelia and spores
- culture on glucose agar of swabs collected in Stuart's transport medium

### Treatment
Anti-fungal agents as directed by manufacturer e.g.:
- nystatin vaginal pessaries one each night for 14 nights *or*
- miconazole 100 mg pessaries 2 each night for 7 nights *or*
- clotrimazole 200 mg pessaries 1 each night for 3 nights *or*
- econazole 150 mg pessaries 1 each night for 3 nights
- the equivalent anti-fungal cream is applied externally
- ketoconazole is best avoided in pregnancy.

If the infection recurs treat possible reservoirs of the organism (e.g. webs of fingers, nail beds, skin folds, or gut) as well as repeating course of vaginal therapy. The partner should be

## 9.0 Maternal and fetal infections

### 9.1 Sexually transmitted diseases

treated with anti-fungal cream. Asymptomatic infections must also be treated during pregnancy because the neonate has little resistance and may become infected.

### Trichomoniasis
This is due to *Trichomonas vaginalis* (TV). It is often associated with and may aid the spread of gonococcal infections. Co-existing genital warts will not respond to treatment until trichomoniasis is eradicated.

### Manifestations
- pruritus
- greenish or brown frothy vaginal discharge.

### Diagnosis
- microscopy of wet smears shows motile flagellated protozoa about the same size as a polymorph leucocyte
- culture of swabs collected in Bushby's brown transport medium.

### Treatment
Metronidazole 200 mg eight hourly for seven days, except in first trimester when strong Penotrane pessaries (one each night for 14 nights) or clotrimazole pessaries (one each night for 12 nights) should be used. Metronidazole should also be given to the male partner. Alcohol should be avoided during treatment because the drug has an antabuse-like effect. If infection recurs double the dose of oral metronidazole and also use suppositories vaginally preceded by antibacterial (e.g. Sultrin) pessaries.

### Gonorrhoea
This is due to *Neisseria gonorrhoea* which attacks columnar and transitional epithelium, e.g. in urethra, paraurethral ducts and glands, endocervix and ano-rectal canal. It is commoner in

## 9.0 Maternal and fetal infections

9.1 Sexually transmitted diseases

women and can cause serious infection in neonates (see page 272). All sexual contacts should be traced and investigated.

### Manifestations
- may be asymptomatic initially
- purulent discharge from urethra or cervix
- bilateral salpingitis may occur in first trimester or after delivery.

Pregnancy predisposes to gonococcal septicaemia and arthritis.

### Diagnosis  T/S
- Swabs from urethra, cervix and anus. Gonorrhoea cannot be definitely excluded until 3 sets of swabs are negative in culture.

Gram negative intracellular and extracellular diplococci are seen on directly stained smears or after culture on modified Thayer-Martin plates. Plates can be inoculated directly or swabs can be transported to the laboratory within 24 hours of collection in Stuart's transport medium. This should be fresh (less than 4 months old) and colourless. Blue Stuart's medium should be discarded.

600 mg ×4

### Treatment
- Penicillin sensitive organisms: procaine penicillin G 2.4 or 4.8 mega units i.m. *and* ampicillin 3 g orally. Probenicid is best avoided in pregnancy.
- $\beta$-lactamase producing penicillin-resistant organisms or penicillin allergy: treat with erythromycin or spectinomycin. Consult venereologist.
- Treatment for septicaemia—Penicillin G 1 mega unit i.m. 4 hourly for ten days or erythromycin.

### Treponemal infections
- *Treponema pallidum* causes syphilis
- *T. pertenue* causes yaws
- *T. carateum* causes pinta.

## 9.0 Maternal and fetal infections

9.1 Sexually transmitted diseases

---

The organisms are indistinguishable morphologically and serologically. Yaws is non-venereal and endemic in Africa, South East Asia, the Caribbean and South Pacific. Its major significance in pregnancy is to give false positive tests for syphilis.

ie. not v. specific

### Syphilis

Primary or secondary syphilis may be transmitted to the fetus and this is more likely after 16 weeks gestation or when the infection is recent. Clinically apparent syphilis is rare in pregnancy but failure to diagnose it can have severe long-term effects on mother and offspring. Routine antenatal screening tests are therefore still necessary.

VTRL.
TPA

### Diagnostic tests for syphilis in pregnancy

*Screening*
RPR (Reiter protein reagin) and VDRL (Venereal disease reference laboratory) tests or VDRL and TPHA (*Treponema pallidum* haemagglutination) tests. The RPR and VDRL tests detect reagin, an antibody-like substance produced early in treponemal infections and some other conditions. The TPHA test indicates past or present treponemal infections.

Further action is indicated if:
- screening tests are positive
- and/or there is a history of contact
- and/or there is clinical suspicion of syphilis.

The screening tests are repeated and, in the UK, blood is sent to the Venereal Disease Reference Laboratory in London or Manchester for repeat VDRL or TPHA as well as FTA (abs) IgM and TPI tests. TPI (*Treponema pallidum* immobilization) is the most specific test but is less sensitive than FTA (abs) and TPHA. It may be negative in early secondary syphilis and remains positive despite treatment. FTA (abs) (fluorescent treponemal antibody (absorbed)) is the most sensitive test for syphilis. It

## 9.0 Maternal and fetal infections

### 9.1 Sexually transmitted diseases

becomes positive early in primary syphilis and remains positive despite treatment. FTA (abs) IgM indicates recent infection but may give a transient false positive infection with herpes. TPHA is less sensitive than FTA (abs) in early syphilis and may give some false positive results.

*specific*

*Biological false positive reactions (BFPR)*
These are six times more common than real infections. FTA (abs) and TPI are negative in BFPR detected by other tests.

Among conditions which may give BFPR are:
- blood transfusions
- leprosy
- chronic nephritis
- leptospirosis
- haemolytic anaemias
- malaria
- hepatic cirrhosis
- post-vaccination
- infectious mononucleosis
- pregnancy
- rheumatoid arthritis
- systemic lupus erythematosus
- Sjögrens syndrome

**Treatment for pregnant women with syphilis**
- Procaine penicillin G 600,000 units i.m. daily for 17 days
- If daily treatment is not possible give benzathine penicillin 1.2 mega units i.m. into both buttocks at intervals of 14 days for three double injections.
- If patient has a **mild (non-anaphylactic) penicillin allergy** she should receive cephaloridine 0.5 G i.m. eight hourly for 21 days as an in-patient.
- If she has a **severe (anaphylactic) penicillin allergy** give erythromycin (base or stearate) 750 mg six hourly for 21 days and treat baby with procaine penicillin G 150,000 units daily for ten days.

**Management of subsequent pregnancies**
It may be best to re-treat women in subsequent pregnancies with procaine penicillin G 600,000 units i.m. daily for 10 days *or* benzathine penicillin 1.2 mega units into both buttocks repeated once more two weeks later.

## 9.0 Maternal and fetal infections

### 9.1 Sexually transmitted diseases

**Congenital syphilis**

The effects of syphilis on the developing fetus can be severe and include:

- intra-uterine death
- intra-uterine growth retardation
- abnormal CNS signs and fits
- damage to eyes and ears
- defective bone growth
- nephritis
- hepatosplenomegaly
- pneumonia
- anaemia
- purpura
- skin rashes

Adequate treatment of the mother before 16 weeks of pregnancy will prevent infection in virtually all cases. Treatment after this time will still be effective in most cases.

*Serological tests in the newborn*

A positive reagin test or FTA IgG is most likely to be due to transplacental passage of antibody from the mother and therefore does not necessarily signify infection in the child. A serological diagnosis is made by noting increasing titres of antibody or a positive FTA IgM in the neonate. If the tests are negative the baby should still be kept under surveillance for three months.

*Treatment of newborn with congenital syphilis*

- procaine penicillin G 150,000 units i.m. daily for 10 days.

**Herpes simplex virus** (HSV)

HSV Type 2 causes 70% of herpetic genital tract infections. Small vulval or vaginal vesicles may become painful ulcers.

**Diagnosis**

By culture in special viral culture medium.

**Treatment**

Acyclovir cream (5%) reduces the duration of signs and symptoms in the non-pregnant and may also be useful during pregnancy. It should be applied 4 hourly for 5 days in the first instance.

## 9.0 Maternal and fetal infections

9.1 Sexually transmitted diseases

**Management**

The fetus has no intrinsic immunity to the virus and therefore vaginal delivery in the presence of active herpes infection is potentially dangerous. About 50% of affected untreated infants die. If labour occurs, or membranes rupture when the disease is active deliver by caesarean section (within 4 hours of membrane rupture). It is not clear if this is necessary if the virus is culturable from the vagina in the absence of signs and symptoms.

Long-term management should include annual cervical smears because of a possible association between HVH infections and caranoma of the cervix.

**Genital warts**

These are caused by Papova (DNA) virus. They tend to regress spontaneously after delivery. Always check for other STD's.

**Treatment**

- apply saturated trichloracetic acid (TCA) using a split swab stick to the wart (not surrounding skin). When wart has turned white apply an anti-infective cream such as Nystaform-HC (continued night and morning). Repeat TCA every three days until warts are cleared
- the number of warts treated depends on their extent and patient comfort
- Podophyllin is best avoided in pregnancy
- electric cautery under local anaesthesia is an alternative (use an anti-infective cream as above).

Follow-up must include regular cervical smears as for HSV infections.

**Non-specific urethritis**

Non-specific urethritis (NSU) can be caused by *Chlamydia trachomatis* (TRIC agent) or possibly *Ureaplasma urealyticum* (formerly *T. mycoplasma*). If the male partner of a pregnant woman has NSU she should be screened for STD and treated

## 9.0 Maternal and fetal infections

### 9.1 Sexually transmitted diseases

with erythromycin along with him. Ophthalmia neonatorium due to TRIC agent is dealt with on page 272.

### Pediculosis pubis
Pediculosis pubis is caused by an infestation from a crab-like insect about 3 mm in diameter. It is strongly associated with other STDs. The eggs (nits) can be seen as dark dots at the base of pubic and perianal hairs.

### Treatment
By gamma benzene hexachloride 1% rubbed into the roots of the body hair. One treatment is usually enough. The partner should also be treated if affected.

### Scabies
Scabies is caused by a mite which burrows into the epidermis where she lays her eggs.

### Symptoms
Itching, particularly at night, and burrows can be seen in affected areas (e.g. the finger webs, the umbilicus and around the nipples). Scratching causes excoriation which can become infected.

### Treatment
By painting the whole body from the jaw to the soles of the feet with gamma benzene hexachloride 1% lotion. This is repeated in 24 hours and the patient bathes and changes clothes in a further 24 hours. The male partner and other members of the family should also be treated.

### Hepatitis
See Chapter 7.10.

## 9.0 Maternal and fetal infections

### 9.1 Sexually transmitted diseases

**Acquired immune defiency syndrome (AIDS)**

This is caused by human T-lymphotropic virus type III (HTLV-III). Pregnant women exposed to HTLV-III may have a greater risk of developing AIDS than the non-pregnant. There is, as yet, no known cure for the disease. It is transmitted by contact with genital and other secretions or blood and blood products of affected individuals. Isolated cases of transplacental transmission have also been reported.

Policies to protect staff looking after pregnant women with AIDS should be worked out in advance with the local Public Health Laboratory Service. Among the main suggested precautions during labour are:

- admission of the woman directly to a designated delivery room containing only essential equipment and furnishings

- contact with as few staff as possible carrying out full barrier nursing

- staff should wear theatre dress with gloves, boots, mask and protective glasses. Gowns over plastic aprons should be worn for delivery (and other aseptic procedures) and when handling the baby

- if electronic fetal monitoring is performed, clean transducers after use with alcohol 70% and chlorhexidine 0.5% and destroy abdominal straps. If FBS is carried out clean the pH meter with hypochlorite 1% after use

- use disposable items as often as possible. Clean all other items with the more appropriate of the above agents

- clean up spilt blood with a mop using hypochlorite 1% (discard the mophead) which should also be added to all excreta 30 minutes before sluicing

- bathe the infant to remove maternal blood

- double bag and label 'infectious risk' all items for disposal or being sent for laboratory analysis.

These suggestions are for guidance only and are not comprehensive.

## 9.0 Maternal and fetal infections

9.2 Rubella

## 9.2 Rubella

Among the congenital defects associated either singly or in combination with maternal rubella are the following:

- General effects: abortion, stillbirth, IUGR, disorders or bone growth.
- Cardiac lesions: multiple and various.
- Neurological defects: mental retardation, cerebral palsy, microcephaly, cataract, microphthalmia, retinitis, deafness.
- Other problems: hepato-splenomegaly, jaundice, thrombocytopaenic purpura.

Once differentiation has taken place a particular organ is usually no longer susceptible, but virus may persist in cataracts and the inner ear leading to progressive disability.

At least 20% of live born children exposed to intrauterine rubella in the first trimester will:

- die within one year *or*
- have a major cardiovascular and ocular defect *and/or*
- be severely deaf.

**Table 9.1.** Risk of congenital defects due to maternal pregnancy rubella.

| Stage in pregnancy (weeks from LMP) | Average risk of severe defect |
|---|---|
| within first 4 weeks | 33% |
| 5–8 weeks | 25% |
| 9–12 weeks | 9% |
| whole of first trimester | 20% |
| 13–16 weeks | 4% |
| 17–30 weeks | 1% |

**Management after maternal exposure to rubella**

Take blood sample for haemagglutination inhibiting (HI) or radial haemolytic (RH) antibodies as soon as possible after exposure. High titres of antibodies within the incubation period

## 9.0 Maternal and fetal infections

9.2 Rubella

---

(14–21 days) suggest previous infection and, therefore, existing protection.
- If there is no antibody or the titre is low take a second sample 25–28 days after exposure for repeat serological tests. A significant increase in antibody titres (four-fold or greater) confirms recent infection.
- Diagnosis can be confirmed by testing for rubella-specific IgM or IgA antibody which are present for 4–5 weeks after the incubation period.

### Management after development of rubella-like illness in a pregnant woman
- take blood for HI antibody titres as soon as possible and again 5–10 days later
- rubella-specific IgM antibody should be looked for if no rise occurs in antibody titres
- only laboratory tests can confirm that a rash is due to rubella.

### Treatment with gamma-globulin
Immunoglobulin does not prevent infection although the clinical manifestations may be suppressed. Its value is therefore doubted but it should be given if the pregnancy is to continue. The recommended dose of gamma-globulin is 1500 mg repeated in one week.

### Rubella vaccination
- Schoolgirls should be vaccinated routinely between ages of 11 and 13 years.
- Carry out routine screening for rubella antibody at booking visit whatever the history of infection or immunization (N.B. this is not the same as diagnosis of active infection described above).
- Non-immune women should be offered vaccination within 7 days of delivery, preferably while they are still in the hospital or GP unit.

## 9.0 Maternal and fetal infections

9.3 Cytomegalvirus

- The vaccine is a live-attenuated virus and should not be used in pregnancy, or during corticosteroid therapy.
- The vaccinated woman should be advised to avoid pregnancy for three months after injection.
- The above precautionary measures are still wise although no fetal harm has been reported in association with vaccination. Thus termination of pregnancy is not routinely indicated in such pregnancies.

### 9.3 Cytomegalovirus (CMV)

- It is the most common congenital infection but is usually subclinical in the mother. 50–60% of European and over 90% of African and Asian women are sero-positive.
- Between 0.3 and 2.2% of newborn infants are reported to excrete virus but 90% of these are asymptomatic at birth.
- CMV infection may account for 10% of mental retardation in children under six years of age.
- Among other consequences are:

**generalized effects**: abortion, stillbirth, IUGR, failure to thrive

**neurological effects**: microcephaly, cerebral palsy, optic atrophy, deafness

**other effects**: thrombocytopaenic purpura, jaundice, pneumonia.

- However, of congenitally infected infants, less than 10% have serious handicaps and only a minority of these could be detected before 28 weeks.
- Congenital infection follows primary infection (75%) or re-infection (25%) of the mother. It is therefore unlike rubella where only primary infection causes problems. The virus is excreted in breast milk.
- Routine screening of pregnant women to detect evidence of primary infection is not clinically useful.
- Only CMV-negative blood should be used for transfusion in seronegative pregnant women and all newborn infants.

## 9.0 Maternal and fetal infections

9.4 Other viral infections

### 9.4 Other viral infections

The possible effects of some other viral infections during pregnancy are given in Table 9.2.

**Table 9.2.** Possible effects of some viral infections in pregnancy.

| Infection | Effect |
| --- | --- |
| Coxsackie and other enteroviruses | Possible association with cardiac, digestive tract and urogenital anomalies. Severe neonatal disease is possible e.g. myocarditis. |
| Influenza | Possible increased abortion risk. Association with lymphopoietic tumours unproven. Maternal disease is more severe in the last trimester. |
| Mumps | No proven effect. Mumps vaccine should not be used in pregnancy. |
| Poliovirus | Possible increased risk of abortion and pre-term delivery. Neonatal poliomyelitis associated with severe maternal polio just before delivery. |
| Morbilli (measles) | Increased risk of abortion and pre-term delivery. |
| Varicella (Chickenpox) | Serious effects are very rare. |

### 9.5 $\beta$-haemolytic streptococcus (BHS)

The genital tract of up to 15% of women is colonized with BHS and their management during pregnancy remains problematical. The infant is always colonized in these circumstances but only 1% will have significant disease. Early 'congenital' disease mimics hyaline membrane disease and neonatal mortality is about 90% (100% if infant < 1500 g). Treatment with penicillin is usually ineffective. The infants in these cases have no passive immunity because their mothers have not developed adequate antibody levels. Even later neonatal disease has a mortality of 30–50%. Culture of high vaginal swabs from all pregnant women and treatment of all carriers (and their partners) with penicillin is neither effective, practical nor advisable. The presence of BHS in the vagina after premature rupture of the

## 9.0 Maternal and fetal infections

### 9.6 Toxoplasmosis

membranes may well be an indication for delivery and prophylactic treatment of the infant.

### 9.6 Toxoplasmosis
This is due to *Toxoplasma gondii*—a protozoan parasite of which cats are the definitive host. Primary infection in pregnancy may lead to congenital toxoplasmosis but 80% of infants are asymptomatic. The incidence in England and Wales is approximately 1 in 20,000 total births; it is ten times more common in France.

The risk of infection is lessened by avoiding raw or partly cooked meats and contact with items contaminated by cat faeces.

Among the potential fetal hazards of maternal toxoplasmosis are:
- generalized effects: abortion, stillbirth
- neurological effects: microcephaly, hydrocephalus, cerebral calcification, microphthalmia, choroid retinitis
- other effects: periostitis, hepatosplenomegaly, purpura, anaemia.

### Diagnosis
Primary toxoplasmosis is usually subclinical but the woman may have a 'flu-like' illness. If a Sabin-Feldman dye test is high ($\geq 1:512$) or IgM fluorescent antibody test is positive an increasing active infection is probable. Parasites may be found in unfixed placental tissue or body fluids (e.g. cerebrospinal fluid). The low incidence cannot justify routine screening throughout pregnancy.

### Treatment
Spiramycin early in the disease may reduce the fetal effects.

### 9.7 Malaria
Malaria is a common cause of high maternal pyrexia in endemic

## 9.0 Maternal and fetal infections

### 9.8 Listeriosis

areas and the diagnosis must also be considered in non-endemic areas among immigrants or tourists returning from endemic areas suffering from pyrexia of unknown origin (P.U.O.) The high pyrexia may result in abortion or pre-term delivery.

Congenital malaria is rare.

**Diagnosis**
Parasites are seen on thick and thin blood smears.

**Treatment**
Chloroquine 800 mg in one dose then 400 mg six hours later. Another 400 mg is given daily for a further 2 days.

### 9.8 Listeriosis

This is due to *Listeria monocytogenes*. Infections are usually sporadic. Dairy products may be involved in some cases because the organism can survive low and high temperature pasteurization. It can cause abortion, stillbirth, and pre-term labour. The infected pre-term fetus may pass meconium as a result and the diagnosis must always be considered when liquor is meconium stained at < 34 weeks. There is a clinical impression that the incidence of problems due to listeriosis in pregnancy is increasing. There may be a history of a flu-like illness a week or two before delivery or it may be asymptomatic. A live born affected infant may develop meningitis, encephalitis, pneumonia, conjunctivitis and petechial and other skin rashes.

**Diagnosis**
By direct culture of the organisms which grow best at 4°C. Placental granulomas may be noted.

**Treatment**
The organism is sensitive to a wide range of antibiotics.

## 9.0 Maternal and fetal infections

9.9 Urinary tract infections

### 9.9 Urinary tract infections

Bacteriuria is significant when there are > 100,000 organisms/ml of cultured urine. The detection of asymptomatic bacteriuria in pregnancy is important because of its association with the delivery of low birth weight infants and the increased risk of pyelonephritis. Routine culture of a mid-stream urine (MSU) sample is necessary at booking for each pregnant woman. *E. coli* is the infecting organism in 90% of cases. Appropriate treatment is guided by the sensitivities of the organism but co-trimoxazole (Septrin, Bactrim) is still best avoided in pregnancy if possible and definitely in the first trimester (see Chapter 16). Repeat the MSU culture after five days of antibacterial treatment.

### Acute pyelonephritis

Clinical picture:
- patient flushed and ill
- rigors
- vomiting
- frequency of micturition and dysuria
- abdominal pain
- high pyrexia
- renal angle tenderness
- pyuria.

Acute pyelonephritis must be differentiated from other causes of an acute abdomen e.g. appendicitis.

### Management of acute pyelonephritis

- maintain adequate fluid intake, if necessary intravenously
- send MSU for culture immediately
- check blood culture if fever high
- tepid sponging for high pyrexia.

**Treatment** (while awaiting culture and sensitivity results:)
**Severe cases.** Pivmecillinam ('Selexid') 200–400 mg 6–8 hourly for 5 days is very effective against most gram negative organ-

## 9.0 Maternal and fetal infections

### 9.9 Urinary tract infections

isms, particularly *E. coli*. It is not effective against *Pseudomonas pyocyaneus,* and it cannot be used if the patient is allergic to penicillin.

**Mild/moderate cases.** Sulphadimidine 2 g stat then 1 g 6 hourly for 5 days.

Among other antibiotics which can be used are:
- ampicillin 500 mg 6 hourly
- cephalexin 500 mg 6 hourly
- nalidixic acid 1 g 6 hourly
- nitrofurantoin 100 mg 6 hourly

Treatment of *P. pyocyaneus* infections requires gentamicin 40 mg 8 hourly and blood levels should be checked daily. Treatment is for 5 days in the first instance. Check another MSU on the third day (mentioning the antibiotic therapy in the request card). MSU samples to be cultured at regular intervals thereafter.

### Recurrence

If the pyelonephritis recurs treat again and consider maintaining antibacterial therapy for the remainder of the pregnancy with, for example, sulphadimidine 1 g bd, nitrofurantoin 100 mg bd, or nalidixic acid 1 g bd.

# 10.0 Some practical problems

10.1 Thrombo-embolism, 147

10.2 Antepartum haemorrhage, 151

10.3 The assessment of fetal welfare, 153

10.4 Intra-uterine growth retardation, 155

10.5 Fetal lung maturity, 158

10.6 Polyhydramnios, 159

10.7 Breech presentation, 160

10.8 Multiple pregnancy, 162

10.9 Unstable lie towards term, 162

10.10 Post-term pregnancy, 163

10.11 Late missed abortion or intra-uterine death, 163

10.12 Dealing with stillbirth or neonatal death, 164

## 10.0 Some practical problems

### 10.1 Thrombo-embolism
Superficial thrombophlebitis does not carry a significant risk of thrombo-embolism (unless it extends to the deep veins). An area of localized inflammation over the vein is acutely tender. Symptomatic relief can be achieved with traditional remedies such as kaolin or glycerine and ichthyol bandages. The end of the bed can also be elevated.

### Deep vein thrombosis (DVT)
The classical signs are oedema, local tenderness, a positive Homan's sign and an increase in the diameter of the affected leg. Most cases are less clear-cut, and some are silent. Because clinical signs are unreliable, and treatment is not without risk, it is important to positively confirm the diagnosis before treatment if at all possible.

### Diagnosis of DVT
Venography is the method of choice during pregnancy. The radio-opaque medium is injected through a vein on the dorsum of the foot. The radioactive fibrinogen uptake test in which $^{125}$I-labelled fibrinogen is incorporated into any thrombus is not recommended in pregnancy. Detection of lack of patency of leg veins using ultrasound is not accurate enough. The main risk from DVT is of pulmonary embolism but if the thrombosis is extensive enough chronic vascular insufficiency of the leg may persist.

Pulmonary embolism is now the commonest cause of maternal death (see page 251).

Among the factors which are associated with an increased incidence of pulmonary embolism are:
- increasing age and parity
- obesity
- confinement to bed

## 10.0 Some practical problems

### 10.1 Thrombo-embolism

- caesarean section (particularly in pre-eclamptic women)
- blood groups other than O
- sickle-cell disease
- suppression of lactation with oestrogen.

The **symptoms and signs** of pulmonary embolism can be missed all too easily. Typically, there is pleuritic pain, haemoptysis, dyspnoea, and varying degrees of hypotension. The diagnosis must also be considered in the presence of a dry cough, a fever of unknown origin, unexplained tachycardia, or bronchospasm without a past history of asthma. The clinical picture is frequently confused with that of an acute pulmonary infection, and there may be no evidence of a preceding DVT.

### Investigation of suspected pulmonary embolus
Chest X-ray may be helpful but can be totally normal. The ECG is usually normal except when the embolus is large and has produced acute *cor pulmonale.* Even these changes may be obscured by the usual ECG changes which occur in pregnancy. Deficient lung perfusion can be detected by a lung scan using the intravenous injection of aggregated human albumin labelled with technetium-99. If it is available this is the investigation of choice. Pulmonary angiography is diagnostic but is a much more invasive technique.

### Management of thrombo-embolism
If symptoms and signs are equivocal and confined to the lower limb it may be justifiable to watch and wait for 24 or 48 hours. If the diagnosis of DVT becomes clearer (or is still equivocal) perform venography.

### 1. Acute therapy
Give heparin 15,000 units i.v. as a bolus injection then 10,000 units six hourly by continuous i.v. infusion for at least 48 hours.

## 10.0 Some practical problems

10.1 Thrombo-embolism

### 2. Long-term antenatal treatment
Heparin can be continued subcutaneously for the remainder of the pregnancy or warfarin can be commenced.

**Subcutaneous heparin regime**. Heparin 7,500 units is injected subcutaneously 12 hourly. It is important to use correct subcutaneous injection technique as follows:
- a 25 gauge, 16 mm needle is used
- fill a 1 ml tuberculin syringe with the required dose of heparin
- raise a skin fold between thumb and forefinger on the anterior abdominal wall. The choice of site will have to vary
- insert the needle to its full length at right angles to the skin
- aspirate to ensure that a blood vessel has not been punctured
- inject over 10 to 15 seconds
- after removal of the needle press a swab firmly over the injection site.

Activated partial thromboplastin times (APTT) are of no value in monitoring the correct dosage for long-term or prophylactic therapy. The best method is to measure plasma heparin levels (antifactor X activity) which should be maintained between 0.2 and 0.6 units/ml. These should be measured twice weekly initially until the dose is stabilized and every two weeks thereafter. This level of heparin does not add to the risk of haemorrhage, even at caesarean section. If labour supervenes the relevant injection of heparin can be withheld: the next dose is given within 2 hours of vaginal delivery or 12 hours of caesarean section. The patient can thereafter continue with subcutaneous heparin for up to six weeks postnatally. The optimum postnatal dose is usually lower than that required antenatally. Alternatively, treatment can begin with warfarin (see below). Heparin injections should continue for 36 hours after the loading dose of warfarin.

Heparin does not cross the placenta or into breast milk. Maternal osteoporosis resulting in vertebral compression

## 10.0 Some practical problems

### 10.1 Thrombo-embolism

fractures can occur after long-term therapy in pregnancy. The anticoagulant effect of heparin can be reversed readily by protamine sulphate.

**Warfarin therapy**
Warfarin sodium 30 mg is given orally as a loading dose (day 1). No more is given until the evening of day 3 when the correct dose is determined by the one-stage prothrombin time in blood taken that morning. This should be kept at 2–2.5 times the control value. The average dose required is 5 mg 12 hourly. METICULOUS CONTROL IS ABSOLUTELY VITAL. Warfarin should not be used in the first trimester and needs to be replaced by subcutaneous heparin three weeks before delivery. If labour supervenes before the change can be made, fresh frozen plasma and vitamin $K_1$, 10 mg should be given to the mother. The baby's prothrombin times must be monitored carefully.

These precautions are necessary because warfarin crosses the placenta. It does not, however, cross in breast milk. Breast-feeding is therefore not contra-indicated and treatment can begin again in the puerperium. Phenindione does cross into breast milk and should not be used. Anticoagulation should be continued for up to three months after delivery.

**Prophylaxis**
The risk of thrombo-embolism occurring in a patient with a past history of thrombo-embolism in pregnancy or while on the oestrogen/progestrogen contraceptive pill is about 12% but the majority occur post-natally. There is therefore a real dilemma as to whether long-term anti-coagulants are justified in such situations. As a general guide:
- One confirmed episode in the past—give infusion of 500–1000 ml of dextran 70 during labour then subcutaneous heparin or warfarin for six weeks. Also treat such women admitted to hospital and confined to bed for another condition.
- Equivocal or dubious history—no specific therapy.

## 10.0 Some practical problems

10.2 Antepartum haemorrhage

- Multiple episodes and/or antithrombin III deficiency—anticoagulation throughout pregnancy and for six weeks afterwards.
- Consider treatment in the puerperium for the obese grande multipara with varicose veins or who has had an operative delivery.

### 10.2 Antepartum haemorrhage
This is defined as bleeding from the genital tract from 28 weeks of pregnancy onwards.

#### Management
- Admit the patient to hospital, by Flying Squad (see Chapter 12.1) if necessary.
- DO NOT PERFORM A VAGINAL EXAMINATION
- Confine the patient to bed until there has been no bleeding for at least 24 hours. A gentle speculum examination can then be performed to exclude a local cause for the bleeding.
- Keep 2 units of blood crossmatched as required.
- Localize the placenta ultrasonically. Because of deficiencies in techniques and errors of intrepretation no method of localization can be said to display the placental site with absolute certainty.
- Monitor placental function and fetal welfare (See chapter 10.3).
- If vaginal bleeding continues it is important to ensure that the blood is maternal rather than fetal. This can be done simply using Apt's test (see below).
- If the placenta covers the internal os the patient should remain in hospital. Ultrasonic scan placental localizations should be repeated at monthly intervals because the placenta may 'migrate' out of the lower segment.
- If the placenta is normally situated and the pregnancy is progressing satisfactorily, the patient can be allowed home. Careful follow-up must continue at the ante-natal clinic.

## 10.0 Some practical problems

### 10.2 Antepartum haemorrhage

- Consider delivery if maternal and/or fetal welfare are being compromised.
- Allow the pregnancy to continue to 38 weeks if possible and then carry out a pelvic examination in theatre. It may not be necessary to do this under general anaesthesia but, at the very least, all should be ready for an immediate caesarean section and the anaesthetist should be present and prepared.
- If the placenta is not palpable, an ARM can be performed and labour induced. The fetal heart rate must be monitored continuously. If the placenta is palpable within the lower segment proceed to caesarean section.
- Elective caesarean section is indicated if, by 38 weeks gestation, the diagnosis of placenta praevia has become certain.

### Placental abruption

The clinical situation will determine when delivery has become necessary. The amount of revealed blood loss may not reflect the severity of the situation and in moderately severe or severe cases a central venous pressure line must be set up to determine the volume of fluids and blood to be transfused. The level of the C.V.P. should be kept at about +4 cm $H_2O$.

If the fetus is still alive FHR monitoring is mandatory and ready recourse should be made to caesarean section to deliver a distressed fetus. A case can also be made for a caesarean section in some cases in which the fetus is already dead. This is a decision to be made by a senior obstetrician and may be justified in the following circumstances:

- the abruption is severe
- the cervix is tightly shut and amniotomy impossible
- there is, as yet, no coagulation defect but if the uterus were not to be emptied quickly the risk of this developing would be high.

The assessment and management of coagulation defects is discussed in Chapter 12.5.

## 10.0 Some practical problems

### 10.3 The assessment of fetal welfare

**Apt's test**
This test is used to distinguish fetal from maternal blood:
- pass a vaginal speculum and obtain a sample of the blood lying there
- half fill two 10 ml test tubes with water
- to one tube add 2 drops of adult blood obtained by pin-prick from a volunteer
- to the other tube add enough of the vaginal sample to match the colour in that containing adult blood
- add enough sodium hydroxide (NaOH) 1% to increase the volume of each tube by 20%
- the tube containing adult blood will change colour from pink to yellow-brown within 2 minutes as the adult haemoglobin is denatured by the alkali
- if the second tube contains a significant proportion of fetal blood it will remain pink for much longer because fetal haemoglobin is relatively resistant to denaturation

### 10.3 The assessment of fetal welfare
This can be considered in three phases of surveillance which increase in intensity as perception of maternal or fetal risk rises.

**Routine ('first phase') screening**
Applicable to all women (usually on a shared care basis) and comprises:
- clinical impression of uterine and fetal size
- serial measurement of fundal height (see page 31)
- daily count of perceived fetal movements (kick chart) from 28 (or 34) weeks. Mothers are asked to count the number of discrete fetal movements beginning at 9 a.m. each day. The time at which the tenth movement is felt is marked on the chart provided by the ante-natal clinic. If less than 10 movements occur in 12 hours they should contact the maternity hospital for advice.

## 10.0 Some practical problems

### 10.3 The assessment of total welfare

None of these tests is sensitive or specific and they therefore cannot be taken as diagnostic of fetal compromise. Clinical assessment of fetal growth misses over half the babies weighing less than the 10th centile, and wrongly suspects IUGR in 5 women for every 2 correctly predicted.

**'Second phase' screening**
Applicable to women in whom 'first phase' tests have deviated from locally accepted norms or in whom other risk factors exist (e.g. see page 48).

Among these tests are:
- ultrasonic assessment of BPD & AC (see page 28)
- biochemical tests of 'placental function' (see page 35)
- antenatal fetal heart rate monitoring. The true value of this method has not yet been fully assessed. Traces are not always easy to interpret. Visual assessments are liable to bias and computerised methods are not yet widely available.

```
┌─────────────────────┐     Acceleration of ≥ 20 bpm
│ CTG trace reviewed  │     occurs (usually in
│ after 5 minutes     │     response to fetal movement)
└─────────────────────┘
         │
   No acceleration
      ≥ 20 bpm                              ┌──────────────────┐
         │                                  │ Normal-reactive  │
         ▼                                  │ trace — repeat   │
┌─────────────────────┐                     │ in one week      │
│ Continue for up to  │   5 or more         └──────────────────┘
│ 40 minutes          │   accelerations in any
└─────────────────────┘   20 minute period,
         │                with each accel. ≥ 15 bpm
  Loss of baseline        and lasting for at least 15 seconds
  irregularity with
  decelerations in
  response to              Any other pattern
  spontaneous
  contractions
         ▼                          ▼
┌─────────────────────┐   ┌──────────────────────┐
│ Review whole        │   │ Repeat test or carry out │
│ situation urgently  │   │ biophysical profile scoring │
│ with a view to      │   │ within 12–24 hours, as │
│ possible delivery   │   │ dictated by clinical │
└─────────────────────┘   │ circumstances        │
                          └──────────────────────┘
```

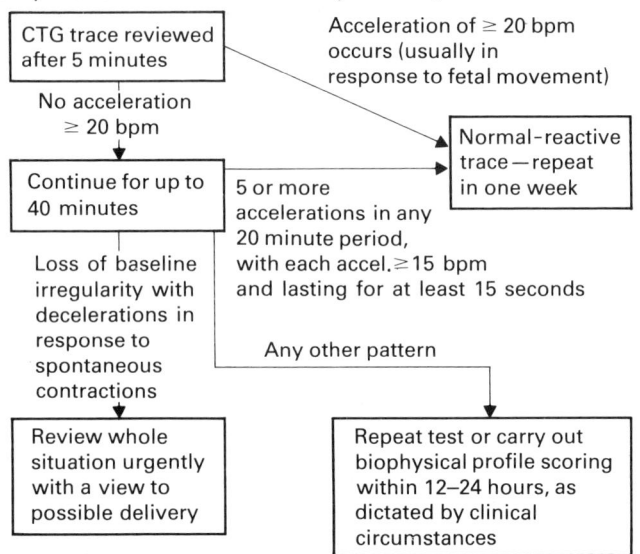

**Fig. 14.** Suggested programme for antenatal FHR recording

## 10.0 Some practical problems

10.4 Intra-uterine growth retardation

Discrete accelerations in response to fetal movements (a 'reactive trace') suggest that the fetus is in good health. Failure to show reactivity early in the trace is not necessarily abnormal because the fetus has 'rest/activity' cycles and the period of rest can be as long as 40 minutes. Baseline irregularity, which is defined on page 218 and should be > 10 bpm is another important feature. However, the earlier the gestation the more unreactive the normal trace is. The time from 28 to 32 weeks is a transitional period for the development of baseline irregularity. DECELERATIONS IN RELATION TO CONTRACTIONS ACCOMPANIED BY LOSS OF BASELINE IRREGULARITY ARE A SERIOUS PROGNOSTIC SIGN.

### Intensive ('third phase') screening
Applicable to women in whom the fetus is thought to be at highest risk on the basis of second phase screening. The main test is biophysical profile (BPP) scoring (Manning *et al.,* 1983) using a fetal heart rate monitor and a real time ultrasound machine (Table 10.1).

It can be achieved within 10 minutes in most cases. The interpretation of the BPP and suggested subsequent management are given in Table 10.2.

Doppler ultrasound measurement of fetal (umbilical or aortic) or uterine (arcuate artery) blood flow as an indicator of fetal well-being is under investigation but has not yet been validated for clinical use.

### 10.4 Intra-uterine growth retardation (IUGR)
The epidemiological definition of IUGR relies on population statistics and is present when the baby weighs less than the 10th (or more stringently the 5th or 3rd) centile for gestational age and sex (see page 26).

This can be misleading in individual cases because:
- the centile charts vary according to the population studied

## 10.0 Some practical problems

### 10.4 Intra-uterine growth retardation

**Table 10.1.** Biophysical profile scoring: technique.

| Biophysical variable | Normal (score = 2) | Abnormal (score = 0) |
| --- | --- | --- |
| 1. Fetal breathing movements (FBM) | At least 1 episode of FBM of at least 30 seconds duration in 30 minutes observation | Absent FBM or no episode of > 30 seconds in 30 minutes |
| 2. Gross body movement | At least 3 discrete body/limb movements in 30 minutes (episodes of active continuous movement considered as a single movement) | 2 or fewer episodes of body/limb movements in 30 minutes |
| 3. Fetal tone | At least 1 episode of active extension with return to flexion of fetal limb(s) or trunk. Opening and closing of hand considered normal tone | Either slow extension with return to partial flexion or movement of limb in full extension or absent fetal movement |
| 4. Reactive fetal heart rate (FHR) | At least 2 episodes of FHR acceleration of > 15 bpm and of at least 15 seconds duration associated with fetal movement in 30 minutes | Less than 2 episodes of acceleration of FHR or acceleration of < 15 bpm in 30 minutes |
| 5. Amniotic fluid (AF) volume | At least 1 pocket of AF that measures at least 1 cm in two perpendicular planes | Either no AF pockets or a pocket < 1 cm in two perpendicular planes |

- some infants below the 10th (or lesser) centile are appropriately grown for that particular mother and therefore healthy

## 10.0 Some practical problems

### 10.4 Intra-uterine growth retardation

**Table 10.2.** BPP scores, interpretation and management.

| Score | Interpretation | Management |
|---|---|---|
| 10 | Normal infant, low risk for chronic asphyxia | Repeat testing at weekly intervals. Repeat twice weekly in diabetics and patient $\geq 42$ weeks gestation |
| 8 | Normal infant, low risk for chronic asphyxia | Repeat testing at weekly intervals. Repeat testing twice weekly in diabetics and patients $\geq 42$ weeks. Oligohydramnios an indication for delivery |
| 6 | Suspect chronic asphyxia | Repeat testing in 4–6 hours. Deliver if oligohydramnios present |
| 4 | Suspect chronic asphyxia | If $\geq 36$ weeks and favourable then deliver. If $< 36$ weeks and lungs immature repeat test in 24 hours. If repeat score $\leq 4$ deliver |
| 0–2 | Strong suspicion of chronic asphyxia | Extend testing time to 120 minutes. If persistent score $\leq 4$, deliver, regardless of gestational age |

- conversely some infants above the 10th centile are growth retarded e.g. if the birth weight lies on the 40th centile when it should have reached the 80th centile then that infant has not reached its full growth potential and is at risk from the same problems as the small baby.

The biological definition of IUGR is, therefore, the failure of the fetus to achieve its full growth potential.

### Aetiology of true IUGR
Among the main causes are:

## 10.0 Some practical problems

10.5 Fetal lung maturity

- genetic, chromosomal
- multiple pregnancy
- congenital malformations
- chronic infections
- maternal smoking

in these cases IUGR is symmetrical i.e. both head and body size are reduced.

- factors affecting placental perfusion e.g. high attitude, maternal disease processes, pre-eclampsia (PET).

In PET the IUGR tends to be asymmetrical i.e. head growth is relatively spared.

The prognosis for infants with IUGR depends on the aetiology, gestational age at delivery and severity of perinatal asphyxia. The particular problem of the growth retarded neonate are discussed on page 261.

### 10.5 Fetal lung maturity

The use of ultrasound to confirm gestational age early in pregnancy and the improvement in neonatal intensive care are among the reasons for the marked decline over the last 5 years in requests for phospholipid analysis of amniotic fluid to assess fetal lung maturity. The *lecithin/sphingomyelin* (L/S ratio) of amniotic fluid obtained by amniocentesis may be outdated less than 15 years after its introduction. Future practise is likely to require assessment of fetal lung maturity in only a few patients with specific indications. In diabetic pregnancies or where the liquor has been collected vaginally after spontaneous rupture of the membranes the best test is detection of *phosphatidylglycerol*. Its presence suggests that the fetal lungs are likely to be mature.

### The 'shake-test'

This is a simple, rapid method for looking at pulmonary surfactant levels which is both easy to perform and compares favourably with the L/S ratio. It is based on the action of phospholipids, and lecithin and sphingomyelin in particular, in

## 10.0 Some practical problems

### 10.6 Polyhydramnios

keeping a ring of bubbles on the surface of increasing dilutions of amniotic fluid.

*Shake test technique*
At least 3 ml of amniotic fluid is required, obtained either by amniocentesis (see page 75), or by vaginal collection either at ARM or after premature rupture of membranes. If the fluid is blood-stained it should be centrifuged in a bench centrifuge at 2000 rpm for 20 minutes. Five test tubes (10 ml) are labelled 1–5 and amniotic fluid and normal saline are added in the following proportions:

| Test tube | 1 | 2 | 3 | 4 | 5 |
|---|---|---|---|---|---|
| Amniotic fluid (ml) | 1.00 | 0.75 | 0.5 | 0.25 | 0.2 |
| Normal saline (ml) | nil | 0.25 | 0.5 | 0.75 | 0.8 |

1 ml of 95% ethyl alcohol is added to each tube and they are then shaken vigorously for 15 seconds. The results are read after the tubes have been left undisturbed for 15 minutes. Only a clear full ring of bubbles is regarded as positive.

*Interpretation of the 'shake-test'*
Findings and their interpretation are listed in Table 10.3.

**Table 10.3.**

| Finding | Interpretation |
|---|---|
| Positive result in 3 or more tubes | Lungs mature |
| Positive result in tubes 1 and 2 | Acceptable lung maturity |
| Positive result in tube 1 | Borderline lung maturity |
| No tubes positive | Lungs immature |

### 10.6 Polyhydramnios

The diagnosis is based on clinical appearances and findings. It is often associated with an unstable lie of the fetus. In the rare

## 10.0 Some practical problems

10.7 Breech presentation

acute cases it may mimic placental abruption. Its cause is often obscure but it can be due to maternal diabetes, twins (especially uniovular), fetal anomaly (e.g. anencephaly, oesophageal atresia), or hydrops fetalis.

In all except minor cases, a GTT should be performed and an ultrasonic scan and/or abdominal X-ray taken to exclude those fetal anomalies amenable to diagnosis.

Antenatal tapping of the excess fluid in severe cases produces only a brief respite and may induce pre-term labour. If labour is induced by amniotomy a controlled release of the liquor must be attempted to minimize the risk of cord prolapse and placental abruption.

Immediately after birth the baby should be tested for oesophageal atresia by passing a soft rubber catheter into the stomach.

### 10.7 Breech presentation

This is the commonest malpresentation occurring in 2–3% of all term deliveries. Management has become more aggressive over the past 10 years with external cephalic version being practiced less and less and elective caesarean section more and more. This policy is not without risk to the mother and is currently being reconsidered.

### External cephalic version (ECV)

ECV is safe for mother and baby in carefully selected patients and reduces the need to consider elective caesarean section.

### Timing of ECV

It is technically easier at 34 weeks (or less) but the malpresentation is more likely to recur and if delivery is urgently necessary the baby is pre-term. It is, therefore, increasingly common to perform ECV around 37 weeks using tocolytic agents to inhibit uterine contractions.

## 10.0  Some practical problems

10.7  Breech presentation

**Protocol for ECV**

Gestational age must be known with certainty and the presentation should be confirmed by ultrasound before proceeding.

*Absolute contraindications*
- multiple pregnancy
- APH (whatever the cause)
- ruptured membranes
- significant fetal anomaly
- caesarean section indicated for other reasons.

*Relative contraindications*
- previous caesarean section
- IUGR
- hypertension
- rhesus iso-immunization
- elderly primigravida
- grande multiparity
- anterior placenta
- obesity.

**Procedure**

ECV is best learned by experience. One technique is as follows:
- perform CTG (see page 000)
- take blood for Kleihauer test (see page 122) before and after ECV and give anti-D immunoglobulin 50 $\mu$g to Rh (D) negative women
- commence i.v. infusion of Ritodrine 50 $\mu$g/min (see page 204)
- apply talcum powder to maternal abdomen
- place woman in lateral position on a couch with her back against the wall and the fetal back upwards
- the seated operator elevates the breech from the pelvis using the edge of one hand
- the other hand turns the fetal head in a forward somersault—

## 10.0 Some practical problems

10.8 Multiple pregnancy

---

(if the fetal back is downwards a backward somersault can be attempted)
- listen to the fetal heart every 2 minutes during the procedure
- each attempt should last no longer than 5 minutes with a minimum of 3 minutes between no more than 3 attempts
- repeat CTG until trace is seen to be normal
- stop Ritodrine infusion.

Breech presentation in relation to labour is discussed on page 192.

### 10.8 Multiple pregnancy

Ultrasound is the standard technique for screening for multiple pregnancy, but up to 10% can be missed by early scan. In addition even if two gestation sacs are seen one may die and be resorbed or present at delivery as a *fetus papyraceous.*

All pregnancy complications occur more frequently in multiple pregnancies and the level of antenatal care provided must reflect this. Iron and folic acid supplements are necessary throughout pregnancy. Pre-term labour is a major risk and the cervix should be examined antenatally at regular intervals to detect too early effacement which may require admission. There is no proven value of routine admission at 26–30, or 30–34 weeks gestation for reducing pre-term labour. Admission should be offered at the first sign of any complication (e.g. pre-eclampsia), or if the mother is excessively tired or cumbersome. Prophylactic oral beta-sympathomimetic drugs have not been proven to reduce the risk of pre-term labour. Fetal growth and well-being should be assessed routinely as in 'phase two' screening (page 154).

On balance, twin pregnancies should not be allowed to proceed much beyond 40 weeks (38 weeks for triplets?)

Delivery in multiple pregnancy is discussed on p. 196.

### 10.9 Unstable lie towards term

If an unstable lie persists to 37 weeks the patient should be

## 10.0 Some practical problems

10.10 Post-term pregnancy

admitted. Causes such as multiple pregnancy, placenta praevia and wrong dates should be excluded. If the lie stabilizes to longitudinal near term, labour can be induced. If the unstable lie persists to 41 weeks gestation the patient should be delivered by caesarean section.

### 10.10 Post-term pregnancy

A pregnancy is considered to be post-term when it extends beyond 293 days (42 weeks) from the onset of the LMP. The extent of fetal risk from this degree of post-maturity is controversial. It is counter-balanced by the risks of induction and of possible errors in dates, leading to delivery of a pre-term infant.

Induction of labour should not be a matter of routine merely because an arbitrary gestational age has been reached in the absence of any other complications.

In general, however, induction may be justified when the patient has reached her EDD+14 days but her feelings in this matter should be considered.

### 10.11 Late missed abortion or intra-uterine death (IUD)

Suspected intra-uterine fetal death can be confirmed by ultrasound or X-ray. The latter may show overlap of skull bones (Spalding's sign) which takes several days to appear and is not a valid sign of death if labour is in progress or the membranes are ruptured. Gas bubbles can also be seen in the heart and great vessels.

If left alone labour will usually start within a month but such a long waiting time is cruel for a woman who knows that the baby she is carrying is dead. In addition, prolonged IUD may occasionally cause a blood coagulation defect in the mother. However, this takes at least four weeks to develop.

INDUCTION OF LABOUR BY AMNIOTOMY IS ABSOLUTELY CONTRA-INDICATED IN THE PRESENCE OF AN IUD because of the risk of introducing micro-organisms into a perfect culture

163

## 10.0 Some practical problems

10.12 Dealing with stillbirth or neonatal death

medium. The resulting intra-uterine infection can be catastrophic.

Oxytocin infusions alone are ineffective; intravenous prostaglandins often have severe side effects and the use of extra-amniotic prostaglandins requires some expertise.

Vaginal prostaglandin $E_2$ gel (as described in Chapter 11.6) or Prostin tables are effective in the management of IUD and their use is the method of choice.

### Programme for dealing with an IUD (Table 10.4)
**Table 10.4.**

|  | Up to 28 completed weeks | After 28 completed weeks |
|---|---|---|
| Dose of prostaglandin $E_2$ | 15 mg | As for routine induction of labour |
| If abortion/delivery has not occurred within 12 hours set up oxytocin infusion | | |
| Dose of oxytocin | Constant 100 mU/min (50 units of oxytocin in 500 ml dextrose/saline at 15 dpm) | As for routine induction of labour. Suggested beginning at 4 mU/min increasing gradually as necessary to 32 mU/min |

Analgesia with Omnopon 15 mg or diamorphine 10 mg should be given as required. Evacuation of the uterus is necessary only when expulsion of the placenta is incomplete.

### 10.12 Dealing with stillbirth or neonatal death

The parents must be treated with the utmost compassion.

They should be encouraged, but not forced, to see their dead child even if disfiguring abnormalities are present. In the UK registration of the birth and death are legally required if the pregnancy has reached 28 completed weeks *or* if the child was born with signs of life before that time. This legislation needs to

## 10.0 Some practical problems

10.12 Dealing with stillbirth or neonatal death

---

be updated as a matter of priority. This is not only because the survival of infants live-born before 28 weeks is around 50% in centres with good neonatal intensive care but also because much unnecessary suffering is caused to grieving parents whose child is stillborn before 28 weeks. *ie. registering imp*

Sympathetic but firm requests must be made for the parents to give permission for autopsy and they must be kept fully informed of any relevant findings. Parents should be given informed assistance with registration and with funeral arrangements. This may be the first time they have faced such a tragic event.

The mother should be given as much privacy as she wishes and be allowed home as soon as medically possible at the most appropriate time for her. Hospital staff frequently find it difficult to come to terms with a stillbirth or neonatal death. They must not isolate the mother physically or emotionally because of their own difficulties.

It may be appropriate to suppress lactation (see page 279) but this should not be automatic. The mother may see lactation as an expression of her grief and that may be helpful for her.

Grief is a normal, natural reaction to such an event and must not be inhibited. Failure to grieve can have long-term psychological consequences.

When the mother goes home her GP and Community Midwife must be informed, first directly and then by letter. The couple should be seen by the obstetrician (and paediatrician in the case of an NND) when all the information on the case is available. Implications for the future must be discussed. The antenatal clinic is not an ideal place for such a visit and the person seeing them must have known them during the pregnancy.

# 11.0 Labour

- 11.1 Preparation, 169
- 11.2 Normal labour, 170
- 11.3 Management of labour (normal pregnancy), 171
- 11.4 Posture during labour, 177
- 11.5 Normal progress in labour, 177
- 11.6 Augmentation of labour, 177
- 11.7 The second stage of labour, 178
- 11.8 Induction of labour, 179
- 11.9 Spontaneous rupture of membranes at term, 183
- 11.10 Analgesia in labour, 184
- 11.11 The bony pelvis and labour, 190
- 11.12 Breech presentation and labour, 192
- 11.13 Labour with malpresentations other than breech, 195
- 11.14 Multiple pregnancy and delivery, 196
- 11.15 Episiotomy and third-degree tear, 198
- 11.16 The third stage of labour, 199
- 11.17 Primary postpartum haemorrhage, 200
- 11.18 Pre-term labour, 201
- 11.19 Instrumental delivery and caesarean section, 207
- 11.20 Intrapartum fetal monitoring, 215

# 11.0 Labour

## 11.1 Preparation for labour

A comprehensive programme of antenatal classes for pregnancy and labour should be organized to begin in mid-pregnancy. They should be coordinated by the midwives and the teaching should be shared among hospital and community midwives, physiotherapists, health visitors and medical staff. Topics for presentation in the preparatory classes for labour might include:

- the signs and symptoms of the onset of labour
- timing and procedure for admission
- basic physiology of labour
- signs of progress in labour
- induction of labour
- breathing and relaxation during labour
- the role of the father during labour
- analgesia
- deviation from normality—definitions and brief description
- indications for and methods of intrapartum fetal monitoring
- normal delivery
- use of obstetric forceps or vacuum extractor
- caesarean section
- the third stage of labour
- the indication for and repair of episiotomy
- immediate care of the newborn baby.

Fathers should be involved in the classes as much as possible.

Plenty of time should be made available for discussion so that anxieties can be expressed and misunderstandings clarified.

A tour of the hospital including a visit to the Delivery Suite should be organized. Audiovisual aids are useful but not essential. One of the major benefits of such classes is to decrease the stress and anxiety understandably associated with labour and the hospital environment.

# 11.0 Labour

11.2 Normal labour

## 11.2 Normal labour

Normal labour is traditionally defined as one in which spontaneous vaginal delivery of the infant occurs within 24 hours of the onset of regular spontaneous contractions. The modern management of labour is primarily concerned with minimizing the risks to mother and baby. The timescale of the above definition is not ideal in practice because the hazards of labour are directly related to its duration, particularly when it exceeds 12 hours.

Labour is characterized by progressive increases in the frequency, duration and strength of uterine contractions. This produces steady effacement and dilatation of the cervix with descent of the presenting part through the pelvis.

The **onset of labour** is taken as that point at which uterine contractions become regular and cervical dilatation begins. It is difficult, however, to time the onset of labour accurately in practice. For example, cervical effacement and some dilatation occur during the last 4 weeks before labour which, therefore, seldom begins as cervical dilatation starts, particularly in multigravidae.

The **first stage of labour** has a latent and an active phase. See Fig. 15 and Table 11.1. The latent phase starts from the onset of

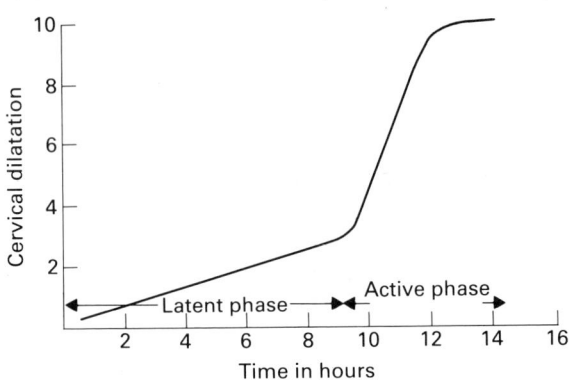

**Fig. 15.** Cervical dilatition time curve.

## 11.0 Labour

11.3 Management of labour (normal pregnancy)

regular uterine contractions and ends when the cervix is 2–3 cm dilated and fully effaced. In the active phase the cervix dilates at a maximum of 3 cm per hour in primigravidae and almost 6 cm per hour in multigravidae. The minimum acceptable rate is 1 cm per hour.

**Table 11.1.** Length of first stage in primigravid and multiparous women.

|  | Mean length in hours (±1 s.d.) | |
| --- | --- | --- |
|  | Primigravidae | Multigravidae |
| Latent phase | 9±6 | 5±4 |
| Active phase | 5±3.5 | 2±1.5 |

### 11.3 Management of labour (normal pregnancy)

It is important that common management guidelines be set down which commence with a clear statement about the diagnosis of the onset of labour.

### Diagnosis of labour

Women should be advised to present themselves to the hospital when regular contractions are occurring and/or the membranes have ruptured or 'show' has appeared.

For confirmation of the diagnosis of labour the following are required:

- Regular contractions occurring with a frequency of $\geq 2$ in 10 minutes and of an intensity which most women would describe as 'painful'.
- Cervical dilatation of at least 3 cm.

If the diagnosis of labour is confirmed the findings are documented at 'zero time' on a partogram (see below) and the woman is admitted to the delivery suite.

If labour is not confirmed she can be admitted to the antenatal ward or allowed to go home as clinical judgement dictates.

## 11.0 Labour

### 11.3 Management of labour (normal pregnancy)

**Monitoring progress in labour**—the use of the partogram
The labouring woman is examined on admission to the delivery suite and at least every 3 hours until full dilatation.

**Cervical dilatation** is marked in centimetres at zero time—the time of admission to the delivery suite—and at every subsequent examination. Alert and action lines may be superimposed on the partogram (as shown in Fig. 16) to help to identify and when indicated correct abnormally slow progress.

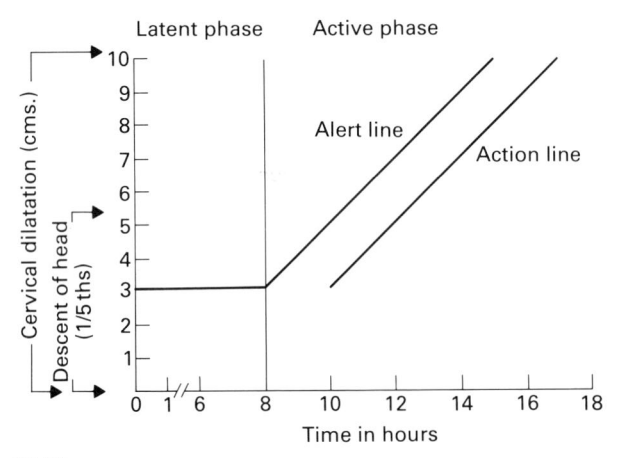

**Fig. 16.** The partogram.

### Descent of the head
Head descent is marked at the same times in fifths palpable above the pelvic brim as shown in Fig. 17. Steady descent of the head should occur.

### Contractions
The frequency, duration and strength of uterine contractions are assessed half hourly and the findings in the last 10 minutes recorded as shown in Fig. 18.

Manual palpation is universally used to evaluate uterine activity

# 11.0 Labour

## 11.3 Management of labour (normal pregnancy)

This is measured abdominally by the amount of Occiput (O) and Sinciput (S) felt.

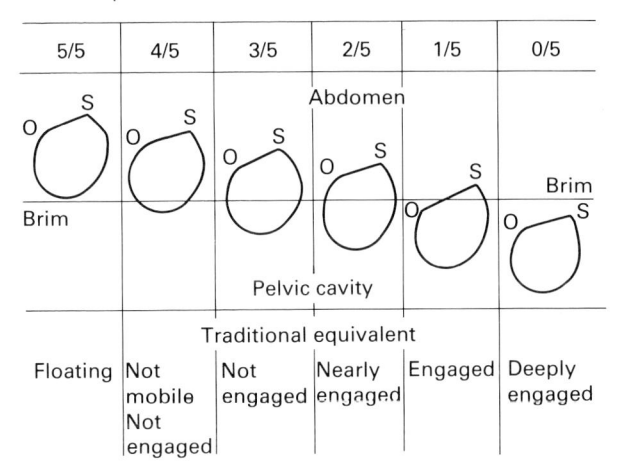

| 5/5 | 4/5 | 3/5 | 2/5 | 1/5 | 0/5 |
|---|---|---|---|---|---|
| (Brim) | | | Abdomen | | Brim |
| | | Pelvic cavity | | | |
| | | Traditional equivalent | | | |
| Floating | Not mobile Not engaged | Not engaged | Nearly engaged | Engaged | Deeply engaged |

**Fig. 17.** Descent of the head in fifths above the pelvic brim.

Frequency. Shade 1 vertical square for each contraction recorded in last 10 mins. of every $\frac{1}{2}$ hr.

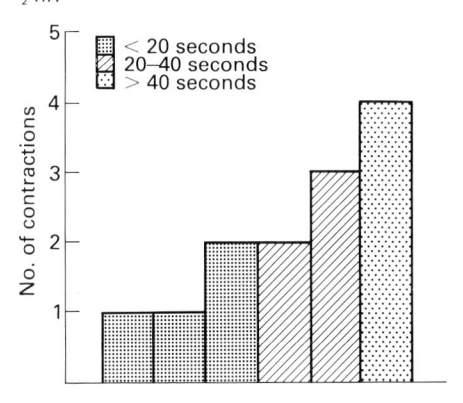

- < 20 seconds
- 20–40 seconds
- > 40 seconds

**Fig. 18.** Contractions.

## 11.0 Labour

### 11.3 Management of labour (normal pregnancy)

and information from external tocography is available when the cardiotocograph is being used.

Among the disadvantages of both of these methods are that:
- they are not quantitative—the true strength of contractions is not measured
- contraction frequency does not correlate with cervical dilatation
- duration of effective contractions varies from one woman to another (though it is usually constant throughout labour in each individual).

The only method which measures pressure directly is the intrauterine catheter but it is 'invasive' and its routine use cannot be justified in normal labour (even in abnormal labour there is resistance to its use). Use of the non-quantitative methods must be accompanied by an awareness of their limitations.

The frequency of contractions should not exceed 1 every 2–3 minutes and at least 1 minute should elapse between them.

The duration of contractions is usually 40–70 seconds. Intrauterine pressure (measured by catheter) between contractions (i.e. uterine tonus) is normally < 10 mmHg and the intensity of effective contractions around 50 mmHg. The active contraction area over a 15 minute period (called the uterine activity integral (UAI) by Steer (see acknowledgements)) is the best correlate with rates of cervical dilatation in the active phase of labour.

### Fetal heart rate

The fetal heart rate (FHR) is charted as beats per minute (bpm). If a continuous recording is not in progress the programme of auscultation is as follows (see Fig. 19);

1  Listen for 15 seconds and multiply by 4.
2  Listen between contractions to obtain baseline rate and chart as a dot.
3  Listen during *and* immediately after contractions and record the lower rate by drawing an arrow down to the level noted.

# 11.0 Labour

## 11.3 Management of labour (normal pregnancy)

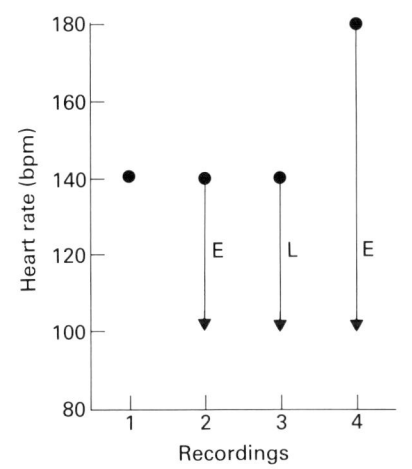

**Fig. 19.** Recording of fetal heart.

4  Decelerations may be early (E) or late (L)
   FHR patterns are discussed more fully on page 218.

### State of the membranes
Controversy still exists over the question of whether membranes should be ruptured or left intact and opinions are as much a matter of belief as scientific fact. The teaching that intact membranes means an intact mother and an intact baby is directly opposed by the view that intact membranes are the greatest single hindrance to normal labour. Their respective advantages are listed in Table 10.4.

### Liquor
The condition of the liquor is noted in the appropriate column by:
- 'C' for clear
- 'M' for meconium-stained
- 'B' for blood-stained
- 'I' for intact membranes.

## 11.0 Labour

11.3 Management of labour (normal pregnancy)

**Table 10.4.**

| Potential advantages of ruptured membranes | Potential advantages of intact membranes |
| --- | --- |
| Meconium staining of the liquor is revealed<br>The fetal head dilates the cervix more efficiently<br>A scalp clip can be applied for fetal heart monitoring | Maternal mobilization is easier<br>• chances of infection are reduced<br>Fetal hypoxia is less likely<br>Hydrostatic pressure is applied equally to the whole fetal surface<br>Rotation of the fetal body and head is not impeded |

The time and manner of rupture are noted by:
- ARM—artificial rupture
- spont—spontaneous rupture.

**Moulding**
Moulding of the fetal skull is assessed at each vaginal examination in relation to the sutures between occipital and parietal plus both parietal bones and can be assigned a score from 0 to +++ as shown below.

*Occipito-parietal and parieto-parietal moulding*

| | |
| --- | --- |
| Cranial bones separate | 0 |
| Bones merely touching | + |
| Bones overlap but can be reduced | ++ |
| Bones overlap and cannot be reduced | +++ |

Excessive moulding (a sum accumulating to 4+ or more) is an important sign of cephalo-pelvic disproportion (CPD) and a sum of 6+ moulding is diagnostic.

Other features charted include the dosage of oxytocin recorded as milliunits per minutes (mu/min) or drops per minute (dpm) (the former is preferable), other maternal medication, blood pressure, pulse, temperature and urinalysis.

## 11.0 Labour

11.4 Posture during labour

### 11.4 Posture during labour
Mobility should be encouraged during the latent phase of labour. In the absence of complications the mother should be allowed to adopt whatever position she finds most comfortable in the active phase. At all times maternal posture should be as upright as possible otherwise placental perfusion may be reduced.

### 11.5 Normal progress in labour
In primigravidae delivery can be expected within 8 hours of the diagnosis of labour and should be achieved within 12 hours. The commonest causes of delay in primigravid labour are inefficient uterine action, occipito-posterior position of the fetal head and (rarely) true cephalo-pelvic disproportion.

Labour is much more rapid in multiparous women and inefficient uterine action is rare.

When an abnormality is noted in the course of labour the following questions should be asked:
- what is the cause of the delay?
- is it correctable (e.g. inefficient uterine action)?
- is delivery by ceasarean section necessary?

### 11.6 Augmentation of labour
THIS POLICY IS ROUTINELY APPLICABLE ONLY TO PRIMIGRAVIDAE not making satisfactory progress in labour. Prolonged labour in a multigravid woman is likely to be due to obstruction. A decision to augment labour in a multiparous woman must be taken only by an experienced obstetrician because her uterus is prone to rupture if oxytocin is used injudiciously. Augmentation must not be applied routinely when obstetric anomalies are present, e.g. breech presentation, multiple pregnancy, or antipartum haemorrhage.

It is indicated in primigravidae when cervical dilatations is less than 1 cm/hr in the active phase of labour.

## 11.0 Labour

11.7 The second stage of labour

- the first step is to rupture the membranes  *or two?*
- if this does not accelerate labour within an hour an intravenous infusion of oxytocin is set up. The regimen is as for the induction of labour described in Chapter 11.8
- the aim is to achieve safe delivery within 8 hours of admission
- 'fetal distress' is dealt with appropriately (see Chapter 11.20)
- caesarean section is carried out on the small number of women undelivered, or in whom delivery is not imminent, within 12 hours of admission to the delivery suite.

### 11.7 The second stage of labour

This begins with full dilatation of the cervix and ends with delivery of the baby. Its average length is 40 minutes in primigravidae and 20 minutes in multiparae. These are not upper limits and, providing there is no evidence of 'fetal distress', intervention is not necessary merely because these times have elapsed.

The second stage has two phases:
- from full dilatation until the presenting part has descended to the pelvic floor (propulsive phase)
- from then until birth of the baby (expulsive phase).

The expulsive phase is recognized by the mother's irresistible desire to bear down and/or the distension of the perineum by the presenting part.

A woman should not usually be encouraged to bear down until she has entered the expulsive phase. If she does she may be exhausted before delivery has occurred and require an otherwise unnecessary instrumental delivery.

If the propulsive phase is prolonged in a primigravida due to inefficient uterine action and *not* cephalo-pelvic disproportions (relative or absolute) Syntocinon can be used as on page 183. Delivery should take place within an hour. This type of delay seems to arise most commonly in association with epidural analgesia (see page 186).

## 11.0 Labour

11.8   Induction of labour

---

### 11.8 Induction of labour

Policies for induction of labour have become more conservative in the last few years after the excesses of the 1970s. The rates are probably still too high in many places and the following cautious advice from Professor Donald is still highly relevant:

'No method of induction is both absolutely certain and safe. One should be as ready to defend the indications for induction as for caesarean section'.

'Any intervention, however apparently trivial, carries with it the responsibilities for the consequences which may be disproportionately severe'.

'The best of paediatric units is no substitute for a healthy uterine environment up to the time of adequate maturity'.

### Indications for elective delivery

The only 2 incontrovertible indications for expediting delivery are when the intrauterine risks are such that the infant will be safer delivered; and when the risk to the mother's health from the continuation of the pregnancy outweighs the risk to the fetus from delivery. If the added risk of labour is unacceptable, delivery should be by caesarean section. Otherwise labour can be induced accompanied by monitoring of maternal and fetal well-being. Decisions as to the optimum moment for delivery remain the most difficult and should always be taken by experienced members of staff. The application of policies outlined on pages 153–155 should assist with such decisions. Social indications rarely constitute adequate reasons for induction of labour. Each situation must, however, be considered on its merits.

Induction of labour is absolutely contra-indicated when:
- the fetal lie is other than longitudinal
- caesarean section has been carried out in a previous pregnancy because of pelvic contraction, a failed trial of labour due to disproportion, or other recurrent cause.
- a tumour occupies the pelvis.

# 11.0 Labour

## 11.8 Induction of labour

Among the relative contra-indications are:
- grand multiparity ($\geq$ para 5)
- previous cervical repair. A previous cone biopsy merits caution.

**Hazards of induction of labour**

**1. Iatrogenic prematurity**
This remains the greatest hazard of induction. Ideally maturity should have been confirmed early in pregnancy by ultrasound scan.

**2. Infection**
Some degree of amnionitis is always detectable within 36 hours of amniotomy but with modern methods of induction-delivery intervals (IDIs) are much shorter than this. There is, therefore, no appreciable risk in practice. The added risk of subacute bacterial endocarditis in women with cardiac disease means that induction is to be avoided in them if at all possible. Induction of labour in cases of intra-uterine fetal death should be carried out without amniotomy because of the serious potential hazard of infection (see Chapter 10.12).

**3. Neonatal jaundice**
There may be an added risk of neonatal hyperbilirubinaemia if the total dose of oxytocin exceeds 20 units. The jaundice is not harmful but the risk must be borne in mind in, for example, such cases as extreme prematurity or rhesus iso-immunization.

**4. Failed induction**
This is the failure to deliver a patient vaginally in whom safe vaginal delivery was initially expected. It therefore not only includes failure to induce effective uterine contractions within 24 hours but also the need to carry out caesarean section for failure to progress (in the absence of disproportion), fetal

## 11.0 Labour

11.8 Induction of labour

distress, infection or cord prolapse. The incidence is not known with certainty but it is still at least 2% of all inductions.

### 5. Additional hazards
In as much as it is possible to compare matched groups of women with spontaneous or induced labour it is suggested that in the latter group labours are longer (particularly the latent phase), the incidence of instrumental delivery and caesarean section is greater, more analgesia is required and Apgar scores in the infants (see Chapter 15) tend to be lower.

### Cervical ripeness
The ripeness or otherwise of the cervix is easy to assess clinically and the cervical state can be given a numerical value using the modified Bishop score (*Obstetrics Gynaecology* **24**, 266, 1964) in Table 11.1. This score correlates closely with the ease of induction of labour.

**Table 11.1.** Modified Bishop score of cervical state.

| Cervical state | Score | | | |
|---|---|---|---|---|
| | 0 | 1 | 2 | 3 |
| Dilatation (cm) | closed | 1–2 | 3–4 | 5+ |
| Length of cervix (cm) | 3 | 2 | 1 | 0 |
| Station of head (cm above ischial spines) | −3 | −2 | −1 | 0 |
| Consistency of cervix | firm | medium | soft | |
| Position of cervix | posterior | middle | anterior | |

If the cervix is 'ripe' (score > 5) induction of labour is likely to be successful. A score of < 5 does not preclude successful induction but in such cases induction is more likely to fail, a longer latent phase of labour is more likely, and a higher total dose of oxytocin will be necessary to achieve optimal uterine activity. Oxytocin infusions are of no value in ripening the cervix

## 11.0 Labour

11.8 Induction of labour

but this can usually be effected by carefully used intravaginal prostaglandins.

In a primigravid woman with an unfavourable cervix (score ≤ 5) two 3 mg PGE$_2$ vaginal tablets can be inserted on the evening before or at 6 am on the morning of induction. The dose for a multiparous women is one tablet (3 mg) on the morning of induction. Frequent uterine contractions of low amplitude are not uncommon. Hyperstimulation of the uterus is rare but can occur. A significant proportion of women with a 'favourable' cervix progress in labour after PG pre-treatment.

If the cervical score remains ≤ 5 despite treatment, another pre-treatment with PGE$_2$ can be carried out after careful consideration. The woman with a persistently unfavourable cervix in whom delivery is definitely indicated should not be subjected to repeated attempts to make the cervix more favourable but may be best delivered by caesarean section.

If prostaglandin pre-treatment is being used in a woman in whom intrapartum fetal heart rate recording is indicated (see page 218) this must begin with the pre-treatment.

**Methods for induction of labour**
The aim is to initiate uterine contractions and then maintain them to delivery. If PG vaginal pessaries are not successful in themselves amniotomy should be performed followed either immediately or 3 hours later if labour has not ensued. Routes of oxytocin administration other than intravenous are contraindicated.

A peristaltic pump (e.g. an Ivac or Tekmar pump) or a syringe pump (Palmer) provide a constant infusion and overcome the wide dose fluctuations which occur with only a gravity fed drip.

The dose of oxytocin required to produce effective uterine contractions is between 4 and 16 millunits per minute (mU/min). Occasionally as much as 32 mU/min are necessary. Careful monitoring of contractions and the fetal heart rate are vital when the higher doses are used.

## 11.0 Labour

### 11.9 Spontaneous rupture of membranes at term

As labour becomes established the uterus becomes more sensitive to oxytocin. This 'stable' phase usually begins at about half dilation (5 cm). From this time the effective dose rate is reduced to about 8 mU/min.

Oxytocin regimes are numerous and whatever scheme is followed the principles remain the same:
- the oxytocin must be given in low doses initially which gradually and steadily increase until effective contractions are produced
- the dose rate must be varied to suit the individual patient
- any hyperstimulation must be detected early.

The dose rate of oxytocin should be expressed as mU/minute rather than drops/minute (dpm).

**Oxytocin regimen**
The infusion begins at a rate of 2 mU/min and doubles every 20 minutes to 32 mU/min. The oxytocin is maintained at the dose rate at which the stable phase of labour is produced (i.e. at which cervical dilation becomes 5 cm). The dose rate at which this usually happens is about 16 mU/min. If the stable phase is not achieved after 30 minutes at 32 mU/min it can be increased to an absolute maximum of 64 mU/min.

*Water intoxication*
The combination of the slight anti-diuretic effect of oxytocin and the infusion of large volumes (over 4 litres) of water has occasionally produced water intoxification. Confusion, and convulsions proceed to coma and even death. The infusion of large volumes of electrolyte free fluid must, therefore, be avoided.

### 11.9 Spontaneous rupture of membranes (SRM) in the absence of labour at term

When SRM occurs in an otherwise normal pregnancy after 37 completed weeks an expectant policy can be adopted:

## 11.0 Labour

11.10 Analgesia in labour

- perform an aseptic speculum examination to confirm SRM and take a high vaginal swab for bacteriological culture
- if SRM is confirmed monitor the FH for at least 1 hour to check fetal well being and exclude cord prolapse or presentation
- transfer to antenatal ward and observe for 24 hours.

Labour will supervene in over 90% of women. Labour can be induced in the remainder by an oxytocin infusion. In some women expectant management can be continued beyond 24 hours but this must be decided individually by an experienced obstetrician.

Delivery will be necessary in some women within 24 hours of SRM. This will usually be clinically obvious but among the indications will be meconium staining of the liquor, antepartum haemorrhage, cord prolapse or presentation, genital tract infection or maternal diabetes.

### 11.10 Analgesia in labour

The mother herself should decide whether she wants pain relief in labour and if so when and how much. Ideally the choice will be open but, in practice, it will be limited by the availability of skilled midwives, obstetricians and anaesthetists. The potential effectiveness and side-effects of the methods should be presented in an unbiased fashion by nursing and medical staff. Guidance about the most effective method may be necessary if the labour is not progressing normally.

No woman in labour should be left alone and the father's presence is to be encouraged.

### Methods for pain relief

Psychological methods such as advocated by the National Childbirth Trust try, by a variety of techniques, to counteract the 'fear-tension-pain' sequence. Antenatal education (see page 00) is an integral part of this process. The woman is taught that the pain of labour is bearable and that, with proper support, she can cope with it. If psychological/relaxation methods prove

## 11.0 Labour

### 11.10 Analgesia in labour

inadequate it is the method, not the mother which has failed. Pain relieving drugs can supplement her own efforts when necessary.

**Opiates**

Opiates are commonly used in analgesia during labour as shown in Table 11.2.

**Table 11.2.**

| Opiate analgesia | Usual i.m. dose |
| --- | --- |
| Pethidine | 50–150 mg |
| Pentazocine | 36–60 mg |
| Papaveretum | 10–20 mg |
| Diamorphine | 5–10 mg |
| Meptazinol | 100 mg |

Intramuscular pethidine in doses of 100–150 mg is the most widely used method of pain relief in the UK. It is often combined with a phenothiazine (see below).

*Advantages of opiates*
- ease of administration
- reasonably rapid effect
- incidence of serious side-effects low
- antagonists available.

*Disadvantages*
- analgesia inadequate in up to 40% of patients
- nausea and vomiting common
- psychic disturbances are also common (e.g. disorientation, confusion and inability to cooperate)
- delayed gastric emptying
- respiratory depression in the neonate (see Chapter 14).

# 11.0 Labour

## 11.10 Analgesia in labour

*Contra-indications*
- previous idiosyncratic reaction
- current use of mono-amine oxidase inhibitors.

*Phenothiazines*
These drugs are most frequently combined with pethidine but usually only for the first dose. They add to the sedative and analgesic effect and decrease nausea and vomiting. They may contribute to maternal and fetal tachycardia. The drugs most commonly used are chlorpromazine, promazine or promethazine in intramuscular doses of 25 to 50 mg.

## Inhalational agents
Nitrous oxide (50%) and oxygen (50%) are best used in the Entonox apparatus. The two gases tend to separate as the ambient temperature falls. Separation is complete by $-7°C$. The main safety factor with this method is self administration. 'Interference' by attendant or partner is avoided.

Inhalational agents seem to be less used than once they were, and their use is usually too late and too hesitant. This is difficult to understand because self-administration is easy, and they can be both highly effective and safe for mother and baby.

## Epidural analgesia
Lumbar epidural analgesia is the most effective method of pain relief available for labour, providing adequate or total analgesia in up to 90% of patients. The incidence of problems is inversely related to the skill and experience of the operator. All staff involved must be competent in the management of patients with epidural blocks and in resuscitation techniques.

*Potential advantages of lumbar route*
- lower dose of anaesthetic agent required

*Potential advantages of caudal route*
- less risk of spinal (dural) tap
- better perineal analgesia and relaxation

## 11.0 Labour

### 11.10 Analgesia in labour

*Potential advantages of lumbar route (cont.)*
- more rapid onset of analgesia
- less risk of infection
- less risk of damage to the rectum
- less risk of trauma to presenting fetal part
- higher overall success rate

*[handwritten: So lumbar usually used.]*

*Possible immediate hazards of epidural analgesia*

**1 Dural tap**—dural puncture with needle or catheter. May lead to spinal headache (see below).

**2 Total spinal**—loss of all sensory and motor function and can include unconsciousness, severe hypotension and apnoea. It results from subarachnoid injection of epidural dose of local anaesthetic agent.

**3 Significant hypotension** may occur if the woman is kept supine after the block is established. It is due to compression of the inferior vena cava by the enlarged uterus. It will be prevented, and can usually be treated, by nursing the patient on her side and by the rapid intravenous infusion of 500–1000 ml of Hartmann's solution which should be given prior to the establishment of the block. Ephedrine 15–25 mg can be given intravenously if other measures are not effective. Other vasoconstrictors are contra-indicated.

**4 Motor paralysis** occurs to a marked degree in some patients especially if concentrated solutions of local anaesthetic are used. This reduces maternal expulsive efforts. Paralysis of the pelvic floor muscles may prevent rotation of the presenting fetal part. Both of these factors contribute to a higher incidence of instrumental delivery in women with epidural blocks.

**5 Toxic reactions** may occur to the local anaesthetic agent due to inadvertent intravenous injection. Before each injection, aspirate the syringe to make sure that a blood vessel has not been punctured.

## 11.0 Labour

11.10 Analgesia in labour

*Possible delayed hazards of epidural block*
- Severe spinal headache may follow accidental dural tap. It is relieved when the patient lies down and can be treated by injecting 10 ml of her own blood into the epidural space ('blood-patch'), or by a slow intra-epidural infusion of 1000–1500 ml normal saline over 24 hours.
- Urinary retention may occur due to blockade of sacral parasympathetic nerves. However, the method and circumstances of the delivery contribute to post-delivery urinary retention more than the epidural does.
- Contrary to general opinion, backache is not caused by epidural analgesia.
- Patches of diminished sensation may persist for some time over the area of distribution of a spinal nerve.
- Sepsis is extremely unlikely if a bacterial filter is interposed between the epidural catheter and the syringe.

*Indications for epidural analgesia in labour*
If epidural analgesia is not available on request, among the circumstances in which it is particularly helpful are:
- incoordinate uterine action
- OP position of the fetal head
- breech presentation
- multiple pregnancy
- pre-term labour
- forceps delivery (especially rotational forceps)
- hypertension
- vaginismus.

Although it can be valuable as part of the intrapartum management of severe pre-eclampsia, the hamodynamic volatility present in this condition make close supervision vital. Epidural analgesia is contra-indicated if pre-eclampsia is associated with significant intravascular coagulation.

## 11.0 Labour

### 11.10 Analgesia in labour

*Contra-indications to epidural analgesia*
- lack of experienced personnel
- infection at site of injection
- bony abnormalities of the spinal column
- coagulation defects/bleeding diatheses/anticoagulant therapy
- hypovolaemia due to haemorrhage
- active neurological disease
- untoward or allergic reactions to local anaesthetic agents.

*Fetal effects*
Epidural analgesia has no significant direct adverse effects on the fetus.

*Guidelines to patient management*
Details of materials and techniques are not considered here (see suggested reading).

- The epidural blockade may be used continuously during labour or as a single injection for operative delivery.
- An intravenous infusion of Hartmann's solution (or some similar fluid) must be set up before insertion of the block (see above).
- Bupivacaine (Marcaine) 0.5, 0.375 or 0.25% is the preferred anaesthetic. Lignocaine (Xylocaine) 1.5–2.0% is a suitable alternative. The dose for the lumbar route is 10–12 ml and for the caudal route 12–18 ml but these must be adjusted to individual requirements. A test dose of 3 ml of 0.5% bupivicaine plain should be injected initially to decrease the risks from accidental dural tap. The patient must be in the horizontal position.
- Maximum analgesia is achieved within 10 to 15 minutes of the full injection.
- It is preferable to defer injection until the cervix is 4 to 6 cm dilated in primigravidae and 3 to 4 cm in multiparous women (the catheter itself can, of course, be inserted much earlier).

## 11.0 Labour

11.11   The bony pelvis and labour

- The patient needs constant observation and, in particular, her BP, pulse, and respiration should be recorded frequently especially in the 30 minutes following each injection of local anaesthetic. The fetal heart rate, uterine contractions and progress in labour must also be charted regularly.
- Analgesia should be maintained by top-up injections, the precise dose and timing of which are chosen to suit the needs of the mother.

*Epidural analgesia and previous caesarean section*
If the obstetrician believes that a patient who has had a caesarean section in a previous pregnancy can be allowed to labour epidural analgesia is not contra-indicated.

Fetal heart rate and, whenever possible, intra-uterine pressure should be observed carefully.

*Local anaesthesia*
**Paracervical block** has no advantages over epidural anaesthesia. Despite its original popularity, the maternal and fetal complications of this technique mean that it has little place in modern obstetric analgesia. The place of **pudendal nerve blockade** is discussed on page 208 as a method of providing analgesia for forceps delivery.

### 11.11   The bony pelvis and labour
Clinical assessment of pelvic dimensions can be performed on all primigravidae at 37 weeks, and should be carried out when clinical suspicion of cephalo-pelvic disproportion (CPD) is present (e.g. high head at term in primigravidae or when the breech presents). It is wise to have ruled out placenta praevia beforehand.

**Clinical pelvimetry**
- A vaginal examination is performed in the routine manner.
- An attempt is made to reach the sacral promontory with the

# 11.0 Labour

## 11.11 The bony pelvis and labour

middle finger. If the pelvis is normal the sacral promontory will not usually be felt.
- The sacrum itself is palpated to note an angulation, straightening, irregularities or false promontories.
- Convergence of the pelvic side walls is then checked for.
- The prominence of the ischial spines and the middle of the sacro-sciatic notches are assessed.
- To assess the outlet the hand is partially removed and the fingers placed in the sub-pubic arch to assess its shape and angulation.
- Finally, the hand is removed and the knuckles of the clenched fist are placed between the ischial tuberosities.
- The patient should be given a description of the findings as the examination progresses.

### The ideal pelvis
- the brim is round and the sacral promontory is not prominent. The angle of inclination is about 55° to the horizontal
- the cavity is shallow with straight, non-converging walls
- the sacrum is smoothly curved
- the sacro-sciatic notches are wide and shallow in the outlet
- the sacrum does not project forwards
- the ischial spines are not prominent
- the pubic arch is wide and domed (like a Norman arch rather than a Gothic arch)
- the sub-pubic angle is a virtual right angle
- the inter-tuberous diameter is wide accommodating 4 knuckles of an average sized hand with ease.

### X-ray pelvimetry
The lateral view is adequate during pregnancy because the brim view involves greater exposure to radiation than can be justified easily. To obtain accurate pelvic measurements the X-ray must be taken so that the femoral head and acetabular margins are superimposed (or very nearly so).

## 11.0 Labour

11.12 Breech presentation and labour

*Information to be gained*
- relationship of presenting part to pelvic brim
- angle of inclination of the brim
- true and obstetric conjugate measurements
- discovery of false sacral promontory
- number of segments in the sacrum and its shape and angle
- width and depth of sacro-sciatic notches
- antero-posterior measurement of mid-pelvis
- antero-posterior measurement of pelvic outlet.

**Indications for X-ray pelvimetry**

*Definite*
- breech presentation at 37 weeks or later
- postnatally after caesarean section for suspected CPD (full pelvimetry possible here)
- at 36–37 weeks in second pregnancy if vaginal delivery is contemplated after caesarean section in first pregnancy when X-ray pelvimetry has not already been performed
- when injury to or disease of the pelvis make contraction possible.

*Possible*
- cephalic presentation with suspected disproportion antenatally or in labour.

|        | Antero-posterior | Oblique | Transverse |
|--------|------------------|---------|------------|
| brim   | 11–11.5          | 12      | 12.5       |
| cavity | 12               | 12      | 12         |
| outlet | 12.5             | 12      | 11–11.5    |

**Fig. 20.** Guide to the average diameters of the normal pelvis (cm).

## 11.12 Breech presentation and labour

The types of breech presentation are:

## 11.0 Labour

### 11.12 Breech presentation and labour

- frank breech (65%)—the thighs are flexed and the legs extended
- full or complete breech (10%)—the thighs and the knees are flexed
- footling or incomplete breech (25%)—one or both feet are lowermost.

Breech presentation is more commonly associated with preterm delivery (see page 201), congenital malformations, multiple pregnancy (see page 193) and cord prolapse (see page 229) than vertex presentations.

It has been argued that breech presentation is indication enough for caesarean section because of the increased perinatal mortality and morbidity (e.g. birth asphyxia and trauma) associated with it. The benefits of this policy in both term and pre-term delivery have not been clearly demonstrated. A more conservative policy is outlined below.

The following must be checked in the assessment for the best method for delivery:
- pelvic dimensions clinically and radiologically at 37 weeks
- BPD, fetal size
- fetal attitude and flexion/extension of fetal head
- exclude major fetal anomalies

} assessed ultrasonically

The **clear indications** for an attempt at **vaginal delivery** are:
- term pregnancy with fetal weight assessed as being 2500–3500 g
- frank breech
- normal pelvic dimensions
- no other complications of pregnancy (e.g. pre-eclampsia)
- normal fetal heart tracing or biophysical profile.

**Definite indications** for **caesarean section** include:
- weight of baby estimated at greater than 3.5 kg
- hyperextension of the fetal head
- any abnormality of bony pelvis
- older primigravida

## 11.0 Labour

11.12 Breech presentation and labour

- intrauterine growth retardation
- bad obstetric history
- previous difficult labour
- failure to progress in first stage of labour
- failure of descent of breech in second stage
- diabetes
- severe pre-eclampsia
- (plus indications which would apply whatever the presentation e.g. fetal hypoxia).

**Possible indications** for **caesarean section** (i.e. an attempt at vaginal delivery must be clearly justified).
- complete or footling breech
- breech presentation plus any other pregnancy complication
- pre-term labour (see page 201)
- uterine anomaly.

Epidural analgesia can be useful in the management of a breech labour. The place of augmentation of labour if uterine action is inefficient is controversial. If oxytocin is used at all it must be under the direction and close supervision of an experienced obstetrician. During labour with a footling or complete breech the membranes should not be ruptured artificially during the first stage. When spontaneous rupture occurs a vaginal examination is necessary to exclude cord presentation.

Induction of labour is best avoided if at all possible in footling or complete breech presentations. The management of vaginal breech delivery is best learned in practice under supervision. The main points are:

- descent of the breech must be progressive in the second stage
- the obstetrician should interfere as little as possible with the delivery
- breech extraction is contra-indicated (except perhaps for a second twin)
- a generous episiotomy is necessary

## 11.0 Labour

11.13 Labour with malpresentations other than breech

---

- great care must be taken in delivery of the after-coming head
- the anaesthetist and neonatal paediatrician must be on hand during the delivery.

One of the hazards of vaginal breech deliveries under 34 weeks is that the after-coming head becomes trapped by the incompletely dilated cervix. The only solution if the fetus is alive is to incise the cervix at 2 and 10 o'clock with episiotomy scissors. This is difficult and can be hazardous for the mother. It must only be done if the head is fully engaged, the cervix > 6 cm dilated and the fetus viable. The incisions should be repaired by an experienced obstetrician.

### 11.13 Labour with malpresentations other than breech

Face and brow presentations are often the end result of a labour in which the vertex presented initially but, due to a flat pelvis, the head extended increasingly during labour. These are secondary malpresentations. Occurrence before the onset of labour constitutes a primary malpresentation.

### Face presentation

This can be diagnosed in labour by detecting the supra-orbital ridges and the alveolar margins. Confusion may arise early in labour between a face and the breech. An attempt at vaginal delivery should be allowed in a patient with a primary face presentation. Spontaneous delivery can occur when the chin is anterior (mento-anterior face presentation). Forceps can be used but the ventouse is totally contra-indicated. Where the chin is posterior (mento-posterior) or if there is any delay in labour, the baby should be delivered by caesarean section.

### Brow presentation

A primary brow presentation may correct itself before labour. A secondary brow presentation is best delivered by caesarean section. Otherwise an obstructed labour may lead to uterine rupture.

195

## 11.0 Labour

### 11.14 Multiple pregnancy and delivery

Delay in the first stage of labour despite good contractions in a multiparous woman may be due to a brow presentation. Diagnosis by vaginal examination is difficult early in labour but later palpation of the supra orbital ridges and the anterior fontanelle is diagnostic. Confirmation can be obtained by erect lateral pelvic X-ray.

**Transverse lie**

*[handwritten: If at 41 weeks, transverse → LUCS (if at 39 or 40?).]*

If the lie is transverse or oblique in labour the fetus must be delivered by caesarean section. In multiple pregnancy external version is possible if a second twin is lying transversely when its amniotic sac is intact after delivery of the first twin. A vaginal delivery is likely under these circumstances.

In a neglected shoulder presentation an arm may well be prolapsed and the baby may be already dead. In these circumstances vaginal decapitation and delivery may be possible but only by an experienced senior obstetrician. Otherwise caesarean section with decapitation *in utero* is less hazardous.

### 11.14 Multiple pregnancy and delivery

Among the conditions relevant to labour and delivery which complicate multiple pregnancy more commonly are pre-term labour, placenta praevia, placental abruption, cord prolapse and malpresentation. In twin pregnancy the presentations (in order of frequency) are:

1 vertex—vertex
2 vertex—breech
3 breech—vertex
4 breech—breech
5 vertex—transverse
6 breech—transverse

**Possible indications for elective caesarean section:**

- first twin presenting as a breech
- pre-term labour (before 34 weeks)
- triplets (?) or higher multiples
- severe pre-eclampsia

## 11.0 Labour

11.14 Multiple pregnancy and delivery

- any indication which would also apply in singleton pregnancies e.g. IUGR, APH.

**Management of twin labour**
- set up i.v. line and crossmatch 2 units of blood
- monitor both fetal hearts continuously
- epidural analgesia can be useful but hypotension must be avoided
- the anaesthetist and two paediatricians should be present for delivery
- once the first baby is delivered check the lie of the second twin. If it is not longitudinal correct it by ECV
- if contractions do not recommence within 15 minutes infuse oxytocin (see page 182)
- when the uterus is contracting rupture the second amniotic sac
- if the cord of the second twin prolapses proceed to ventouse extraction (if presentation is cephalic) or breech extraction. The latter can be carried out under epidural (if already in place) or general anaesthesia
- the interval between delivery of the first and second twin should be no more than 20 minutes.

The risk of PPH is increased, therefore syntometrine (1 ampoule i.m. or i.v.) should be given after delivery of the second twin when the presence of a third baby has been excluded.

After delivery the placentae and membranes should be examined to determine if twins of the same sex are uniovular or binovular. In uniovular twins the septum between the two sacs consists only of two layers of amnion (i.e. it is monochorionic); in binovular twins the two sacs are separated by both the amnion and chorion of one fetus then the chorion and amnion of the second (dichorionic). This discrimination is not always easy to the naked eye and histological confirmation may well be necessary. Among the other methods for determining zygosity are hand and footprints, blood groups or tissue typing.

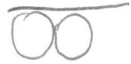

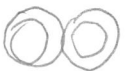

## 11.0 Labour

11.15 Episiotomy and third-degree tear

### 11.15 Episiotomy and third-degree tear

The need for an episiotomy is a matter for experienced clinical judgement. It should never be carried out merely because it is routine. Among the possible indications for an episiotomy will be:

- when a perineal tear appears inevitable otherwise
- in cases of fetal distress late in the second stage
- many forceps deliveries
- pre-term delivery
- breech delivery
- failure to advance because of perineal rigidity.

Too frequent recourse to episiotomy suggests bad management of the second stage of labour. An episiotomy must be:

- performed at the correct time—incise too early and unnecessary blood loss will result
- carried out and repaired with adequate local or regional anaesthesia
- made with sharp scissors in the correct place—a mediolateral episiotomy is preferred to the midline incision in the UK. Whatever is used it must start in the midline
- repaired properly within as short a time of delivery as possible.

Adequate supervision must be given to those not practised in the technique. Medical students must not be allowed to suture episiotomies without personal guidance from an experienced operator. The apex of vaginal wound must always be included in the first (continuous) suture. For a large, fleshy episiotomy or ragged tear, non-absorbable sutures, e.g. silk, cannot be bettered for the skin incision.

**Third degree tears** must be repaired in theatre under general anaesthesia by an experienced obstetrician. The rectum then the anus are first repaired with interrupted catgut sutures (knots towards the gut lumen). If necessary the vagina and rectum should be dissected apart in the upper part of the tear. The torn

## 11.0 Labour

11.16 The third stage of labour

---

ends of the sphincter are then localized and sutured. The residual second degree tear is repaired routinely.

### After-care
- the mother should be given a low residue diet for one week
- liquid paraffin is *not* recommended
- then use a proprietary preparation e.g. Normacol to soften the faeces; or
- after 5 days instil a small quantity of olive oil into the rectum with a soft rubber catheter to soften any faeces.

If the repair breaks down due to sepsis or poor technique another attempt must not be made until all local sepsis has been eradicated. Some surgeons leave further repair for up to 4 months.

### 11.16 The third stage of labour

This begins with delivery of the baby and ends when the placenta is expelled. Active management of the third stage involving the i.m. injection of syntometrine (syntocinon 5 units: ergometrine 0.5 mg) with delivery of the anterior shoulder has become routine and 'normal' over the past twenty years in the UK. The justification for this policy was the significant maternal mortality associated with PPH in the 1950s.

It is now being reconsidered because:

- policies appropriate 10 or 20 years ago are not necessarily still indicated in the 1980s
- the routine use of oxytocins before delivery of the infant is completed is not practiced anywhere other than the UK and it is not proven that this practice is more effective than administration after the birth of the baby
- an undiagnosed second twin can be severely compromised
- the placenta can become trapped due to cervical spasm. 'Fiddling' with the unseparated placenta also contributes to this
- ergometrine can cause sudden and severe hypertension.

## 11.0 Labour

11.17 Primary postpartum haemorrhage

Properly controlled studies are required to reassess this routine practice.

Whatever policy is adopted signs of placental separation must be awaited before any attempt is made to deliver the placenta by maternal effort or controlled cord traction.

### 11.17 Primary postpartum haemorrhage

This is defined as the loss of 500 ml of blood or more within 24 hours of delivery.

The incidence of primary PPH varies from 2–8% among hospitals. An incidence of 6–8% is certainly too high and although the reasons are not always clear it is likely that meddlesome interference with the third stage is a factor.

### Management

- give ergometrine 0.5 mg i.v. (no more than 1 mg of ergometrine should be given within a 4 hour period)
- call the Obstetric Flying Squad (see page 227) if the patient is at home or in an isolated GP Unit. The placenta should be removed before transferring the patient to hospital
- set up an intravenous infusion and crossmatch two units of blood
- give screened Group O Rh-D negative, Kell negative blood if the patient is shocked
- empty the bladder by urethral catheter
- determine whether the placenta is or is not delivered
- if the placenta is not delivered but is separated, rub up a uterine contraction and deliver the placenta by controlled cord traction (CCT)
- if the placenta is unseparated or cannot be delivered by CCT (e.g. the cord has been broken) arrange for an experienced obstetrician to carry out manual removal under general, or pre-existing epidural, anaesthesia. Pethidine 50 mg and diazepam 10 mg can be used intravenously to produce basal narcosis but

## 11.0 Labour

11.18 Pre-term labour

should only be used if alternative more adequate anaesthesia is not available
- if the placenta is delivered rub up a contraction to reduce uterine atony and check the completeness of the placenta. If it is incomplete explore the uterus as above. If it is complete examine the vagina and cervix for lacerations. The patient must be in the lithotomy position and good lighting is essential. Analgesia must be adequate for the examination and repairing any lacerations
- if the bleeding persists set up an infusion of oxytocin (Syntocinon) 20 units in 500 ml dextrose/saline. Check that the blood is clotting (see page 00 for coagulation defects) and explore the uterus to exclude rupture
- bimanual compression of the uterus will help to control bleeding if other measures fail or are not available
- internal iliac artery ligation or hysterectomy may be necessary on rare occasions. Although such extreme action must not be resorted to too readily, unnecessary delay may cost the patient her life
- manual removal of the placenta is also indicated in the absence of bleeding if it remains unseparated after 1 hour.

### 11.18 Pre-term labour
This is defined as regular, painful, uterine contractions accompanied by effacement and dilatation of the cervix after 20 and before 37 completed weeks of pregnancy. Pre-term labour accounts for 5–10% of all deliveries but causes 85% of neonatal deaths.

**Maternal or fetal causes of spontaneous pre-term labour** in general order of importance:
- multiple pregnancy
- ante-partum haemorrhage
- intra-uterine growth retardation
- cervical incompetence

## 11.0 Labour

11.18 Pre-term labour

**Table 11.3.** Main contributory factors to per-term delivery.

|  | Incidence |
| --- | --- |
| Spontaneous onset of labour—cause unknown | 40% |
| Spontaneous onset due to recognized conditions of mother or fetus (except multiple pregnancy) | 25% |
| Associated with multiple pregnancy | 10% |
| Elective delivery | 25% |

- amnionitis (true incidence unknown)
- congenital uterine anomaly
- diabetes
- polyhydramnios
- pyelonephritis
- general infections.

+ previous pre term
+ unknown -

### Prediction of risk of pre-term labour
Several scoring systems have been developed in an attempt to predict the risk of pre-term labour. None has proved superior to clinical judgement. The strongest association is with pre-term delivery in a previous pregnancy.

There is no evidence that cervical cerclage early in pregnancy reduces the incidence of pre-term delivery or improves neonatal survival even in women with histories suggestive of cervical incompetence.

### Management of pre-term labour
This is dependent on 5 main factors:

1  The state of the membranes. Attempts to inhibit pre-term labour are unlikely to be successful if the membranes are ruptured.

2  Dilatation of the cervix. Labour is likely to progress despite attempts to stop it if cervical dilatation is more than 4 cm.

3  Gestational age. The earlier in gestation that pre-term labour supervenes, the more strenuous efforts to stop it should be.

# 11.0 Labour

## 11.18 Pre-term labour

Labour is usually allowed to progress if the estimated fetal weight is over 2000 g.

4 The cause of pre-term labour. Treatment of a simple cause (e.g. pyelonephritis) may be enough to stop contractions. If the cause is prejudicing fetal welfare, delivery is indicated rather than suppression of labour. The baby must be delivered in as healthy condition as possible. Caesarean section should, therefore, be considered from 27 weeks onwards and/or when fetal weight is estimated at over 1000 g but it cannot be automatically assumed that this is the best method for delivery.

5 The availability of neonatal intensive care facilities. If adequate facilities are not immediately available, transfer of the patient to the nearest neonatal intensive care unit must be considered. Neonatal paediatricians must be kept fully informed about all cases.

### Treatment of pre-term labour

In up to 50% of patients contractions will stop spontaneously and the pregnancy will continue to term without any treatment whatsoever. The clinical problem is to discern correctly those in whom treatment is indicated. One possible quide is the presence or absence of 'fetal breathing' movements assessed by real-time ultrasound over a maximum of 45 minutes. If fetal breathing movements can be seen it suggests that the pre-term labour is likely to subside spontaneously.

### Beta-sympathomimetic drugs

Beta-sympathomimetic drugs suppress uterine activity but even if their use is associated with a significant prolongation of pregnancy it does not necessarily follow that the baby will benefit. Once more, each case must be considered on its merits and in discussion with neonatal paediatric colleagues.

The use of salbutamol and ritodrine hydrochloride are described below. The infusions can be regulated by an infusion pump or by the rate of the drip in drops/minute.

## 11.0 Labour

11.18 Pre-term labour

### Salbutamol
3 ml (3 mg) is diluted in 500 ml dextrose/saline. The initial dose rate is 10 drops per minute for 15 minutes. This is increased by 10 drops per minute every 15 minutes until contractions cease or side-effects are troublesome (see table below).

**Table 11.4.** Potential side effects of beta-sympathomimetic agents.

| Side effect | Stop infusion if: |
| --- | --- |
| Maternal tachycardia | > 130 beats/minute |
| Hypotension | SPB fails > 20 mmHg |
| Fetal tachycardia | FH increases > 20 beats/minute |
| Palpitations | |
| Headache | |
| Visual disturbances | These become severe |
| Nausea, vomiting | |

Once labour is inhibited maintain the infusion rate for 4 hours then reduce it gradually by 5 drops half hourly. During the infusion observe maternal pulse and fetal heart rate every 5 minutes while the dose is increasing; then half hourly while infusion continues. Maternal temperature is taken 4 hourly and hyperkalaemia must be excluded if the infusion continues for longer than 24 hours.

### Ritodrine hydrochoride
See Table 11.5.

**Table 11.5.** Suppression of labour with ritodrine HCl.

| Required dose ($\mu$g/min) | No. of 5 ml (50 mg) ampoules per 500 ml dextrose/saline | Rate of infusion (ml/min) |
| --- | --- | --- |
| 50 | 1 | 0.5 |
| 100 | 1 | 1.0 |
| 150 | 1 | 1.5 |
| 200 | 2 | 1.0 |
| 300 | 2 | 1.5 |
| 400 | 3 | 1.5 |

## 11.0 Labour

11.18 Pre-term labour

The initial dose is 50 $\mu$g/min gradually increasing by 50 $\mu$g/min every 10 minutes until contractions cease or the maternal pulse is 130–140 beats per minute. The infusion should be continued for 12–48 hours after contractions have ceased. The effective dose is usually between 150 and 350 $\mu$g/min.

Oral ritodrine HCl 10 mg every 2 hours can be given for 24 hours then 10–20 mg every 4–6 hours (maximum 120 mg daily) for as long as is thought desirable.

Intravenous therapy can be restarted if pre-term labour recurs, but probably only for a further two episodes, after which no further treatment should be given.

Prophylactic oral beta-mimetics have not yet been shown to be effective in the prevention of pre-term labour.

### Contra-indications to beta-mimetic drugs
- ante-partum haemorrhage
- severe pre-eclampsia
- cardiac disease or thyrotoxicosis
- treatment with anti-hypertensive drugs (risk of myocardial infarction) tricyclic antidepressants or MAOIs
- any other situation in which prolongation or pregnancy may be hazardous to mother and/or baby.

**Pulmonary oedema** due to right heart failure is a rare but serious complication associated with intravenous beta-mimetics usually when glucocorticoids have also been administered.

Extreme caution should also be exercised if the patient has **diabetes mellitus** (blood sugar levels must be monitored during treatment), or is being treated with corticosteroids or potassium depleting diuretics.

**Prostaglandin-synthetase inhibitors** (e.g. indomethacin, naproxen sodium or mefanamic acid)
The risk of intra-uterine closure of the ductus arteriosus contra-indicates the use of these drugs in the treatment of pre-term labour.

## 11.0 Labour

11.18 Pre-term labour

**Glucocorticoid therapy** and the prevention of respiratory distress syndrome (RDS)

Although it remains true that glucocorticoids given to the mother can induce production of pulmonary surfactant in the lungs of the immature fetus, there has, over the last few years, been a gradual but definite change in attitude towards their use for the prevention of RDS. In some centres they are hardly ever prescribed and among those in which their use is still advocated the numbers treated have decreased and the indications have become more stringent.

Among the possible reasons for this are:

- the incidence of RDS due to hyaline membrane disease has fallen spontaneously
- the results achieved by neonatal intensive care have continued to improve dramatically
- controlled studies of the value of glucocorticoid therapy could show benefit in only a proportion of those treated
- high doses of steroids (even for a short period of time) cannot be assumed to be free of side-effects.

The potential benefit of glucocorticoid therapy must, therefore, be carefully considered in each case. Treatment is with betamethasone or dexamethasone in doses of 4 mg, 8 hourly intramuscularly for 48–72 hours. Glucocorticoid therapy is of no value after 34 weeks gestation and is probably best avoided at any time in severe pre-eclampsia.

### Mode of delivery in pre-term labour

Delivery by caesarean section for women in pre-term labour before 34 weeks has not been clearly demonstrated to be beneficial to the baby (even when presenting by the breech). Studies suggesting that caesarean section is necessary have included cases in which the outlook was so bad that caesarean section was positively contra-indicated (e.g. pre-term labour at 24–26 weeks) and those in which vaginal delivery was precipitate. The poor outcome in these cases born vaginally has

## 11.0 Labour

### 11.19 Instrumental delivery and caesarean section

biased the results in favour of caesarean section. Not only that but caesarean section at early gestations and with infants < 1000 g can be hazardous for the mother and is not necessarily safer for the baby.

If the fetus is viable, it should be delivered by the route assessed as being least likely to cause trauma or hypoxia in that case. This may mean caesarean section but not necessarily so. The indications for caesarean section are stronger but not absolute in pre-term labour associated with multiple pregnancy and breech presentation.

*Note*: pre-term labour is unpredictable and the woman may become fully dilated quickly and silently.

**Premature rupture of membranes without uterine contractions**
This can be managed conservatively before 34–36 weeks gestation unless intrauterine infection is present or likely to develop. A high vaginal swab should be taken at a sterile speculum examination on admission. If any significant organisms are cultured (particularly beta-haemolytic streptococci) delivery should be expedited and the neonatal paediatricians alerted. A normal CTG tracing at admission helps to rule out cord prolapse or presentation.

Any intrauterine infection must be treated vigorously and expeditiously. If contractions develop it is probably best to let labour proceed (unless delivery by caesarean section is indicated).

### 11.19 Instrumental delivery and caesarean section
The techniques for delivery by obstetric forceps and the vacuum extractor (ventouse) and for caesarean section are best taught by example and learned by experience.
The following features need to be emphasized.

#### Conditions for the proper use of forceps
- a legitimate indication must be present

## 11.0 Labour

### 11.19 Instrumental delivery and caesarean section

- the presentation must be suitable i.e. vertex, face (mento-anterior) or after-coming head in a breech delivery
- there must be no cephalo-pelvic disproportion. Moulding of the fetal skull must not be excessive (see page 176).
- the head must be engaged. Ideally no part of the fetal head should be palpable per abdomen and if more than 1/5 can be palpated, VAGINAL DELIVERY MUST NOT BE CONTEMPLATED
- the position of the head must be known
- the cervix must be fully dilated
- analgesia must be adequate
- the bladder must be empty
- the uterus must be contracting.

The same conditions apply to the proper use of the ventouse except that it may be used before the cervix has reached full dilatation. The ventouse must not be considered as a soft-option when adverse features are present or the position of the fetal head is unknown.

### Analgesia for instrumental delivery

**Perineal infiltration** alone is suitable for episiotomy, and low outlet deliveries using Wrigley's forceps or the ventouse. 10–15 ml of 1% lignocaine are injected fan-wise from the midline at the fourchette.

**Pudendal nerve block** is useful for midcavity forceps and some ventouse deliveries. It does not provide sufficient analgesia for rotational forceps. The transvaginal route is recommended for insertion of the block. A 15 cm, 17 gauge needle is attached to a 20 ml syringe containing 1% lignocaine without adrenalin. A specially designed guarded needle is available which keeps the sharp tip within the shaft of the guard until it is at the spine. Even at its fullest extent the needle tip only protrudes a few millimetres from the guard.

### Insertion technique

- The index and middle finger of the hand opposite to that in

## 11.0 Labour

### 11.19 Instrumental delivery and caesarean section

which the block is being inserted are placed in the vagina.
- When they reach the ischial spine the shaft of the needle is placed in the groove between the fingers.
- The needle penetrates the skin just below the ischial spine.
- At this point the line of the needle shaft is about 45° to the horizontal. It is now moved to lie paralled to the table.
- After aspiration to ensure that the tip has not penetrated a blood vessel, 10 ml of local anaesthetic is injected.
- This is repeated on the other side and then perineal infiltration is performed with a further 8–10 ml of 1% lignocaine.

**Epidural anaesthesia**
See Section 11.10. Epidural anaesthesia is ideal for all instrumental deliveries, but is also suitable for elective caesarean sections and those emergency section in which an existing epidural block is affording good analgesia. Its insertion to carry out emergency caesarean section is far from ideal, but in some communities this is necessary because of lack of anaesthetic staff. This form of analgesia is optimal for rotational forceps.

General anaesthesia in obstetrics is the province of experienced anaesthetic staff specifically trained in obstetric anaesthesia. Between 1979 and 1981, 13% of maternal deaths in England and Wales were due to anaesthetic difficulties. This showed no change compared with the previous triennium. Skilled help must also be available to help the anaesthetist in theatre e.g. to apply cricoid pressure properly.

The major cause of general anaesthetic deaths were:
- inhalation of stomach contents
- difficulty with endotracheal contents — intubation?
- misuse of drugs
- accidents with apparatus
- inadequately trained anaesthetists
- failure to monitor intra-operatively.

## 11.0 Labour

11.19 Instrumental delivery and caesarean section

**Guidelines for the proper use of general anaesthesia** (GA)
The anaesthetist must be experienced. Skilled help must be available in theatre to, for example, apply cricoid pressure properly. A cuffed endotracheal tube *must* be used. To reduce risk from inhalation of stomach contents the stomach should be empty. If the stomach is thought to be full, its contents must be aspirated through a naso-gastric tube.
Antacids must be given to raise gastric PH.

*Antacid therapy*

All patients should be given 30 ml, 0.3 M sodium citrate orally as an antacid during labour.

For elective caesarean section whether under general or epidural anaesthesia one suggested regimen is given in Table 11.6.

**Table 11.6.**

| Time of operation | a.m. | p.m. |
|---|---|---|
| Give ranitidine 150 mg orally | the night before: | at 6.00 on the day |
| Give ranitidine 150 mg orally | at 6.00 on the day: | at 12.00 on the day |

Give 30 ml 0.3 M sodium citrate orally just before leaving the antenatal ward *and* again in the anaesthetic room.

For emergency caesarean sections under general or epidural anaesthesia give 30 ml 0.3 M sodium citrate orally *and* ranitidine 50 mg i.v. as soon as the decision to proceed is made. A further 30 ml of sodium citrate is given just before induction of general anaesthesia.
(The management of inhalation of acid stomach contents is discussed in Chapter 12.7)

**Indications for instrumental delivery**
Only a general guide is possible because each case must be

## 11.0 Labour

11.19 Instrumental delivery and caesarean section

dealt with on its merits. Again, there can be no substitute for experience.

- maternal conditions in which (prolonged) expulsive efforts may be detrimental, e.g. cardiac and respiratory disease, severe pre-eclampsia or eclampsia
- fetal distress in the second stage
- prolapse of the cord in the second stage
- failure to advance in the second stage (see page 178).

*epi dural*

### The use of forceps

#### Face to pubes delivery with forceps

In certain cases it may be preferable to deliver the head with the occiput still posterior. This requires great judgement and must be carried out with even greater care.

Potential indications are as follows:

- the head is directly occipito posterior (OP) and deeply engaged
- the pelvis has a narrow transverse diameter, inhibiting rotation but still allowing delivery safely.

#### Forceps to the after-coming head (ACH) in a breech delivery

This is the method of choice for delivery of the ACH because of the degree of control the operator can exercise. Sudden delivery of the head may be associated with intracranial trauma.

#### Forceps in the delivery of low birth weight infants (< 2500 g)

The use of forceps in pre-term delivery and for other low birth weight (LBW) infants is based on the false premise that the forceps protect against intraventricular haemorrhage. However, this is not caused by trauma but is related to prolonged hypoxia particularly in RDS. Lift-out forceps neither protects against nor induces birth trauma in LBW infants. Their use is therefore optional. Rotational forceps are more dangerous for LBW infants and they must be used judiciously if at all.

## 11.0 Labour

### 11.19 Instrumental delivery and caesarean section

**Trial of forceps**

In an important sense each forceps delivery is a trial of forceps. This term, however, is confined to those situations in which it is likely, but not entirely certain, that vaginal delivery by forceps will be successful. If it is likely that forceps delivery will not be successful, it must not even be attempted. The patient should be delivered by caesarean section. A trial of forceps must be carried out by an experienced obstetrician in a theatre fully prepared for immediate caesarean section.

**The use of the ventouse**

The patient's expulsive efforts are used to assist delivery. The fetal head must be at least at the level of the spines. Vaginal delivery is said to be feasible from a cervical dilatation of 5 cm but this is not generally recommended. The instrument is most useful in the delivery of women with cardiac disease (the legs do not need to be placed in the lithotomy position) and for a second twin (if it is cephalic).

The largest possible of the 4 cups should be used. A vacuum of $-0.2$ kg/cm$^2$ is applied initially and, after checking that no cervix or vagina is caught within the cup, the vacuum is increased by $-0.2$ kg/cm$^2$ every two minutes to $-0.8$ kg/cm$^2$.

If delivery is not imminent after pulling on the ventouse during three contractions the attempt must cease and the patient be delivered by caesarean section.

**Caesarean section**

This procedure must not be carried out without good reason. Although it is a relatively safe operation under modern conditions there were 80 and 87 maternal deaths following caesarean section in England and Wales in the years 1976–78, and 1979–81 respectively. These represent a mortality rate of 0.7 and 0.5 respectively per 1000 caesarean sections during these years. The operation also has a significant effect on the remainder of the woman's obstetric career.

## 11.0 Labour

### 11.19 Instrumental delivery and caesarean section

**Table 11.7.** Causes of death after caesarean section in England and Wales 1976–78 and 1979–81 (number and percentage).

| Immediate cause of direct death | 1976–78 | 1979–81 |
|---|---|---|
| Haemorrhage | 8 (10) | 7 (8.0) |
| Pulmonary embolism | 9 (11.2) | 7 (8.0) |
| Sepsis and paralytic ileus | 8 (10.0) | 4 (4.6) |
| Hypertensive diseases of pregnancy | 12 (15.0) | 13 (14.9) |
| Anaesthesia | 18 (22.5) | 19 (21.8) |
| Other direct causes | 6 (7.5) | 9 (10.3) |
| Associated diseases | 19 (23.8) | 28 (32.2) |
| Total | 80 | 87 |

Indications and techniques will not be discussed in detail here. They can be found elsewhere and are, of course, best learned by experience. The transperitoneal lower segment caesarean section (LSCS) quite properly accounts for virtually all of the sections in modern practice.

### Potential indications for a classical upper segment caesarean section

- when the membranes have ruptured and liquor has drained away with the fetus trapped in a transverse lie
- in some cases of anterior placenta praevia when the lower segment is excessively vascular. A LSCS is, however, usually possible
- when a structural abnormality or space-occupying lesion (e.g. a fibroid) makes the lower segment approach impossible
- if hysterectomy is scheduled at the same time
- when the patient is already dead or moribund and rapid delivery of the baby is vital

## 11.0 Labour

### 11.19 Instrumental delivery and caesarean section

- a modern variant of the operation using a vertical incision starting in the lower segment but extending into the upper segment may be necessary if caesarean section is being performed at or before 28 weeks gestation. This is because the low segment is narrow and has not yet formed properly. Under these circumstances the transverse lower segment incision carries a greater risk of extension into the uterine vessels towards the ureters.

Most maternity units should be able to offer epidural anaesthesia for elective caesarean sections for those women who wish it and in whom it is not contra-indicated (see page 186).

Among the advantages of epidural anaesthesia are:
- the mother is awake and sees the child at delivery
- the father can usually be there also and they can both hold the baby
- consciousness is not impaired during the immediate recovery phase
- there are fewer post-operative problems (e.g. coughing, pyrexia, vomiting) and less pain than after GA
- breast feeding and mobilization can start early.

Among the disadvantages are:
- the procedure takes longer
- sometimes anaesthesia is not complete. (The patient should be fully prepared for GA should that become necessary.)

### Delivery in subsequent pregnancies

Caesarean section will be necessary in subsequent pregnancies if the cause is recurrent (e.g. CPD) or if the mother has already been delivered by this route on two or more occasions. After a first caesarean section puerperal X-ray pelvimetry is helpful in decisions regarding future management. In any case in which subsequent vaginal delivery is contemplated the normality of the pelvis must be beyond question.

Oxytocin must be used judiciously and under careful super-

## 11.0 Labour

11.20 Intrapartum fetal monitoring

vision in labours following previous delivery by caesarean section. The use of epidural anaesthesia has been discussed in Chapter 11.8.

After successful vaginal delivery and if an epidural block is in place a digital examination of the lower segment should be carried out to ascertain the integrity of the old scar.

### 11.20 Intrapartum fetal monitoring

The purpose of intrapartum monitoring is to act as a screening test for fetal hypoxia. The effect of hypoxia on the fetus depends on its reserves of glycogen. Thus, a growth retarded fetus will be affected earlier and to a greater degree than a well nourished fetus. Hypoxia may be reversible (e.g. due to maternal hypotension or uterine overactivity) or irreversible (e.g. due to placental insufficiency or occlusion of the umbilical cord).

#### Effects of hypoxia

Anaerobic glycolysis produces an accumulation of lactate. The fetus therefore develops a metabolic acidosis. The fetal $P_{CO_2}$ rises causing a respiratory acidosis. The blood pH drops due to both effects. There may in addition, be effects on the fetal heart rate (FHR).

The main sign is the onset of decelerations. The traditional diagnosis of 'fetal distress' depended predominantly on simply observable FHR changes. In fact, the term 'fetal distress' is misleading and unhelpful. Half of all babies delivered by forceps or caesarean section because of 'fetal distress' are not hypoxic; and half of the most hypoxic babies do not exhibit 'fetal distress'.

#### Methods of intra-partum monitoring

Because hypoxia can produce changes in FHR and pH the measurement of these remains the basis of modern intra-partum monitoring.

## 11.0 Labour

11.20 Intrapartum fetal monitoring

### 1. Intermittent recording of FHR using a fetal stethoscope

The best technique for this is described on page 174. It should only be applied to low risk patients with no obstetric abnormalities. More intensive monitoring as described below should be started if the FHR is over 160 bpm, under 120 bpm, decelerates during or after a contraction, or becomes irregular. The appearance of meconium in the liquor also indicates the necessity for continuous FHR monitoring.

### 2. Continuous recording of the FHR

The signal used to trigger the monitor should, whenever possible, be the fetal EGC obtained from an electrode on the fetal scalp or buttock. The alternatives are an ultrasound transducer or occasionally a microphone, placed on the maternal abdomen.

The fetal heart monitor measures the interval between paired beats, converts it into 'beats/minute' (bpm) and registers this on the chart recorder.

Uterine activity is usually assessed by a strain gauge transducer strapped to the maternal abdomen over the fundus of the uterus in the midline. When necessary actual uterine pressure can be recorded more accurately by an intra-uterine pressure catheter.

The combined print-out of continuous FHR and uterine activity is known as a **cardiotocograph** (CTG).

Continuous recording of the FHR is a screening technique which facilitates the detection of fetal hypoxic stress. It is not, of itself, diagnostic. Even when the most ominous fetal heart pattern is present (see below) only 50% of the babies have a low Apgar score (see page 257) at birth. Continuous FHR recording must therefore be backed up by measurement of fetal scalp pH. This has been clearly stated for over 10 years. Despite this the number of units where this policy is followed is small. This is one of the contributory factors in the unacceptably high (and rising) caesarean section rate.

## 11.0 Labour

### 11.20 Intrapartum fetal monitoring

*Indications for continuous FHR monitoring in labour*
There is no clear indication that it is beneficial to continuously monitor the FHR in all women during labour.

The following gives a guide to those 'high-risk' categories in which continuous FHR monitoring during labour is clearly indicated:

*Antepartum problems*
- Primigravidae over 30 years of age
- grande multiparity
- multigravidae aged 40 or more
- suspected IUGR
- pre-eclampsia
- history of APH during this pregnancy
- bad obstetric history
- diabetes
- hypertension
- twins
- Rh iso-immunization
- oligohydramnios
- reduced fetal movements
- abnormal antenatal FHR tracing

*Intrapartum abnormalities*
- FHR > 160 or < 120 bpm
- meconium-stained liquor
- prolonged labour
- epidural anaesthesia
- augmentation of labour
- pre-term labour
- supine hypotension
- breech presentation

### Interpretation of FHR tracings in the first stage of labour
The whole clinical situation must be considered. Tracings should be marked with the patient's name, date and time of starting. Significant events e.g. vaginal examination, insertion of an epidural block or FBS should also be marked. It is useful for each unit to make its own collection of normal and abnormal tracings and display them on a board in the labour ward. The following is a guide to the characteristics of normal and abnormal traces and of the action which should be taken. There is no substitute for personal experience and it is not possible to indicate definitely the appropriate course of action from a particular FHR pattern (or even FBS) alone.

# 11.0 Labour

## 11.20 Intrapartum fetal monitoring

### 1. Normal pattern
- a rate between 120 and 160 bpm
- no significant change in rate during uterine contractions
- baseline irregularity (previously called beat-to-beat variability) of 5 or more bpm. Tracings obtained using an ultrasound transducer may show less baseline irregularity than those from a scalp clip. Traces obtained by ultrasound are, therefore, more difficult to interpret.

This suggests that the fetus is in good health. Nothing further is indicated.

### 2. Loss of baseline irregularity
- the FHR has a variability of less than 5 bpm
- loss of irregularity is the feature most commonly associated with fetal hypoxia
- the fetal pH should be determined if the pattern persists or if other adverse features (described below) are present
- maternal drug administration (e.g. pethidine) can affect baseline irregularity.

### 3. Baseline bradycardia
- FHR of less than 120 bpm.

This is an adverse feature only if it is accompanied by loss of baseline irregularity and/or decelerations (complicated bradycardia). Turn the patient on her side, give oxygen and determine the fetal pH.

### 4. Baseline tachyrardia
- FHR of 160 bpm or more
- the fetal pH should be determined if the tachycardia is persistent or accompanied by decelerations or loss of baseline irregularity.

### 5. Acceleration pattern
- an increase in FHR at the start of a contraction returning to

## 11.0 Labour

## 11.20 Intrapartum fetal monitoring

baseline during or at the end of the contraction.
This is evidence of a good fetal circulatory responsiveness and is normal.

### 6. Early deceleration (Type 1 dip)
- the deceleration begins with the onset of the contraction
- it returns to the baseline rate by the end of the contraction
- it is usually, but not necessarily, of low amplitude (< 40 bpm).

This pattern may be due to head compression but may be an early sign of cord compression or hypoxia due to placental insufficiency. If the pattern deteriorates into variable or late decelerations the fetal pH should be determined.

### 7. Variable deceleration
- the deceleration appears at a variable time during the contraction
- its shape is irregular with an amplitude of more than 50 bpm.

If it appears consistently with each contraction it is likely that fetal hypoxia is developing. The fetal pH should, therefore, be measured especially if it is accompanied by other adverse features or if the pattern persists after turning the patient on her side.

### 8. Late deceleration (Type 2 dip)
- a deceleration lowest point of which is past the peak of the contraction i.e. there is a lag time. The greater the lag time the more serious its significance: the most ominous pattern is of shallow late decelerations accompanied by loss of baseline irregularity and tachycardia. A fetal pH measurement is mandatory.

### Dip area
It has been suggested that the degree of fetal hypoxia correlates well with the cumulative amplitude and duration of decelerations. A dip area of more than 200 beats in any 20 minute

## 11.0 Labour

11.20 Intrapartum fetal monitoring
---

period suggests hypoxia and is an indication for fetal pH measurement.

### Normal uterine contractions (as displayed by the CTG)
- 3–4 contractions every 10 minutes
- a duration of up to 75 seconds ⎫
- baseline tone of 5–12 mmHg ⎬ measurement by intra-uterine catheter
- peak pressure between 30 and 60 mmHg ⎭

Maternal bearing down and respirations cause a multi-spike appearance of contractions during the second stage.

### FHR in the second stage of labour
Fetal heart rate patterns are complex in the second stage of labour. Brief profound decelerations are not uncommon but prolonged bradycardia must not be ignored.

### Fetal blood sampling
The indications for this procedure have been described above. The equipment required is shown below:
- pH meter
- cold light source (for the amnioscope)
- ethyl chloride spray
- antiseptic lotions and cream
- silicone jelly
- small magnet with iron 'fleas' to stir the sample.
  Sterile pre-packed tray:
- a range of amnioscopes
- long forceps to hold swabs
- a long-handled blade holder
- a 2 mm guarded disposable blade (Rocket) to fit the holder
- 2 pre-heparinized glass capillary tubes
- 2 rubber mouthpieces to fit the tubes
- cotton wool balls and dental swabs.

The pH meter should be kept running at all times. It must be

# 11.0 Labour

## 11.20 Intrapartum fetal monitoring

serviced and standardized regularly because the pH readings can drift causing errors during clinical use. It should be calibrated with standard buffers at pH 7.48 and 6.84 respectively each time. The machine is checked again using the buffer at pH 7.48. If the reading obtained is not within 0.05 pH units of the standard, the meter is unreliable and should be serviced before being used.

Samples are obtained from the fetal scalp (or buttocks in a breech presentation). The procedure is not difficult but practice is necessary for the consistent collection of good samples.

### Technique
The technique is as follows:
- explain to the mother what is happening and why
- the operator should wear sterile gown and gloves
- place the patient in the left lateral position and wash and drape her routinely. (If the lithotomy position is used the patient should be tilted 10–15° to one side to prevent caval obstruction by the uterus)
- assess cervical dilatation and the level of the presenting part in the pelvis. An FBS should be obtainable if the cervical dilatation is $\geq 3$ cm
- use the shortest, widest amnioscope which will pass through the cervix. Take care to totally exclude the cervix from view. Fit the light source to the amnioscope
- the fetal scalp (or buttock) is cleaned and dried and a smear of silicone jelly applied
- an assistant sprays the area on view with ethyl chloride for 10 seconds. The resultant hyperaemia facilitates collection of the sample
- stab the presenting part once with the guarded 2 mm blade
- collect a 15 cm column of blood by capillary action into one tube. If necessary facilitate collection by gentle suction using the mouthpiece. It is important to exclude air bubbles from the sample because they affect the validity of the readings obtained.

## 11.0 Labour

11.20 Intrapartum fetal monitoring

Fill the second capillary tube similarly if possible
- insert the iron 'fleas' into the samples and mix the heparin with the blood by moving them up and down the tube with the magnet
- an assistant takes the samples immediately to the previously prepared pH meter
- ensure that the fetal scalp has stopped bleeding before removing the amnioscope. Pressure from a dental swab for 2–3 minutes is usually effective.

**Table 11.8.** Interpretation of fetal scalp sample

| pH | Interpretation | Action |
|---|---|---|
| pH > 7.25 | normal | allow labour to proceed |
| pH 7.20–7.25 | borderline | repeat |
| pH < 7.20 | abnormal | deliver |

### Other methods of assessing fetal welfare in labour

#### 1. Fetal ECG patterns
This information is fed into the monitor whenever a scalp clip is used to pick up the signal. A computer is necessary to eliminate irrelevant electrical activity but modern electronics are making this easier. Depression of the ST segment is an index of hypoxia. This method is not generally available as yet.

#### 2. Measurement of lactate in fetal scalp sample
The upper limit of normal for lactate in the fetal scalp during labour is 3.0 mmol/l. Its measurement adds nothing more than the scalp pH in the diagnosis of fetal hypoxia.

### Significance of meconium staining in the liquor
Meconium is present in the liquor of about 15% of all deliveries at term and up to 40% when the pregnancy is past term. Its significance as an indicator of 'fetal distress' has been over-

## 11.0 Labour

### 11.20 Intrapartum fetal monitoring

emphasized. It is as likely to be due to normal fetal gastrointestinal ~~mortality~~ motility as hypoxia. Gross staining is more likely to be significant. Whatever the extent meconium staining indicates the necessity for continuous FHR monitoring and fetal scalp pH measurement.

Aspiration by the baby of liquor heavily stained with meconium causes a severe pneumonia which can prove fatal.

A paediatrician (or someone trained in neonatal resuscitation procedures) should be present at deliveries where meconium staining of the liquor is present or likely (i.e. when there is 'fetal distress'). The mouth and nasopharynx should be aspirated to remove all meconium after delivery of the head but, if possible, before complete expulsion of the child. If this is not possible the infant should be taken as quickly as possible to the resuscitation table set up in the same room for ease of access and immediate aspiration carried out under direct laryngoscopic vision. All of these babies should be intubated and meconium aspirated from the trachea and main bronchi.

**Management of fetal hypoxia**
Strenuous efforts have been made to treat intra-uterine hypoxia by maternal infusion of e.g. bicarbonate and glucose. The latter may be positively harmful and the former has no proven beneficial effect whatsoever.

The best management of fetal hypoxia is its early detection and the prompt, safe removal of the fetus from its hostile environment. When a baby is delivered by forceps or caesarean section because of 'fetal distress' a double clamped segment of umbilical cord should be taken so that the pH (and if possible other blood gases) can be checked. Fetal blood within the cord will maintain its pH for up to 30 minutes. This procedure is not only of value to the paediatrician but also helps to indicate if the decision to intervene was appropriate.

# 12.0 Obstetric emergencies

- 12.1 The obstetric Flying Squad, 227
- 12.2 Cord prolapse, 229
- 12.3 Impacted shoulders, 230
- 12.4 Eclampsia, 231
- 12.5 Coagulation defects, 234
- 12.6 Amniotic fluid embolism, 235
- 12.7 Gastric aspiration (Mendelson's syndrome), 236
- 12.8 Uterine rupture, 236
- 12.9 Broad ligament haematoma, 238
- 12.10 Utrine inversion, 238
- 12.11 Morbid adherence of the placenta, 239

## 12.0 Obstetric emergencies

### 12.1 The Obstetric Flying Squad

This is a mobile team comprising obstetrician, midwife and anaesthetist equipped to resuscitate the patient in her home before she is transferred to hospital. The GP should call the Flying Squad if a pregnant (or recently pregnant) woman requires urgent admission to hospital and needs, or is likely to need, resuscitation before or during transfer.

Among the main reasons for calling the Flying Squad are:

- antepartum haemorrhage
- postpartum haemorrhage
- retained placenta
- severe pre-eclampsia and eclampsia
- haemorrhage due to inevitable abortion
- ectopic pregnancy

Clear information about the procedure for calling the Flying Squad must be available to all GPs and community midwives.

If, in cases such as the above, services of the Flying Squad are not requested during the initial referring call to the hospital, they must be volunteered by the person receiving the call.

The constitution of, and the equipment carried by, the Flying Squad will be determined by the area of its responsibility, the state of the roads and transport facilities. Ideally, an ambulance should transport the team to the patient's home and then return with the patient to the hospital. The use of local taxis or privately owned cars is not recommended. Medical and nursing staff must clarify with their Health Authority the situation regarding insurance cover during such duties. The table below gives some guide as to the drugs and equipment which might need to be carried. The final composition must be determined by local requirements.

## 12.0 Obstetric emergencies

### 12.1 The Obstetric Flying Squad

**Equipment of Obstetric Flying Squad**

- portable anaesthetic machine

- laryngoscope
- endotracheal tubes
- airways
- portable suction apparatus

- selection of i.v. cannulae
- intravenous fluid and blood-giving sets
- selection of syringes (2–30 ml) and an insulin syringe
- selection of venepuncture needles
- spirit-impregnated 'Mediswabs'

- set of delivery instruments in a bowl
- pelvic examination pack
- sterile gowns, hand towels, drapes and gloves
- plastic cord clamps
- variety of sterile dressings and swabs

- bottles for blood samples (serum and plasma)
- adhesive dressings
- plastic bags for placenta and rubbish
- scissors
- sticky labels for specimens
- paper and pen

- sphygmomanometer
- stethoscope
- fetal stethoscope
- thermometer
- torch
- portable drip stand
- bottle holders
- arm splint
- mouth wedge
- urinary catheter and drainage bags

- 2 units Group O Rh D-negative screened blood
- dextrose 5%—500 ml
- normal saline—500 ml
- Hartmann's solution (or equivalent) 500 ml×2
- plasma 500 ml×2
- pethidine 100 mg 2 ampules
- morphine 15 mg 2 ampoules
- Syntometrine×2 ampoules
- ergometrine 0.5 mg 2 ampoules
- hydrocortisone
- diazepam
- frusemide
- aminophylline
- digoxin
- promazine
- adrenalin
- insulin
- thiopentone
- water for injection

- neonatal resuscitation equipment
- mucus extractors (2)
- incubator readily available

## 12.0 Obstetric emergencies

### 12.2 Cord prolapse

In general, the team should confine operative intervention to such things as manual removal of the retained placenta. The woman should not be moved until her SBP is at least 100 mmHg (unless bleeding is uncontrollable e.g. ectopic pregnancy).

The following is a practical guide to the steps to be taken on arrival at the patient's home:
- the senior member of the team takes charge and quickly reviews the whole scene
- check vital signs
- ensure airway patency
- set up intravenous line and take blood for cross match
- take appropriate action to arrest any haemorrhage
- give relevant medication, e.g. oxygen, morphine
- check health of infant
- check uterine fundus and note whether placenta is retained or not
- if it is retained prepare to remove it
- if it is delivered check its completeness.

The situation should now be coming under control and arrangements should be made for whatever further action is appropriate (e.g. transfer to hospital).

### 12.2 Cord prolapse

Cord presentation discovered before rupture of membranes is an indication for immediate caesarean section. The risk is that the prolapsing cord will become compressed and occluded. Handling of the cord may also cause it to go into spasm. If the cord has prolapsed emergency measures attempt to keep the presenting part from occluding it.

Depending on the circumstances the following can be tried (all together if required):
- displace the presenting part with the examining hand
- if possible drop the head end of the bed or stretcher
- fill the bladder with 500–750 ml of normal saline using a size 16 Foley catheter which is clamped and kept in place

## 12.0 Obstetric emergencies

### 12.3 Impacted shoulders

- if all but the first are impossible (e.g. if she is at home) get the patient into the knee-elbow position
- try to keep the cord within the vagina
- if the cervix is fully dilated delivery should be effected by forceps (cephalic presentation) or breech extraction (breech presentation) if the presenting part is low enough in the pelvis. Otherwise, caesarean section is indicated
- if the cervix is not fully dilated and the baby is still alive carry out an immediate caesarean section: in a well-organized unit it should be possible to deliver the baby within 15 minutes of the prolapse being noted.

### 12.3 Impacted shoulders

This complication, which can be a nightmare, is associated with large and often postmature babies.

**Procedure**

Place patient in lithotomy position with pillow under her buttocks which should be over the edge of the bed. A large episiotomy is vital. Draw the head backwards (trying not to damage the brachial plexus) while an assistant provides firm, suprapubic pressure. Try to digitally rotate the anterior shoulder under the symphisis.

Experience with symphisiotomy may allow it to be used at this point (N.B.: Previous experience is vital). If this is not possible general anaesthesia is now required. Further attempts must be made to deliver the anterior shoulder. It may be possible to rotate the shoulders so that the original posterior shoulder, now anterior, can be delivered. Failure at this stage means that the baby's chances are very poor and it may already be dead. Cleidotomy (division of the clavicle with strong scissors) will allow delivery of the dead child.

## 12.0 Obstetric emergencies

12.4 Eclampsia

### 12.4 Eclampsia

The maternal death rate due to eclampsia has not improved over the last 10 years and 6–7 women die each year in England and Wales of this complication. The perinatal mortality rate is approximately 15%. The clinician is taken by surprise far too often because its onset is insidious and should be pre-empted.

The **symptoms and signs** of impending eclampsia are as follows:

- unusual headache—Persistent, severe, generalized (but may be occipital or frontal)
- visual disturbance e.g. blurring, flashes or spots, photophobia
- restlessness, agitation
- epigastric pain, nausea and vomiting
- sudden severe hypertension and proteinuria
- fluid retention with reduced urine output
- hyper-reflexia and ankle clonus
- retinal oedema, haemorhages and even papilloedema.

Women of non-Caucasian origin tend to develop eclampsia at lower blood pressures and are at increased risk of death from complications of hypertensive diseases of pregnancy.

The four priorities in eclampsia (actual or impending) are:

- prevention or control of convulsions
- control of the hypertension
- maintenance of maternal fluid and acid-base balance
- delivery of the infant.

### Control and prevention of convulsions

The methods still used most commonly in the UK are either intravenous diazepam or chlormethiazole. Intramuscular diazepam has no anti-convulsant action and is therefore of no value in this context. The regimen for **diazepam** is to give 10 mg i.v. as a bolus injection then 40 mg in 500 ml dextrose 5% at 60 dpm until the fits are controlled and/or the patient is sleepy. Consciousness is not lost completely but the fetus is affected

## 12.0 Obstetric emergencies

### 12.4 Eclampsia

(sometimes seriously) by the drug at birth and for some time afterwards. This is the most serious drawback of this method because there is no antidote available to counteract the fetal effects.

The regimen for **chlormethiazole** is to give a 0.8% solution i.v. at 60 dpm until the fits are controlled and/or the patient is sleepy. This drug does not depress the mother's cough reflex or respiratory centres, but it is not such an effective anticonvulsant as diazepam or phenytoin.

**Phenytoin sodium** is effective in the management of the generalized tonic-clonic seizures of epilepsy and has no sedative action on the central nervous system. It should therefore be eminently suitable in the treatment or prevention of eclampsia. 500 mg parenteral phenytoin sodium is diluted in 200 ml 0.9% saline (*not* 5% dextrose to avoid crystallization). This is infused intravenously over 1–2 hours and can be repeated for another 1 or 2 doses as is clinically indicated. Too rapid an infusion (> 50 mg/min) may produce bradycardia, arrhythmias and hypotension. Once made up the solution must be used within 6 hours otherwise it will crystallize. The intramuscular route is not suitable. The drug can be continued orally after delivery as a single or 2 divided doses of 150–300 mg per day.

Intravenous and intramuscular **magnesium sulphate** has retained its popularity in the USA. It controls convulsions and reduces blood pressure to some extent but in reducing neuromuscular irritability it causes cerebral depression. The margin of safety is not large. Respiratory depression can be reversed by calcium gluconate 10 ml of a 10% solution i.v. The regimen for magnesium sulphate is to inject 4 g i.v. (20 ml of a 20% solution) over 5 minutes. This is followed immediately by 5 g i.m. (10 ml of a 50% solution) deeply into each buttock. Thereafter 5 g is given i.m. into alternate buttocks 4 hourly as long as knee jerks are present, respirations are more than 6 per minute and at least 100 ml of urine has been excreted since last dose. Treatment is continued until 24 hours after delivery.

## 12.0 Obstetric emergencies

## 12.4 Eclampsia

*Status eclampticus* is best treated by curarization and intermittent positive pressure ventilation.

### Control of hypertension
Severe hypertension requires treatment whether eclampsia is impending or not to reduce the risk of cerebral haemorrhage. This is discussed fully on page 000 but, in general, hypotensive drugs are indicated when the SBP is $\geq$ 170 mmHg or the DBP $\geq$ 110 mmHg hydralazine 10 mg i.m. can be given but the maximum effect may not be achieved for up to 40 minutes. The dose can be repeated if the blood pressure is not controlled within that time. Alternatively hydralazine or labetalol can be given intravenously as follows:

**Table 12.1.**

|  | Hydralazine | Labetalol |
| --- | --- | --- |
| **Initial 'stat' dose:** | 5 mg | 10 mg |
| **Infusion** (using paediatric soluset with IVAC drip counter) | | |
| Dextrose 5% 100 ml plus | 50 mg (5 mg/ml) | 200 mg (2 mg/ml) |
| Commence at 10 dpm | 5 mg/hour | 20 mg/hour |
| Double the dose every 30 minutes until the BP is controlled* | | |
| **Maximum dose** 80 dpm | 40 mg/hour | 160 mg/hour |

*DBP 90–100 mmHg—maintain infusion rate
DBP 70–89 mmHg—halve infusion rate
DBP < 70 mmHg—stop infusion and recommence as necessary
N.B.: the side-effects of parenteral hydralazine (vomiting, headache, tremors) may mimic impending eclampsia.

### General management of the patient with eclampsia
Patency of the airway must be maintained and oxygen should be given as necessary. A urinary catheter should be inserted to monitor urine output. Disorders of electrolyte balance must be investigated and corrected. Any disseminated intravascular coagulation should be managed as described below.

## 12.0 Obstetric emergencies

12.5 Coagulation defects

### Obstetric management
Delivery by caesarean section is the method of choice but only when the eclampsia and hypertension are under control.

If eclampsia supervenes when the patient is well advanced in labour vaginal delivery may be possible but this decision must be made by a consultant obstetrician. FHR monitoring is obligatory in these circumstances.

### 12.5 Coagulation defects
The main causes of coagulation defects in pregnancy are:
- placental abruption
- retention of a dead fetus (see page 163)
- amniotic fluid embolism (see page 235)
- endotoxic shock.

The principles of management of hypovolaemic or endotoxic shock should be familiar to all medical practitioners and are dealt with elsewhere (see suggested further reading).

### Diagnosis
- the patient may be bleeding heavily and the blood fails to clot properly
- **clot observation test**

Take a 5 ml sample of blood into a round bottomed 10 ml glass tube. Note the time taken and keep the blood sample in a pocket. Observe each minute for clot formation. It should clot within 5–6 minutes and remain stable for a further 30 minutes. Failure to clot strongly suggests a significant coagulation defect

- the platelet count will be markedly reduced
- these crises may occur suddenly and at inopportune moments. Complex clotting investigations are therefore hardly ever of practical value even if they are available. A haematologist should, however, be consulted wherever possible.

### Management
- the coagulation defect is usually self-limiting if the stimulus producing it is removed

## 12.0 Obstetric emergencies

### 12.6 Amniotic fluid embolism

- therefore in placental abruption and IUD THE UTERUS SHOULD BE EMPTIED AS QUICKLY AS POSSIBLE
- for basic management of placental abruption see Chapter 10.2
- the transfusion of fresh blood is ideal. If this is not available transfuse as much fresh blood as possible alternating with fresh frozen plasma (FFP) and, if possible, platelets; 1 litre of whole blood or FFP contains 3 g of fibrinogen
- for every 5 units of citrated bank blood transfused, 10 ml of calcium gluconate should be given to counteract the anticoagulant effect of the citrate
- heparin should only be given in these circumstances after specific instructions and guidance from a haematologist
- excessive fibrinolysis is virtually never the main problem and fibrinolytic drugs are not necessary (except when specifically indicated and under expert guidance as above).
- avoid plasma expanders, e.g. dextran which reduce platelet aggregation and dilute remaining clotting factors.

This plan has been simplified greatly but contains the principles which may be life-saving in what can be a frightening and complex clinical situation.

### 12.6 Amniotic fluid embolism

This produces profound shock, cyanosis, dyspnoea and a severe coagulation defect. It is still a significant cause of maternal death in labour or postpartum. Amniotic fluid embolism is proportionately more common in induced labour. Precipitate labour, hypertonic uterine action, injudicious use of oxytocin and uterine rupture are frequent antecedent factors.

#### Management
The first objective is to prevent immediate death from pulmonary vascular obstruction
- oxygen must be given, initially by mask
- endotracheal intubation and ventilation may be necessary so call an anaesthetist urgently

## 12.0 Obstetric emergencies

12.7 Gastric aspiration (Mendelson's syndrome)

- inject hydrocortisone 1000 ml 1–2 hourly i.v.
- give heparin 5000 units i.v. to reduce intravascular coagulation in the pulmonary vessels.

### 12.7 Gastric aspiration (Mendelson's) syndrome
This is due to the deep inhalation of liquid, acid and irritant gastric contents during general anaesthesia. It accounts for half of the obstetric anaesthetic deaths. Those practising obstetric anaesthesia must be skilled in its prevention, recognition and treatment. Steps to prevent it are discussed on page 210.

### Clinical presentation
Cyanosis, tachycardia, bronchospasm, pulmonary oedema, and deepening shock in relation to general anaesthesia. It may be confused with pulmonary oedema secondary to mitral stenosis, cardiac failure or amniotic fluid embolism.

### Management
- tilt the patient head down
- turn her on one side and aspirate the pharynx
- give oxygen
- inject aminophylline 250 mg and hydrocortisone 1000 mg i.v. and repeat as necessary
- suck bronchial tree clear through a bronchoscope (under GA)
- prescribe broad-spectrum antibiotics

### 12.8 Uterine rupture
This caused 14 maternal deaths in England and Wales in 1976–78 but only 4 in 1979–81. The commonest antenatal cause is a previous caesarean section scar, often classical. Instrumental delivery, intrauterine manipulation, the inappropriate use of oxytocin to augment labour (e.g. in multiparous women or obstructed labour) and previous cervical surgery are among the other causative factors. Avoidable factors are present in most cases.

## 12.0 Obstetric emergencies

### 12.8 Uterine rupture

**Signs and symptoms**
- severe bursting pain (which will even break through an epidural block). However the patient may only complain of some lower abdominal discomfort
- unexplained tachycardia
- variable amount of vaginal bleeding (sometimes catastrophic)
- fainting and ensuing shock
- cessation of contractions
- disappearance of the presenting part from the pelvis
- profound fetal bradycardia.

The possibility of an unrecognized rupture must be considered when, for example:
- bleeding continues after delivery despite a well-retracted uterus
- when a cervical laceration has been noted and sutured but haemorrhage persists and the patient is becoming shocked
- there is unexplained shock.

All of these are more relevant if she has had an instrumental delivery or previous caesarean section.

**Management**
- cross-match 6 units of blood and begin transfusion with Group O Rh negative, screened blood
- carry out the least extensive surgery compatible with the patient's immediate health and future welfare. The choice between repair of the uterus and total or sub-total hysterectomy must be taken by a consultant obstetrician
- take great care to identify the ureters and exclude them from any sutures
- prescribe broad spectrum antibiotics.

**Future pregnancies**
Sterilization should be discussed with the patient. If she decides against it close observation is required during any future preg-

## 12.0 Obstetric emergencies

12.9 Broad ligament haematoma

---

nancy and delivery should be by elective caesarean section at 38 weeks.

### 12.9 Broad ligament haematoma

This presence of a broad ligament haematoma must be suspected in a recently delivered woman who has unexplained tachycardia and hypotension but no excessive vaginal bleeding.

As the haematoma enlarges it will cause pain and excessive tenderness on the affected side. The uterus will tend to be deviated to the opposite side. Action is often necessary on suspecion rather than certain diagnosis.

Decisions regarding the necessity for laparotomy should be taken by an experienced obstetrician. Maternal death is too common in this condition, usually due to failure to suspect the diagnosis and delays in proceeding to laparotomy.

### 12.10 Uterine inversion

This is fortunately a rare, but profoundly shocking complication of the third stage. It is often caused by injudicious cord traction with an atonic uterus and fundal insertion of the placenta. The inversion may not be complete and therefore not immediately visible. Diagnosis is by vaginal examination.

#### Management

Try immediately to reduce the inversion. Call assistance and get an intravenous line established. Initiate 'anti-shock' measures.

Removal of a still-attached placenta is only to be carried out by a very experienced obstetrician under general anaesthesia once any shock has been corrected.

The following hydrostatic method for reduction is usually effective:

- attach 1 or 2 litres of warm saline to cystoscopy tubing such as the Uromatic Y-type TVR administration set (Travenol)
- the inverted uterus is held within the vagina using the right

## 12.0 Obstetric emergencies

### 12.11 Morbid adherence of the placenta

hand which is also holding the free end of the tubing
- an assistant occludes the vagina using the labia to encircle the operator's hand
- two litres of warm saline are infused rapidly and the even hydrostatic pressure exerted usually reduces the inverted uterus.

### 12.11 Morbid adherence of the placenta
*(placenta accreta)*

This is fortunately a rare occurrence and its management is the province of a senior obstetrician. As much of the placenta as possible is removed and the uterus is packed. Transfusion will be necessary. Severe degrees of *placenta accreta* will require hysterectomy.

# 13.0 Perinatal and infant mortality

**13.1 Perinatal and infant mortality, 243**

## 13.0 Perinatal and infant mortality

### 13.1 Perinatal and infant mortality

**Definitions**

**Stillbirths** late fetal deaths: after 28 completed weeks of gestation.

**Perinatal deaths** stillbirths and deaths in the first week of life.

**Neonatal deaths** deaths in the first 28 days of life.

**Postneonatal deaths** deaths at ages over 28 days and under 1 year.

**Infant deaths** deaths at ages under 1 year.

Stillbirths and perinatal deaths are recorded per 1000 live and stillbirths, the other categories are recorded per 1000 live births.

**Live birth**—the WHO definition of live birth is "the complete expulsion or extraction from its mother of a product of conception, irrespective of the duration of the pregnancy, which, after such separation, breathes or shows any other evidence of life, such as beating of the heart, pulsation of the umbilical cord or definite movement of voluntary muscles".

This takes no account of the important practical problem of fetal viability. As yet there is no record of any infant surviving if born before 25 weeks *and* weighing under 500 g. Some survivors have been reported at 23 weeks but only when the birthweight was over 500 g.

The 28 weeks lower limit used in the UK is in urgent need of revision because up to 50% of infants liveborn before 28 weeks survive. Some countries include in their perinatal mortality figures births from 20 or 22 weeks and deaths up to 28 days after birth.

National perinatal mortality statistics should include infants with birthweight $> 500$ g. If birthweight is not available the gestational age should be at least 22 completed weeks or the crown-heel length at least 25 cm.

Table 13.1 shows the dramatic fall in the PMR in England and Wales in the last 50 years.

## 13.0 Perinatal and infant mortality

13.1 Perinatal and infant mortality

**Table 13.1.**

| Period | PMR | Period | PMR |
|---|---|---|---|
| • 1931–5 | 62.5 | • 1971–5 | 21.0 |
| • 1941–5 | 48.6 | • 1976–8 | 16.7 |
| • 1951–5 | 37.6 | • 1981 | 11.8 |
| • 1961–5 | 29.4 | • 1982 | 11.3 |
|  |  | • 1983 | 10.4 |

These overall or 'crude' rates are not good indicators of the standard of perinatal care and should not be used to provide league tables of 'good' or 'bad' hospitals, districts or regions. If the success or failure of health care provision is to be compared between regions in the same country, or between nations, the data need to be broken down into birthweight and casual groups so that like can be compared with like.

Different countries and different parts of the same country have varying birthweight distributions, proportions of multiple births, and incidences of congenital malformations which invalidate comparisons of crude mortality rates. International comparisons are further confounded by differing definitions and methods of data collection. There are no national statistics available for perinatal morbidity or subsequent handicap, nor is there any agreed definition of handicap. The OPCS monitor (Ref VS and DH3—see suggested further reading) provides regular reviews of the statistics for England and Wales.

### Causes of death

Table 13.2 gives details of perinatal, neonatal, and infant mortality for England and Wales in 1981. It is derived from OPCS DH3 84/3.

This tabulation follows the recommendations of the ninth revision of the International Classification of Diseases (ICD). It is far from ideal from the perinatal point of view because it does not specifically address some of our main clinical problems e.g.

## 13.0 Perinatal and infant mortality

### 13.1 Perinatal and infant mortality

**Table 13.2.** Mortality rates.

|  | Perinatal | Neonatal | Infant |
|---|---|---|---|
| All causes | 11.8 | 6.6 | 10.9 |
| Infections and parasitic diseases | 0.0 | 0.0 | 0.2 |
| Diseases of respiratory system | 0.1 | 0.2 | 1.0 |
| Congenital anomalies | 2.5 | 2.1 | 2.1 |
| Anencephalus and similar anomalies | 0.5 | 0.1 | 0.1 |
| Spina bifida | 0.3 | 0.3 | 0.5 |
| Other CNS anomalies | 0.3 | 0.1 | 1.0 |
| Cardiac anomalies | 0.4 | 0.6 | — |
| Conditions originating in perinatal period | 9.1 | 3.9 | 4.1 |
| Maternal conditions | 1.1 | 0.2 | — |
| Complications of placenta, cord or membranes | 2.9 | 0.1 | — |
| Other complications of labour and delivery | 0.2 | 0.1 | — |
| Immaturity and unspecified low birth weight | 0.7 | 0.7 | — |
| Birth trauma | 0.2 | 0.2 | — |
| Intrauterine hypoxia and birth asphyxia | 1.0 | 0.4 | — |
| Respiratory distress syndrome | 0.9 | 1.0 | — |
| Other respiratory conditions of fetus and newborn | 0.5 | 0.5 | — |
| Infections specific to perinatal period | 0.1 | 0.1 | — |
| Fetal and neonatal haemorrhage | 0.2 | 0.0 | — |
| Haemolytic disease | 0.1 | 0.0 | — |
| Sudden infant death syndrome (cause unknown) | — | — | 1.6 |
| External causes of injury and poisoning | 0.0 | 0.0 | 0.3 |

unexplained intrauterine or neonatal death. The first priority is to gather data to help us to understand why 60% of our perinatal mortality occurs among normal infants of over 1000 g birthweight.

### Cause of perinatal mortality (and morbidity)

The following alternative classification has been suggested by Professor Whitfield, Queen Mother's Hospital, Glasgow:

## 13.0 Perinatal and infant mortality

13.1 Perinatal and infant mortality

Spontaneous pre-term delivery
IUGR
Unexplained IUD
Unexplained NND
Intra-partum asphyxia (specify cord accident or breech presentation)
Trauma
Hypertension (specify pre-eclampsia)
APH—placental abruption; placenta praevia; other
Maternal disease (excluding hypertension)
Fetal malformation—detectable; not detectable
Haemolytic disease
Infection
Other

Data collected in this manner would be of much greater value as an audit of perinatal care.

### Factors influencing perinatal and infant mortality

#### 1. Birthweight
Although infants of birthweight < 2500 g comprised only 6.6% of all births in 1981, 48% of all stillbirths and infant deaths occurred within this group.

Almost half of all births of infants weighing < 1500 g resulted in stillbirth or infant death. Above 1500 g mortality rates fall dramatically with increasing birthweight, reaching their lowest between 3500 and 3999 g. Rates rise again slightly among infants > 4000 g.

#### 2. Social class and legitimacy
Table 13.3 shows that perinatal and infant mortality rise as social class falls and are higher among illegitimate births. The figures are for England and Wales in 1981.

**Table 13.2.** Mortality and live births (assessed from a 10% sample) for England and Wales 1981 (from OPCS DH3 84/3).

| | All weights | Under 2,500 | Under 1,500 | 1,500– 1,999 | 2,000– 2,499 | 2,500– 2,999 | 3,000– 3,499 | 3,500– 3,999 | 4,000 and over | Not stated |
|---|---|---|---|---|---|---|---|---|---|---|
| **Numbers** | | | | | | | | | | |
| Stillbirths | 4,207 | 2,497 | 1,250 | 657 | 590 | 559 | 432 | 216 | 122 | 381 |
| Perinatal | 7,521 | 4,435 | 2,521 | 997 | 917 | 867 | 721 | 391 | 198 | 909 |
| Neonatal | 4,176 | 2,294 | 1,477 | 413 | 404 | 476 | 452 | 262 | 107 | 585 |
| Postneonatal | 2,709 | 556 | 156 | 129 | 271 | 619 | 770 | 511 | 121 | 132 |
| Infant | 6,885 | 2,850 | 1,633 | 542 | 675 | 1,095 | 1,222 | 773 | 228 | 717 |
| Livebirths | 634,492 | 39,549 | 4,724 | 7,477 | 27,348 | 114,753 | 236,191 | 164,578 | 50,609 | 28,812 |
| **Rates** | | | | | | | | | | |
| Stillbirths | 6.6 | 59.4 | 209.2 | 80.8 | 21.1 | 4.8 | 1.8 | 1.3 | 2.4 | 13.1 |
| Perinatal | 11.8 | 105.5 | 422.0 | 122.6 | 32.8 | 7.5 | 3.0 | 2.4 | 3.9 | 31.1 |
| Neonatal | 6.6 | 58.0 | 312.7 | 55.2 | 14.8 | 4.1 | 1.9 | 1.6 | 2.1 | 20.3 |
| Postneonatal | 4.3 | 14.1 | 33.0 | 17.3 | 9.9 | 5.4 | 3.3 | 3.1 | 2.4 | 4.6 |
| Infant | 10.9 | 72.1 | 345.7 | 72.5 | 24.7 | 9.5 | 5.2 | 4.7 | 4.5 | 24.9 |

## 13.0 Perinatal and infant mortality

13.1 Perinatal and infant mortality

**Table 13.3.**

| Social class | | PMR | Infant mortality |
|---|---|---|---|
| | All | 11.8 | 10.9 |
| | All legitimate | 11.3 | 10.2 |
| I | Professional occupations | 8.2 | 7.7 |
| II | Intermediate occupations (e.g. most managers and senior administrators) | 9.7 | 7.9 |
| IIIN | Skilled occupations (non-manual) | 9.8 | 8.5 |
| IIIM | Skilled occupations (manual) | 11.7 | 10.3 |
| IV | Partly-skilled occupations | 13.2 | 12.6 |
| V | Unskilled occupations or unemployed | 15.5 | 15.8 |
| | Illegitimate | 15.1 | 15.2 |

### 3. Maternal age and parity

The PMR is lowest between the ages of 25 and 29 years. It climbs steadily thereafter being increased three-fold by 40–44 years of age. Teenage mothers are also at greater risk.

The lowest death rate is associated with the second child. Mortality doubles to the fourth and fifth children and has trebled by the sixth and seventh. However, there is a social class effect here also because working class women account for proportionately more teenage mothers and highly parous older women than do middle class women. In addition, lethal congenital malformations are more common in older than younger women.

### 4. Multiple births

Mortality is higher in multiple than singleton births.

### 5. Smoking

It has been suggested that smoking adds between 3 and 8 deaths/1000 births to the PMR but this is difficult to verify because of the complex inter-relationship between smoking, social class and maternal age.

# 14.0 Maternal mortality

**14.0 Maternal mortality, 251**

## 14.0 Maternal mortality

### 14.0 Maternal mortality

The traditional definition of maternal mortality used in the UK is death of the mother occurring during pregnancy or labour, or as a consequence of pregnancy within one year of delivery or abortion. The International Federation of Gynecology and Obstetrics (FIGO) definition excludes deaths more than 42 days from delivery or abortion and it is this definition which is used in the data given below derived from the Confidential Enquiry 1979–81. Deaths are divided into those directly attributable to the pregnancy, indirect deaths resulting from a condition which preceded or developed during pregnancy the effect of which was not directly due to but was aggravated by the pregnancy, and unrelated or 'fortuitous' deaths.

Deaths are also related to the number of mothers delivered (*maternities*) rather than the number of births. The addition of legal terminations produces an estimate of *'conceptions'*. The further addition of hospital admissions for miscarriages and ectopic pregnancies produces an estimated figure for the total number of *pregnancies* (recognised to be an under-estimate).

Table 14.1 shows some statistics for maternal mortality for England and Wales between 1951 and 1981.

Tables 14.2 and 14.3 show the numbers and main causes of direct maternal deaths in England and Wales between 1970 and 1981.

**Table 14.1.** Some Statistics of Maternal Mortality and births 1951–1981 (England & Wales).

| Numbers of Maternal Deaths | 1951 | 1961 | 1971 | 1981 |
|---|---|---|---|---|
| Total | 686 | 345 | 168 | 57 |
| Abortions | 107 | 54 | 27 | 3 |
| Direct Obstetric Deaths | 419 | 220 | 106 | 43 |
| Indirect Obstetric Deaths | 160 | 71 | 35 | 11 |
| Maternal Mortality Rate per 100,000 total births | 98.9 | 41.7 | 21.1 | 8.9 |
| Total Births (Thousands) | 694 | 827 | 793 | 639 |

**Table 14.2.** Causes of direct maternal deaths. Numbers and percentages 1970–1981. (Late deaths excluded).

|  | 1970–1972 No (%) | 1973–1975 No (%) | 1976–1978 No (%) | 1979–1981 No (%) |
|---|---|---|---|---|
| Hypertensive diseases of pregnancy | 47 (13.8) | 39 (17.2) | 29 (13.4) | 36 (20.4) |
| Pulmonary embolism | 52 (15.3) | 33 (14.5) | 43 (19.8) | 23 (13.0) |
| Anaesthesia | 37 (10.9) | 22 (9.7) | 27 (12.4) | 22 (12.5) |
| Ectopic pregnancy (excluding anaesthetic deaths) | 34 (10.0) | 19 (8.4) | 21 (9.7) | 20 (11.4) |
| Amniotic fluid embolism | 16 (4.7) | 14 (6.1) | 11 (5.1) | 18 (10.2) |
| Haemorrhage | 27 (7.9) | 21 (9.3) | 24 (11.1) | 14 (8.0) |
| Abortion (excluding anaesthetic deaths) | 71 (20.9) | 27 (11.9) | 14 (6.4) | 14 (8.0) |
| Sepsis, excluding abortion | 30 (8.8) | 19 (8.4) | 15 (6.9) | 8 (4.6) |
| Ruptured uterus | 13 (3.8) | 11 (4.8) | 14 (6.4) | 4 (2.2) |
| Other direct causes | 13 (3.8) | 22 (9.7) | 19 (8.8) | 17 (9.7) |
| All deaths | 340 (100%) | 227 (100%) | 217 (100%) | 176 (100%) |

Table 14.3. Direct maternal deaths by cause, rates per million pregnancies 1970–81. (Late deaths excluded).

| | 1970–72 | 1973–75 | 1976–78 | 1979–81 |
|---|---|---|---|---|
| Hypertensive diseases of pregnancy | 17.2 | 16.5 | 12.7 | 14.7 |
| Pulmonary embolism | 19.0 | 13.9 | 18.9 | 9.4 |
| Anaesthesia including deaths associated with operations for abortion and ectopic pregnancy | 13.5 | 12.7 | 12.3 | 9.0 |
| Ectopic pregnancy | 12.4 | 8.9 | 9.2 | 8.2 |
| Amniotic fluid embolism | 5.8 | 6.3 | 4.8 | 7.4 |
| Haemorrhage | 9.9 | 8.9 | 10.5 | 5.7 |
| Abortion | 26.0 | 10.1 | 6.1 | 5.7 |
| Sepsis, excluding abortion | 11.0 | 8.0 | 6.6 | 3.3 |
| Ruptured uterus | 4.8 | 4.6 | 6.1 | 1.6 |
| Other direct causes | 4.8 | 5.9 | 7.9 | 7.0 |
| All deaths | 124.3 | 95.9 | 95.2 | 72.0 |

## 14.0 Maternal mortality

14.0 Maternal mortality

Although these results are better than for other triennia, substandard care still contributed to a significant proportion. For example, substandard care contributed to the majority of anaesthetic deaths, 12 of 14 deaths from haemorrhage, and 3 of 4 from ruptured uterus.

The death rate from Caesarean section fell but more women died following delivery by that method in 1979–81 (87) than in 1976–78 (80). Emergency Caesarean section carried a death rate of 80 per 100,000 compared to 20 per 100,000 for an elective procedure.

# 15.0 The neonate

**15.0 The neonate,** 257

**15.1 Apgar score,** 257

**15.2 Resuscitation,** 258

**15.3 Babies in need of 'special care',** 261

**15.4 Routine examination of the baby at birth,** 262

**15.5 Assessment of gestational age,** 263

**15.6 Routine discharge examination,** 269

**15.7 Some neonatal problems,** 270

**15.8 BCG vaccination,** 272

**15.9 Screening for PKU,** 273

**15.10 Screening for congenital hypothyroidism,** 273

**15.11 Detection of cystic fibrosis,** 274

## 15.0 The neonate

### 15.0 The neonate
Most babies are born in good condition and require nothing more than to be given to the mother.

### 15.1 Apgar score
A guide to the baby's condition at birth is given by the Apgar score, which is illustrated in Table 15.1 below and should be carried out at 1 and 5 minutes after birth.

**Table 15.1.**

| Sign | Score | | |
|---|---|---|---|
| | 0 | 1 | 2 |
| Heart rate | Absent | Slow below (100) | Over 100 |
| Respiratory effort | Absent | Slow; irregular | Good; crying |
| Muscle tone | Limp | Some flexion of extremities | Active motion |
| Response to catheter in nostril (tested after propharynx is clear) | No response | Grimace | Coughs or sneezes |
| Colour | Blue; pale | Body pink; extremities blue | Completely pink |

If a baby fails to take a breath within 1 minute of birth, active resuscitation may be required, but this will depend on events over the next 2 minutes. If after 3 minutes the baby is white rather than blue, has a slow ($< 80$ bpm) or falling heart rate, and is not breathing ASSISTED VENTILATION IS URGENTLY NECESSARY. An Apgar score which is falling or is under 7 at 5 minutes after birth also suggests some degree of birth asphyxia. If the baby is gasping, the lungs will usually be expanded and normal respiration initiated as long as the airway is clear.

## 15.0 The neonate

15.2 Resuscitation

### 15.2 Resuscitation
Midwives, obstetricians and anaesthetists as well as paediatricians should familiarize themselves with the resuscitation equipment. Personnel skilled in endotracheal intubation must be readily available at all times in all maternity units.

All staff involved with delivering labouring women whether in consultant or GP units, must become skilful in the practice of resuscitation by bag and mask. Errors in placement of an endotracheal tube due to lack of experience are dangerous. Intubation can, however, be practised on a specially designed plastic model or dead babies, progressing to actual resuscitation under supervision.

The priorities in resuscitation are
1 maintenance of body temperature
2 clearance of airways
3 establishment of ventilation (with or without administration of oxygen).

### Plan of action
**1** Measure time from delivery with a stop-clock.

**2** If the baby has not gasped by 1 minute after delivery aspirate mouth and nostrils gently with a mucus trap. Vigorous suction with a catheter in the nasopharynx causes reflex bradycardia and apnoea and is therefore harmful.

**3** If the apnoea continues but the baby's heart rate is over 80 bpm and stable or rising it is not unreasonable to await events. The first gasp may be expedited by flicking the baby's feet or by applying intermittent positive pressure ventilation (IPPV) by face mask. The mask must be held firmly over the baby's face and the chin must be elevated to lift up the tongue.

**4** If the baby's heart rate is less than 80 bpm and falling or if spontaneous gasping is not followed quickly by regular respiration commence bag and mask resuscitation immediately. If the operator is skilled in intubation this should be carried out. DO

## 15.0 The neonate

### 15.2 Resuscitation

NOT allow the baby to suffer prolonged hypoxia during attempts at resuscitation.

**5** Inspect the cords with a laryngoscope and aspirate secretions or meconium under direct vision.

**6** Intubate using an endotracheal tube (with a shoulder on it) attached to a Y-piece adaptor or a 15 mm connector.

**7** Attach one side limb of the Y-adaptor to oxygen flowing at 2 litres/minute or attach the 15 mm connector to the resuscitation bag. The pressure release valve should be set at 30–35 cm $H_2O$. The patent limb of the adaptor is occluded until the oxygen pressure reaches 20–25 cm $H_2O$. The thumb is then released for 2 seconds and this is repeated regularly and rhythmically at a rate of about 30 ventilations per minute.

Spontaneous respiration should be established for at least 5 minutes before the endotracheal tube is removed; and the baby's condition must be stable before he is moved from the delivery suite.

**Maintenance of the body temperature** is the single most important part of resuscitation. Cold stress increases oxygen consumption and thus significantly reduces the length of time for which apnoea can be tolerated without risk of neurological damage. Even if the baby's temperature is normal he or she may undergo significant cold stress if the skin remains wet or if there is no radiant heater. Delivery rooms should be at 24°C. Radiant heaters above resuscitation trolleys should be left switched on all the time. The neonate should be dabbed dry quickly. Wrapping the baby in a Silver Swaddler (Lewis Woolf Griptight Ltd. Birmingham) will prevent radiant heat loss but should not be used under a radiant heater. The baby's chest needs to remain accessible. If necessary the baby should be transferred to a pre-heated incubator as soon as his condition is stable.

Correction of acidosis will occur once the baby is warm and adequately ventilating. The infusion of hypertonic alkali solutions is no longer recommended during initial resuscitation.

## 15.0 The neonate

15.2 Resuscitation

It can be helpful to double clamp the umbilical cord at delivery in high risk cases using the short closed section to check umbilical vein and artery pH and blood gases.

Narcotic and respiratory depression is a real possibility if opiate analgesics have been given to the mother within 4 hours of delivery. Treatment is by naloxone 0.02 mg/kg body weight by deep i.m. injection. A further dose may be needed after 3–4 hours because of the short half-life of naloxone.

**Cardiac arrest**
Cardiac arrest requires prompt action comprising
- rapid intubation preceded by suction
- external cardiac massage
- IPPV with 100% oxygen
- intracardiac adrenalin (0.2 ml 1/10,000 solution).

**Indication for the presence of neonatal paediatrician (or equivalent) at delivery**
- all caesarean sections
- all instrumental deliveries
- pre-term delivery
- IUGR
- APH
- breech delivery
- polyhydramnios
- meconium staining of the liquor
- multiple pregnancy
- severe rhesus iso-immunization
- maternal history of diabetes, thrombocytopaenia, myasthenia, thyrotoxicosin, drug abuse
- known or suspected fetal anomaly
- suspected amnionitis.

If at all possible two members of the paediatric staff should attend multiple births or delivery $\leq$ 32 weeks.

## 15.0 The neonate

15.3 Babies in need of 'special care'

### 15.3 Babies in need of 'special care'

Babies should not be separated from their mothers without good cause and indiscriminate admission to special care units is to be discouraged. Most babies needing 'special care' can stay with their mothers on transitional care wards provided that adequate levels of trained staff (especially nurses) can be maintained.

The following babies are likely to require admission to the special care unit:
- after prolonged resuscitation
- birth weight less than 2000 g
- gestational age less than 36 weeks
- persisting respiratory problem
- some severe congenital anomalies
- all ill babies.

The mother and father should be given the opportunity to see and hold the baby before transfer if at all possible.

Among the groups of babies who, although requiring close observation, should normally be allowed to go with their mother (providing the listed precautions are observed) are:

**1. Intra-uterine growth retardation** (as long as birthweight is $\geq$ 2000 g)

#### Necessary observations
- check blood sugar level with a reagent strip (e.g. Dextrostix) within 2 hours of birth and repeated before 3-hourly feeds
- ensure early feeding—at 2 hours or earlier—of expressed breast milk. The baby may also be put to the breast.
- review at 24 hours. If the reagent strip reads 2 mmol/l or less after a feed inform the paediatrician
- measure plasma glucose and feed again. If it is less than 1 mmol/l transfer the baby to the special care unit for more frequent feeds and Dextrostix tests.

## 15.0 The neonate

15.4 Routine examination of the baby at birth

### 2. Babies born at 36–37 weeks gestation
- blood sugar levels should be measured within 2 hours of birth and before feeds for the first 24 hours
- temperature should be recorded 6-hourly
- the baby should be re-examined at 12 hours or earlier if necessary.

### 3. Febrile babies
After a review of maternal history (e.g. maternal pyrexia or antibiotic therapy) a full examination should be carried out. Babies who are otherwise well should have swabs taken and gastric aspirate microscopy carried out. Their temperature should be checked hourly for six hours. They should be transferred to the special care unit if symptoms arise, pyrexia persists beyond six hours, or if microscopy of the gastric aspirate shows > 10 white cells/high powered field and/or organisms on Grain staining.

### 15.4 Routine examination of the baby at birth
This should be carried out within two hours of delivery to answer the following questions:
1. Is the baby pre-term or small-for-dates?
2. Are cyanosis, anaemia or jaundice present?
3. Is there any evidence of birth trauma?
4. Are there any congenital malformations? e.g.
   - excessive salivation suggesting oesophageal atresia
   - respiratory difficulties raising the possibility of infection, aspiration or diaphragmatic hernia
   - cleft palate
   - exomphalos or abdominal tumours
   - imperforate anus
   - spina bifida
   - abnormal genitalia
   - single umbilical artery or single transverse palmar crease (pointing to less obvious but more serious anomalies)

## 15.0 The neonate

15.5 Assessment of gestational age

- Down's syndrome or other possible chromosomal abnormalities.

### 15.5 Assessment of gestational age

Gestational age can be assessed independently from knowledge of menstrual age by, for example, the Dubowitz scoring system (Fig. 21) which combines neurological with physical criteria of maturity. The total score is translated into an estimate of gestational age using the graph shown in Fig. 22. This helps greatly in the classification of low birthweight infants into preterm or growth-retarded categories.

#### Neurological criteria (notes)
(N.B.: If the score for an individual criterion differs on the two sides of the baby, take the mean.)

*Posture*
This is observed with infant quiet and in supine position. Score 0: Arms and legs extended; 1: beginning of flexion of hips and knees, arms extended; 2: stronger flexion of legs, arms extended; 3: arms slightly flexed, legs flexed and abducted; 4: full flexion of arms and legs.

*Square window*
The hand if flexed on the forearm between the thumb and index finger of the examiner. Enough pressure is applied to get as full a flexion as possible, and the angle between the hypothenar eminence and the ventral aspect of the forearm is measured and graded according to diagram. (Care is taken not to rotate the infant's wrist while doing this manoeuvre.)

*Ankle dorsiflexion*
The foot is dorsiflexed onto the anterior aspect of the leg, with the examiner's thumb on the sole of the foot and other fingers behind the leg. Enough pressure is applied to get as full flexion

**Table 15.2.** Dubowitz scoring: physical (external) criteria.

| External sign | Score 0 | 1 | 2 | 3 | 4 |
|---|---|---|---|---|---|
| Oedema | Obvious oedema hands and feet; pitting over tibia | No obvious oedema hands and feet; pitting over tibia | No oedema | | |
| Skin texture | Very thin, gelatinous | Thin and smooth | Smooth, medium thickness. Rash or superficial peeling | Slight thickening. Superficial cracking and peeling especially hands and feet | Thick and parchment-like; superficial or deep cracking |
| Skin colour (infant not crying) | Dark red | Uniformly pink | Pale pink; variable over body | Pale. Only pink over ears, lips, palms or soles | |

| | | | | | |
|---|---|---|---|---|---|
| Skin opacity (trunk) | Numerous veins venules clearly seen, especially over abdomen | Veins and tributaries seen | A few large vessels clearly seen over abdomen | A few large vessels seen indistinctly over abdomen | No blood vessels seen |
| Lanugo (over back) | No lanugo | Abundant; long and thick over whole back | Hair thinning especially over lower back | Small amount of lanugo and bald areas | At least half of back devoid of lanugo |
| Plantar creases | No skin creases | Faint red marks over anterior half of sole | Definite red marks over more than anterior half; indentations over less than anterior third | Indentations over more than anterior third | Definite deep indentations over more than anterior third |
| Nipple formation | Nipple barely visible; no areola | Nipple well defined; areola smooth and flat diameter < 0.75 cm | Areola stippled, edge not raised diameter < 0.75 cm | Areola stippled, edge raised diameter > 0.75 cm | |
| Breast size | No breast tissue palpable | Breast tissue on one or both sides > 0.5 cm diameter | Breast tissue both sides; one or both 0.5–10 cm | Breast tissue both sides; one or both > 1 cm | |

## 15.0 The neonate

### 15.5 Assessment of gestational age

| Neurological sign | Score 0 | 1 | 2 | 3 | 4 | 5 |
|---|---|---|---|---|---|---|
| Posture | | | | | | |
| Square window | 90° | 60° | 45° | 30° | 0° | |
| Ankle dorsiflexion | 90° | 75° | 45° | 20° | 0° | |
| Arm recoil | 180° | 90–180° | < 90° | | | |
| Leg recoil | 180° | 90–180° | < 90° | | | |
| Popliteal angle | 180° | 160° | 130° | 110° | 90° | <90° |
| Heel to ear | | | | | | |
| Scarf sign | | | | | | |
| Head lag | | | | | | |
| Ventral suspension | | | | | | |

**Fig. 21.** Neurological criteria.

## 15.0 The neonate

### 15.5 Assessment of gestational age

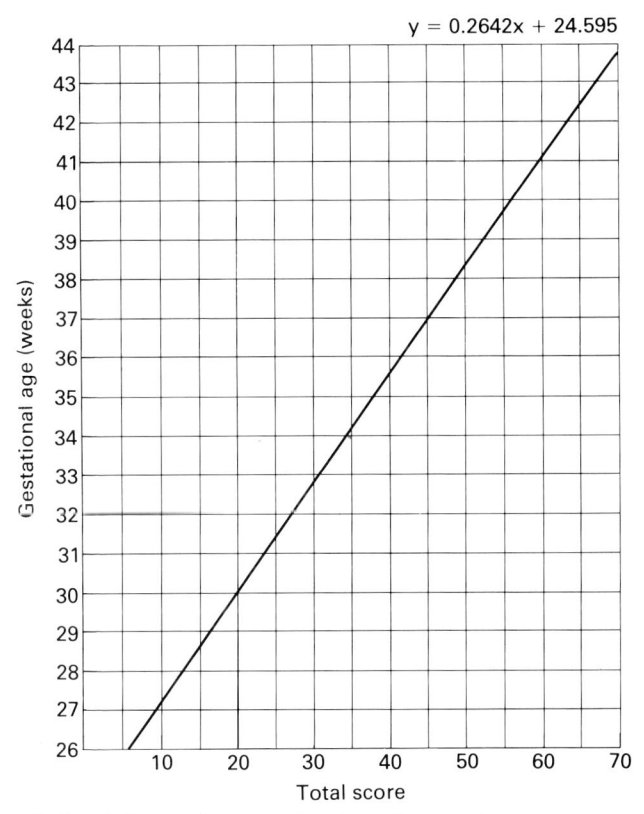

$y = 0.2642x + 24.595$

**Fig. 22.** Graph for reading gestational age from total score.

as possible, and the angle between the dorsum of the foot and the anterior aspect of the leg is measured.

*Arm recoil*

With the infant in the supine position the forearms are first flexed for 5 seconds, then fully extended by pulling on the hands, and then released. The sign is fully positive if the arms return briskly to full flexion (Score 2). If the arms return to incomplete flexion or the response is sluggish it is graded as

## 15.0 The neonate

### 15.5 Assessment of gestational age

Score 1. If they remain extended or are only followed by random movements the score is 0.

*Leg recoil*
With the infant supine, the hips and knees are fully flexed for 5 seconds, then extended by traction on the feet, and released. A maximal response is one of full flexion of the hips and knees (Score 2). A partial flexion scores 1, and minimal or no movement scores 0.

*Popliteal angle*
With the infant supine and his pelvis flat on the examining couch, the thigh is held in the knee-chest position by the examiner's left index finger and thumb supporting the knee. The leg is then extended by gentle pressure from the examiner's right index finger behind the ankle and the popliteal angle is measured.

*Heel to ear manoeuvre*
With the baby supine, draw the baby's foot as near to the head as it will go without forcing it. Observe the distance between the foot and the head as well as the degree of extension at the knee. Grade according to diagram. Note that the knee is left free and may draw down alongside the abdomen.

*Scarf sign*
With the baby supine, take the infant's hand and try to put it around the neck and as far posteriorly as possible around the opposite shoulder. Assist this manoeuvre by lifting the elbow across the body. See how far the elbow will go across and grade according to illustrations. Score 0: Elbow reaches opposite axillary line; 1: Elbow between midline and opposite axillary line; 2: Elbow reaches midline; 3: Elbow will not reach midline.

## 15.0 The neonate

15.6 Routine discharge examination

*Head lag*
With the baby lying supine, grasp the hands (or the arms if a very small infant) and pull him slowly towards the sitting position. Observe the position of the head in relation to the trunk and grade accordingly. In a small infant the head may initially be supported by one hand. Score 0: Complete lag; 1: Partial head control; 2: Able to maintain head in line with body; 3: Brings head anterior to body.

*Ventral suspension*
The infant is suspended in the prone position, with examiner's hand under the infant's chest (one hand in a small infant, two in a large infant). Observe the degree of extension of the back and the amount of flexion of the arms and legs. Also note the relation of the head to the trunk. Grade according to diagrams.

### 15.6 Routine discharge examination
All babies should be examined before going home to assess progress from birth, exclude malformations or traumatic lesions missed earlier, identify any superficial infections and to reassure the mother. The examination should take place with the mother present in a warm room (24°C), on a warm surface, using warm hands. The baby must be handled gently.

The following should be checked:
- the baby's general appearance
- superficial infections (and other lesions) of eyes, mouth, umbilicus, nails
- heart for murmurs
- abdomen (N.B. the liver is normally 1–2 cm palpable)
- male genitalia for hypospadias, undescended testes, herniae and hydrocoeles
- female genitalia for vaginal discharge, fused labia, enlarged clitoris
- hips for congenital dislocation and feet for talipes (See below).

## 15.0 The neonate

15.7 Some neonatal problems

### 15.7 Some neonatal problems

**Congenital dislocation of hips** (CDH)
The routine examination for CDH is illustrated in Fig. 23.

If the hips are dislocated or dislocatable the baby should be treated in an abduction splint for 8–12 weeks and referred to a paediatrician or orthopaedic surgeon.

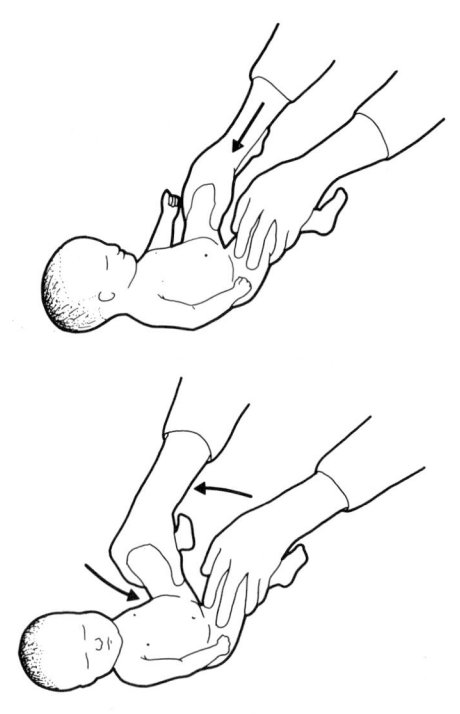

**Fig. 23.** Examination for CDH.

### Talipes equinovarus
An orthopaedic opinion should be sought and the parents reassured by pictures of 'before and after' treatment.

## 15.0 The neonate

### 15.7 Some neonatal problems

**Cleft palate**
Babies with cleft palates commonly have great difficulty with feeding, and are at high risk of aspirating milk into the lungs. They should be nursed with the mother on a transitional care ward and expert help given to establish breast or bottle feeding. An orthodontic plate is a priority to help with feeding and to maintain normal alveolar shape. Feeding may be easier with a long ('lamb's') teat or spoon-shaped teat. Pictures of 'before and after' treatment should be shown to the parents.

**Jaundice**
In term babies who become jaundiced the date of onset of jaundice, method of feeding, the mother's blood group and any history of perinatal trauma should be checked. The baby can stay with the mother under most circumstances.

If the initial bilirubin is greater than 250 $\mu$mol/l the proportion of direct bilirubin should be determined. Send the baby's blood for grouping, Coomb's test, full blood count (including reticulocytes) and differential white cell count.

Phototherapy should be considered if the bilirubin level is greater than 300–350 $\mu$mol/l depending on the age, state of hydration and feeding, and rate of change of bilirubin. Levels > 200 $\mu$mol/l within 48 hours of birth require prompt investigation. At the time of starting phototherapy, (or earlier if indicated) urine should be taken for microscopy and culture and checked for reducing substances. Blood should be sent for haemagglutinins and haemolysins, thyroid function studies and a glucose 6-phosphate dehydrogenase assay.

There is no hard and fast rule about the level of bilirubin at which a baby may be allowed home. The doctor must use his or her discretion and be satisfied that the baby has been adequately investigated and the bilirubin level is stable or falling. It is however essential to inform the GP by telephone of the baby's discharge and send him a summary letter thereafter. Follow-up must be organized.

## 15.0 The neonate

15.8 BCG vaccination

### Ophthalmia neonatorum
This is still a notifiable disease and when it occurs is liable to cause severe eye damage if not treated promptly and adequately. It is defined as 'any purulent discharge from the eyes of an infant starting within 21 days of birth'. Marked inflammation and swelling of the conjunctivae are accompanied by a yellow-green purulent discharge. Conjunctival smears should be taken for culture and plated on to or placed in the following media:
- Thayer-Martin plates for *Neisserin gonorrhoea*
- Stuart's transport medium for other organisms
- sucrose-phosphate-serum medium in a plastic container (placed in liquid nitrogen) for *Chlamydia trachomatis* i.e. TRIC agent.

**Treatment** should be in consultation with an ophthalmologist and bacteriologist or venereologist.

### N. gonorrhoea
Flood eyes with benzyl penicillin eye drops 1 mega unit/ml and repeat after 15 minutes. Continue after feeds for 3 days, plus procaine penicillin 300,000 units i.m. daily for 3 days. If the organism is penicillin-resistant apply framycetin eye drops 0.5% every minute for 15 minutes then after each feed for 3 days.

### Other bacteria
Apply chloramphenicol eye ointment 1% after each feed until the inflammation has cleared.

### TRIC agent
Apply chlortetracycline eye ointment 1% after each feed for two weeks plus erythromycin 12 mg/kg orally three times a day.

### 15.8 BCG vaccination
BCG should be given to newborn children in families known to have had tuberculosis, whatever the type and however long

ago, and children of *all* Asian immigrant families. (Tuberculosis is still widespread in the Asian communities even amongst those who have been in the country for some years.)

If the mother has tuberculosis, discuss the case with a consultant in respiratory diseases before delivery (see Chapter 7.8). In general if the mother's sputum is positive for tuberculosis the baby should be isolated and BCG given. It may be necessary to arrange special care for the baby. If the mother's sputum is negative but she is being treated, give the baby isoniazid-resistant BCG.

## 15.9 Screening for phenylketonuria (PKU)

Phenylketonuria has been discussed in Chapter 6.2. Its incidence in the UK is 1 in 10,000 live births. The Guthrie test or an alternative for PKU should be carried out routinely between 7 and 14 days after delivery.

After cleaning and pricking the heel of the baby, apply the blood to the centre of the ring on the absorbent paper of the test card. The whole area enclosed by at least two rings must be saturated. If the Guthrie bacteriological test is used it should be postponed if the baby is on antibiotics. A chromatographic method is now widely used and this is not affected by antibiotics.

## 15.10 Screening for congenital hypothyroidism

Congenital hypothyroidism causes mental retardation unless it is treated early. Without a screening programme for its detection only 40% of cases will be diagnosed by 3 months of age. The incidence of primary hypothyroidism detected by screening programmes is about 1 in 4400 live births (c.f. PKU above) in the UK.

Testing can be carried out on a saturated dried blood filter paper spot at between 2 and 5 days after delivery. Most programmes either measure TSH alone or thyroxine and TSH. Alternatives to the dried blood spot are tests on cord blood serum or capillary serum from a heel prick on day 5.

## 15.0 The neonate

15.11 Detection of cystic fibrosis

### 15.11 Detection of cystic fibrosis

As noted on page 67 cystic fibrosis (CF) is the commonest severe autosomal recessive genetic disease among white people (frequency approx. 1:1600 live births).

The specific biochemical defect is still not known but the effects of the condition are:
- abnormally salty sweat
- deficient pancreatic exocrine secretions causing azotorrhoea and steatorrhoea
- predisposition to severe and chronic lung infections.

In addition to a positive family history, symptoms which require exclusion of CF are:
- neonatal meconium ileus
- failure to thrive
- recurrent chest infections.

Diagnosis is based on the NaCl content and osmolality of sweat. The traditional 'Gibson-Cooke' pilocarpine sweat test requires the collection of at least 200 $\mu$l of sweet. The production of this amount in neonates is neither easy nor safe so the test is not appropriate for infants under 6–8 weeks of age. Other techniques have been developed which require smaller samples of sweat. One such is described by Carter *et al.,* (1984), *Arch. Dis. Child* **59**, 919–922. Over 99% of CF homozygotes have sweat Na and Cl concentrations greater than 60 and 70 mmol/l respectively. Sweat osmolality in a group of affected neonates has been noted to be 255–345 mmol/kg compared with 87–123 mmol/kg for normal neonates.

The potential value of routine screening of all neonates for CF is controversial. No clear benefit from early diagnosis has as yet been demonstrated but it has been suggested that pre-symptomatic diagnosis would be beneficial because:
- teaching of postural drainage can start early (but not all affected infants are at risk of developing chronic lung infections)
- an appropriate diet can be instituted
- pancreatin replacement therapy can begin

## 15.0 The neonate

15.11 Detection of cystic fibrosis

- mild respiratory infections can be taken seriously.

Currently the most promising screening test (which can either be used routinely or on suspicion) relies on the detection of elevated immuno-reactive trypsin (IRT) in a blood sample (e.g. the same sample as is taken for PKU screening). Blood IRT is elevated early in the course of the disease before severe pancreatic damage causes it to fall. A small number of neonates exhibit innocent transient hypertrypsinaemia so a second blood sample is taken if the IRT level in the first is $> 80\ \mu g/l$. A sweat test is indicated if the level is still 80 $\mu g/l$ in the second test. Heeley *et al.* (1984—see suggested further reading) have found only 1 false negative test from 70,000 infants screened—a sensitivity of 98%.

If an infant has meconium ileus IRT testing should be carried out before laparotomy because this causes levels to fall temporarily. Testing in the UK can be carried out at the Regional Neonatal Screening Laboratory, Dept. of Clinical Chemistry, Peterborough District Hospital, England (Dr A.F. Heeley).

# 16.0 The puerperium

16.0 The puerperium, 279

16.1 Infant feeding and suppression of lactation, 279

16.2 Puerperal pyrexia, 282

16.3 Secondary postpartum haemorrhage, 283

16.4 Prevention of Rh-D sensitization and rubella vaccination, 283

16.5 Family planning advice, 284

16.6 Postnatal exercises, 284

16.7 Discharge from hospital, 285

16.8 Postnatal visit, 285

## 16.0 The puerperium

### 16.0 The puerpurium
The puerperium is the period of time over which the genital tract returns to normal after childbirth. Traditionally it is said to last for 6 weeks.

### 16.1 Infant feeding and suppression of lactation
The average amount of breast milk ingested by a normal full term infant during its first day of feeding is said to be 20 ml/kg body weight and this is what artificial feeding should aim to provide. Thereafter feeds are increased by 20 ml/kg each day until a maximum of 150 ml/kg is achieved on day 7. The infant regains his or her birthweight by day 7–10 and should thereafter gain 30 g/day for the next 100 days.

**Breast-feeding** is to be encouraged because:
- it promotes bonding between mother and baby
- the fat and protein in breast milk are more readily digested and absorbed than those in cow's milk
- colostrum and breast milk contain antibodies which provide the infant with passive immunity to many infections
- gastro-enteritis is rare among breast-fed babies
- milk allergies are avoided
- it is safe, cheap and simple
- overfeeding is virtually impossible
- the risk of hypocalcaemia with convulsions is reduced
- uterine involution is promoted
- the incidence of subsequent breast cancer is reduced.

### Some points about breast-feeding
- If the nipple is partially inverted Waller design plastic shields may be used over the latter part of pregnancy
- the baby can be put to each breast shortly after, or within, a few hours of birth
- a small but increasing amount of colostrum will be obtained for the first 36–48 hours and the suckling will stimulate subsequent milk production.

## 16.0 The puerperium

### 16.1 Infant feeding and suppression of lactation

- by day 3 the feeding will be either on demand or 3–4 hourly. (The natural demand cycle is usually about 4 hourly.)
- 'rooming in' of babies with mothers at night makes demand feeding easier, though no mother should be made to feel guilty because she does not want the baby with her at night
- some mothers wish the baby to be alongside them in their own bed. Although this is a marvellous idea in theory it must be pointed out that should any accident befall the baby during the night the responsibility for this would lie with the hospital. The practice must therefore be gently but firmly discouraged, unless a safety bed-rail can be provided
- it is sometimes 'Granny' who influences her daughter against breast-feeding so that she herself can participate in the ritual of feeding
- if the baby seems still to be hungry after a feed or there is progressive weight loss, a 24-hour period of test feeding may be carried out. The baby should be weighed without changing before and after each feed
- if the amount of each feed is lacking, and the baby's position at the breast is correct, he can either be put to the breast more frequently or additional (complementary) artificial feeds can be given. Complementary feeding is rarely necessary within the first 5 days of life and should only be used thereafter when thought to be absolutely necessary
- the only major contra-indications to breast-feeding are serious illness in the mother (e.g. tuberculosis) and certain drugs described in Chapter 17
- sore nipples can be protected by nipple shields but the milk flow is reduced by their use. Almost always the solution is to correct the baby's position at the breast
- mothers whose babies are in the special care nursery should be encouraged to express their milk so that it can be used to feed their own baby until they can breast-feed.

## 16.0 The puerperium

16.1 Infant feeding and suppression of lactation

### Enhancement of lactation
If the 'let-down' of milk is insufficient it can be enhanced by oxytocin given through a nasal spray. Oxytocin is placed in a spray bottle at a concentration of 40 $\mu$/ml. One 'puff' in each nostril (total 3 units oxytocin) just before feeding or expression is effective and does not alter the composition of the milk.

### Bottle feeding
This is dealt with in the Child Health Pocket Consultant and is not considered in detail here. It is however important to reassure the mother that a failure to breast-feed is not going to harm her child.

### Suppression of lactation
The use of oestrogens to suppress lactation is no longer justified. They are not particularly effective, there is a high incidence of rebound engorgement after they are stopped, and they predispose to secondary PPH and thrombo-embolism.

Firm support of the breasts with a good bra, plenty of warm bathing of the breasts, and adequate analgesia for any initial engorgement, are all that is necessary in the vast majority of cases.

In those women in whom clinical judgement suggests that suppression of lactation is necessary, bromocryptine 2.5 mg 8-hourly for 10 days is a very effective treatment.

The expression of milk from engorged breasts merely encourages further milk production.

### Mastitis
Acute intramammary mastitis arises as a result of failure of milk withdrawal from a lobule. It can frequently be resolved by getting the baby to empty the breast by continued feeding. Cold compresses ease the discomfort. If there is no improvement within 24 hours, antibiotics should be given to prevent abscess formation.

## 16.0 The puerperium

16.2 Puerperal pyrexia

Infective (or epidemic) mastitis may be due to *Staphylococcus aureus* carried by the baby. The inflammation is usually at the areolar margin. Treatment is with one of the newer penicillins to which the organism is sensitive.

### Breast abscess
This is a rare but preventable condition. Antibiotics are only helpful when given early, otherwise they tend to delay full resolution of the inflammation. Surgical drainage under general anaesthesia is the treatment of choice for an established abscess. A radial incision should be used and an appropriate small drain inserted. The incision must not leave an ugly scar.

### 16.2 Puerperal pyrexia
This is defined as a temperature of 38°C on any occasion in the first 14 days after delivery of miscarriage. Its notification is no longer legally compulsory.

No pyrexia should be ignored in the puerperium but a slight fever is not uncommon within the first 24 hours of delivery. After this time the commonest causes (in order of importance) are:
- urinary tract infection
- genital tract infection
- breast infection
- deep vein thrombosis
- respiratory infection
- other non-obstetric causes.

After a full clinical examination (including breasts and legs) the following investigations should be carried out in all women with puerperal pyrexia:
- MSU for microscopy and culture
- cervical and high vaginal swabs (HVS)
- blood culture
- sputum culture (if possible).

After the samples have been sent to the laboratory, and if the clinical situation warrants it, antibiotic therapy can be started

# 16.0 The puerperium

## 16.3 Secondary postpartum haemorrhage

perhaps using ampicillin 500 mg orally 6-hourly with metronidazole 400 mg orally 8-hourly. Treatment can be modified as necessary when the results of investigations are available.

### 16.3 Secondary postpartum haemorrhage

The lochia are mainly blood for the first few days after delivery; for the next 7–10 days they are sero-sanguinous usually remaining clear thereafter for up to 6 weeks.

Secondary postpartum haemorrhage is defined as excessive blood loss from the genital tract more than 24 hours after delivery. If it occurs within a few days of delivery it is likely to be due to retained placental fragments or blood clot. Thereafter it is often associated with intra-uterine infection.

#### Management

If the bleeding has been slight and there is no evidence of infection the patient needs no more than to be kept under observation. Treatment with oral ergometrine is of doubtful value.

Evacuation of the uterus under general anaesthesia is indicated if:

- an ultrasound scan suggests the presence of retained products
- heavy bleeding persists
- the uterus is larger than expected and tender and the cervix is open.

Two units of blood should be cross-matched and the uterus must be evacuated under general anaesthesia with the greatest of care using a sharp curette. The uterus is very easily perforated at this stage of involution.

### 16.4 Prevention of rhesus sensitization and rubella vaccination

The use of anti-D immunoglobulin 100 $\mu$g to prevent the sensitization of rhesus negative women is discussed in Chapter 8.

## 16.0 The puerperium

16.5 Family planning advice

---

They 'lying-in' period is also the best time to immunize women who are not already immune to rubella. They must be advised to avoid further pregnancy for at least 3 months.

### 16.5 Family planning advice
Any large maternity unit should have at least one full time member of the nursing staff whose sole responsibility it is to provide family planning advice within the hospital, particularly to women in the post-natal wards.

For a woman who wishes to breast-feed, the combined oestrogen-progestogen pill is probably not the best contraception. It may reduce lactation to some slight extent and is also minimally excreted in breast milk. For lactating women the progestogen-only pill ('the mini-pill') can be taken until the baby is weaned. The combined pill can then be taken.

For non-lactating women a barrier method may be best until menstruation starts or until the puerperium is complete (whichever is the sooner). After this time their preferred method can be used.

An IUD is best fitted at the post-natal visit.

For some multiparous women puerperal tubal ligation on day 2 through a mini-laparotomy is worthwhile. It must have been fully discussed, preferably antenatally, and the husband must be in full agreement. The written consent of the woman is obligatory and of the husband advisable. The ease of interval laparoscopic tubal occlusion and the number of women who regret tubal ligation in the immediate puerperium are making the latter procedure less popular than it was.

Sexual relations can begin whenever the couple feel it is appropriate. Husbands must be made to understand that a lack of sexual interest on the part of the wife is not unnatural for some weeks after delivery.

### 16.6 Postnatal exercises
The physiotherapy department will actively instruct women on

the appropriate exercises; they should be encouraged to carry them through for at least 6 weeks. The main purpose is to strengthen the abdominal and pelvic floor muscles.

## 16.7 Discharge from hospital

The length of stay should be flexible, compatible with home circumstances, and the amount of help available for the mother at home. A stay of 5–7 days is adequate after most normal or instrumental deliveries; 8–10 days after a caesarean section.

An accurate, legible discharge summary must be provided quickly for the GP and the midwife and any special problems communicated to them by telephone. The mother should be informed that a midwife will call on her the day after discharge and will hand over her care to the health visitor at an appropriate time.

## 16.8 The postnatal visit

This occurs 6 weeks after delivery and the two main practical purposes of this visit are to carry out a cervical smear and provide further contraceptive advice. Few women need to return to hospital for a postnatal visit. Those who have had a caesarean section may be advised to return so that the result of postpartum X-ray pelvimetry, and policies for future deliveries can be discussed.

Couples whose baby was stillborn or died neonatally should return for a full discussion but not to a clinic where they will be required to mix with pregnant women or those with babies (see Section 10.13).

# 17.0 Prescribing during pregnancy and lactation

**17.0 Prescribing during pregnancy and lactation, 289**

## 17.0 Prescribing during pregnancy and lactation

- most drugs cross the placenta and are excreted in breast milk
- in the first trimester there is a theoretical risk of congenital malformations, although few drugs have been conclusively proven to cause them
- fetal growth and development can be affected by drugs taken during the second and third trimesters
- some drugs given close to term or during labour can affect the neonate
- such seemingly innocuous treatment as ointment applied to the nipples may be harmful if ingested by the infant.

Among the principles for prescribing during pregnancy and lactation are:

- drugs should only be prescribed for a pregnant woman when the indications are clear and specific and the expected benefit to the mother is greater than the risk to the fetus
- if at all possible avoid all drugs in the first trimester (even non-prescription drugs)
- prescribe drugs which have been well tried in pregnancy in preference to newer preparations
- use the smallest effective dose for the shortest therapeutic time.

Table 17.1 is a selective guide to prescribing during pregnancy and lactation, in addition to the guidance given in the relevant chapters. It must not be assumed that drugs not mentioned in the table are safe.

**Table 17.1.**

| Drug | Effect | Comment |
|---|---|---|
| **Anti-emetics** (cyclizine, prochlorperazine, promethazine etc.) | No proven teratogenic effects despite many years of usage | Avoid if possible on basis that all drugs are best avoided in pregnancy. Often used during labour to counter nausea associated with opiate analgesics |
| **Anti-infective agents** | | |
| tetracyclines | Causes permanent staining of deciduous teeth and reversible depression of bone growth. (Occasional severe fatty degeneration of maternal liver when given parenterally) | Avoid during pregnancy, lactation and in children up to 7 years of age |
| chloramphenicol | Inhibits protein synthesis and may cause collapse, grey cyanosis and death in neonates. Maternal aplastic anaemia rare | This 'grey syndrome' has *not* occurred if the mother is given the drug. Use an alternative if possible. This potential complication has virtually condemned an otherwise very useful inexpensive antibiotic |
| sulphonamides | The antibacterial effect depends on interference with folic acid synthesis. They compete with bilirubin for binding sites on albumin, giving a theoretical risk of kernicterus | No effects noted over many years of usage. May cause haemolysis in glucose 6-phosphate dehydrogenase (G6PD) deficiency. No cases of kernicterus reported |

| Drug | | |
|---|---|---|
| co-trimoxazole (Bactrim, Septrin) | The trimethoprim component also inhibits folic acid metabolism. See above for the sulphonamide component | Use alternative if possible. Definitely avoid during first trimester |
| aminoglycosides (streptomycin, kanamycin, gentamicin) | All are ototoxic but eighth nerve damage is rare even after long-term streptomycin. No nephrotoxicity reported | If used in severe infections the therapeutic balance is in their favour |
| rifampicin | May increase risk of bleeding in neonate | Isoniazid and ethambutol are drugs of choice but rifampicin can be used if a more potent drug is required. Give neonate vitamin K1 |
| metronidazole (Flagyl) | Interferes with inosinic acid, an important nucleic acid precursor | Theoretical objections only since no effects reported. Best to avoid in first trimester |
| Ketoconazole (Nizoral) | Can cause liver damage | Choose another anti-fungal agent in pregnancy |
| chloroquine | Causes fetal retinal damage after high doses | Use as antimalarial but not for other purposes (e.g. rheumatoid arthritis) |
| vaccines | Live viral vaccines may infect fetus ∴ avoid rubella, smallpox, measles, live oral polio and yellow fever vaccinations | Killed viruses are not contraindicated. Avoid rubella vaccination in children of pregnant women |

### Analgesics

| | | |
|---|---|---|
| salicylates | Possible association with some congenital abnormalities. Platelet dysfunction and diminished factor XII in fetus | Avoid during first trimester. Excessive doses may cause haemorrhage in neonates |

| Drug | Effect | Comment |
|---|---|---|
| indomethacin, naproxen sodium, mefenamic acid | Prostaglandin synthetase inhibitors | May cause intrauterine closure of ductus arteriosus. Avoid during pregnancy |
| **Opiates** | | |
| morphine, heroin | Cross placenta and into breast milk, causing respiratory depression and unresponsiveness | Hazards well recognized. Withdrawal symptoms can be fatal in babies born to addicts (see page 000) |
| **Psychotropic drugs** | | |
| chlorpromazine | Prolonged high doses may cause fetal retinal damage. No problems noted at normal dosage | All phenothiazines cross in breast milk but no significant ill-effects have been noted |
| monoamine oxidase inhibitors (MAO) | Contra-indicated in pregnancy | See page 000 |
| diazepam (Valium) | Crosses placenta and into breast milk: can cause low Apgar score, apnoeic spells, hypotonia, reluctance to feed, and impaired response in stress | Infant may be depressed at birth and for several days afterwards or be sedated by suckling |
| chlordiazepoxide (Librium) | Crosses placenta and to some extent into milk. Adverse reports are rare, but may cause similar depression to diazepam | Use judiciously |
| lithium carbonate | Crosses placenta and is excreted in milk | Could alter fetal electrolyte balance and may cause goitre. Use only if indications are unequivocal |

## Hypnotics

| | | |
|---|---|---|
| nitrazepam (Mogadon) | Crosses placenta and into breast milk | May interfere with interpretation of antenatal cardiocography or sedate breast-fed infant |
| dichlorphenazone (Welldorm) | Excreted in milk | Mild sedation of breast-fed baby. The routine use of hypnotics is not recommended |
| barbiturates | Crosses placenta very quickly | Severe respiratory depression at birth. Contra-indicated except as anticonvulsants |

## Anticonvulsants

| | | |
|---|---|---|
| barbiturates with primidone or phenitoin | Cases occasional vitamin K deficiency type of coagulation defect with serious haemorrhage in infants. Congenital malformations increased (see page 000) | Drugs are of obvious value and prophylactic Vitamin K is important in mother or neonate (see page 000) |

## Anticoagulants

| | | |
|---|---|---|
| warfarin, sodium, phenindione | Causes fetal anticoagulation via placenta. Phenindione is excreted in milk. (Heparin does not cross placenta or into milk) | Phenindione is contraindicated. Indication for warfarin therapy must be good and careful control is VITAL. Stop 4 weeks before expected delivery and substitute heparin. Breast-feeding is not contraindicated with warfarin (see page 000) |

## Steroids

| | | |
|---|---|---|
| corticosteroids (systemic) | Fetal adrenal function not impaired, but increased perinatal mortality has been noted | Risk is small enough to justify treatment if indication is good |

*Table 17.1 continued*

| Drug | Effect | Comment |
|---|---|---|
| **Sex steroids** | | |
| oestrogens, progestogens | Masculinization of female fetus noted after maternal treatment with 19 norprogestogens, testosterone and diethylstilboestrol (DES). May be due to fetal target organ deficiency or error in steroid metabolism. DES also implicated in causing clear cell adenocarcinoma of vagina in offspring of mothers treated in early pregnancy | Hormonal pregnancy test MUST NOT be used. The use of DES is contraindicated. The slight excretion in breast milk does not contraindicate postpartum use of oral contraceptives, but lactation may be slightly suppressed |
| **Antihypertensive therapy** (and see pages 86–88) | | |
| reserpine | Noradrenaline depletion may upset thermal equilibrium in neonate. Fetal bradycardia, lethargy, depression of Moro reflex and mucous membrane engorgement can also occur | The mucous membrane engorgement may cause nasal obstruction and threaten life in the neonate. This drug is therefore contra-indicated |
| hexamethonium | Fetal ganglion blockade may cause neonatal hypotension and paralytic ileus | Use alternative hypotensive drugs |
| thiazide diuretics | Chronic hypokalaemia? Thrombocytopaenia. Cross in breast milk | Used too readily in pregnancy. Avoid during lactation |
| enalapril maleate (Innovace) | Teratogenic in mice | Avoid in pregnancy |

| | | |
|---|---|---|
| propranolol | Crosses placenta and can cause prolonged beta-adrenergic blockade. May adversely affect fetal cardiac output | Valuable in primary cardiomyopathies, paroxysmal tachycardia). Cannot be recommended for hypertension in pregnancy. Avoid if possible |
| diazoxide (Eudemine) | Crosses placenta. May cause neonatal alopecia and hyperglycaemia | Oral use not recommended |

## Thyroid drugs
(see page 000)

| | | |
|---|---|---|
| iodides ($^{131}$iodine) | Crosses placenta and into breast milk with ease. Goitre and hypothyroidism may result. Avoid during pregnancy and lactation | Some proprietary 'cough bottles' contain large quantities of iodides. Iodine containing contrast media may raise the maternal PBI for some years and can affect the fetus |
| carbimazole, propylthiouracil | Cross placenta and into milk → goitre hypothyroid | Breast feeding is not necessarily contraindicated (see page 102) |
| **Local anaesthetics** | Readily crosses the placenta. Excess doses may cause fetal methaemoglobinaemia. Indirect effect of maternal regional anaesthesia causing hypotension | Recommended doses must not be exceeded |

Antidiabetic agents

| | | |
|---|---|---|
| chlorpropamide, tolbutamide | Cross placenta | Best avoided in pregnancy (see p. 93) |

*Table 17.1 continued*

| Drug | Effect | Comment |
|---|---|---|
| **Cytotoxic drugs** | | |
| methotrexate, cyclo-phosphamide | Crosses placenta and into milk. Causes growth retardation and may affect fetal gonads | Avoid if possible, but in some instances maternal and fetal survival may depend on them. Breast-feeding contraindicated |
| **Miscellaneous** | | |
| ergotamine | Can cause fetal limb deformities (Poland anomaly) if used in high does in early pregnancy<br><br>Potential contractile effect on uterus. Crosses in milk and may cause vomiting, diarrhoea and unstable blood pressure in infant | Use alternative therapy for migraine during pregnancy and lactation |

## 17.0 Prescribing during pregnancy and lactation

17.0 Prescribing during pregnancy and lactation

- iodides and $^{131}$iodine
- ketoconazole
- live viral vaccines (rubella, smallpox, measles, polio and yellow fever)
- methotrexate for psoriasis
- mono-amine oxidase inhibitors
- oral hypoglycaemic agents
- oral progestagens
- phenindione
- reserpine
- tetracyclines.

### 2. Drugs best avoided

| In first trimester | Throughout pregnancy | During lactation |
|---|---|---|
| antacids | amiodarone | |
| iron supplements | clofibrate | chloramphenicol |
| metronidazole | co-trimoxazole | laxatives |
| salicylates | diazoxide | |
| sodium valproate | diuretics | |
| | enalapril | |
| | ergotamine | |
| | hypnotics | |
| | iodide cough mixtures | |
| | probenecid | |
| | propranolol | |
| | prostaglanden-synthetase inhibitors | |

## 17.0 Prescribing during pregnancy and lactation

17.0 Prescribing during pregnancy and lactation

**3. Drugs to be used under specialist supervision** (and only with unequivocal indications)

anticonvulsants
anti-thyroid drugs
aminoglycoside antibiotics
cytotoxic drugs
hypotensive agents
lithium carbonate
systemic corticosteroids
warfarin sodium

# Appendixes

**Suggested further reading, 301**

**Abbreviations, 303**

**Conversion tables, 304**

**Useful addresses, 305**

# Appendixes

## Suggested further reading

'Antenatal Diagnosis of Genetic Defects' Eds. A. B. Gerbie, *Clinics in Obstetrics and Gynaecology,* 7: No. 1, W.B. Saunders, 1980.

*Benefits and Hazards of the New Obstetrics* Ed. T. Chard and M. Richards, Spastics International Medical Publications, 1977.

*British National Formulary* No. 11, British Medical Association and Pharmaceutical Society of Great Britain, 1986.

*Clinical Physiology in Obstetrics* Eds. G. V. P. Chamberlain and F. E. Hytten, Blackwell Scientific Publications, London, 1980.

*Contemporary Obstetrics* G. Chamberlain, Butterworths, 1984.

*Diagnostic Indices in Pregnancy* F. E. Hytten and T. Lind, Documenta Geigy, 1973.

*Effectiveness and Satisfaction in Antenatal Care* Eds. M. Enkin and J. Chalmers, Spastics International Medical Publications, 1982.

*Fetal and Maternal Medicine* Eds. E. J. Quilligan and N. Kretchmer, John Wiley, 1980.

*Fetal Physiology and Medicine* R. W. Beard and P. W. Nathanielsz, Butterworths, 1984.

*Medical Disorders in Obstetric Practice* Ed. M. de Swiet Blackwell Scientific Publications, 1984.

*The New Genetics and Clinical Practice* D. J. Weatherall, Nuffield Provincial Hospitals Trust, 1982.

'Obstetric Anaesthesia and Analgesia' *Clinics in Obstetric Gynaecology,* 9: No. 2, W.B. Saunders, 1982.

*Pre-eclampsia—the Hypertensive Disease of Pregnancy* by I. MacGillivray, W.B. Saunders, 1983.

*Pre-natal Diagnosis* Eds. C. H. Rodeck and K. H. Nicolaides, John Wiley and Sons Ltd., 1984.

Prescribing in Pregnancy *Clinics in Obstetrics and Gynaecology,* 8: No. 2, W.B. Saunders, 1986.

*Pre-term Labour* Eds. M. G. Elder and C. H. Hendricks, Butterworths 1981.

# Appendixes

Suggested further reading

*Progress in Obstetrics and Gynaecology,* Vols 1–5, Ed. J. Studd, Churchill Livingstone 1981–5.

*Recent Advances in Perinatal Medicine,* Vol III, p. 41, Ed. M. L. Chiswick, Churchill Livingstone, Edinburgh.

*Report on Confidential Enquiries into Maternal Deaths in England and Wales* 1979–81, HMSO, 1986.

*Report of the RCOG Working Party on Routine Ultrasound Examination in Pregnancy* RCOG, 1984.

'The Small Baby' *Clinics in Obstetrics and Gynaecology,* Ed. P. W. Howie and N. B. Patel, II: No. 2, W.B. Saunders, 1984.

The value of blood trypsin measurement by RIA in the early diagnosis of cystic fibrosis. Heeley A. F., Heely M. E., Richmond S. W. J. In: *'Progress in Perinatal Medicine—Biochemical and Biophysical Diagnostic Procedures.'* Eds. A. Albertini and P. G. Crosignani, Excerpta Medica, Amsterdam, pp. 195–203, 1983.

# Appendixes

## Abbreviations

| | |
|---|---|
| ACH | Aftercoming head (in breech presentation) |
| AFT | Alpha-feto protein |
| ARM | Artificial rupture of membranes (amniotomy) |
| BPD | Biparietal diameter |
| CF | Cystic fibrosis |
| CPD | Cephalo-pelvic disproportion |
| CTG | Cardiotocograph |
| DBP | Diastolic blood pressure |
| DVT | Deep vein thrombosis |
| $E_1$ | Oestrone |
| $E_2$ | Oestradiol 17$\beta$ |
| $E_3$ | Oestriol |
| EDD or EDC | Expected date of delivery (or confinement) |
| FBS | Fetal blood sample |
| FHR | Fetal heart rate |
| GTT | Glucose tolerance test |
| hCG | Human chorionic gonadotrophin |
| hPL | Human placental lactogen |
| HVS | High vaginal swab |
| IPPV | Intermittent positive pressure ventilation |
| IUCD | Intra-uterine contraceptive device |
| IUD | Intra-uterine death |
| IUGR | Intra-uterine growth retardation |
| IUT | Intra-uterine transfusion |
| LMP | Last menstrual period |
| LSCS | Lower segment caesarean section |
| L/S | Lecithin-sphingomyelin ratio |
| MSU | Midstream specimen of urine |
| NND | Neonatal death |
| NTD | Neural tube defect |
| OA | Occipito anterior |
| OP | Occipito posterior |
| OT | Occipito transverse |
| PET | Pre-eclamptic toxaemia |

## Appendixes

Conversion tables

| | |
|---|---|
| PKU | Phenylketonuria |
| PMR | Perinatal mortality rate |
| POP | Persistent occipito posterior |
| PPH | Post-partum haemorrhage |
| RDS | Respiratory distress syndrome |
| SB | Stillbirth |
| SBP | Systolic blood pressure |
| STD | Sexually transmitted disease |

## Conversion tables

**Weight conversion tables, metric to imperial (1000 g = 1 kg, 16 oz = 1 lb)**

| g | lbs | oz | g | lbs | oz |
|---|---|---|---|---|---|
| 500 | 1 | 1½ | 3000 | 6 | 10 |
| 600 | 1 | 5 | 3100 | 6 | 13½ |
| 700 | 1 | 8 | 3200 | 7 | 1 |
| 800 | 1 | 11½ | 3300 | 7 | 4½ |
| 900 | 1 | 15½ | 3400 | 7 | 7½ |
| 1000 | 2 | 3 | 3500 | 7 | 11½ |
| 1100 | 2 | 7 | 3600 | 7 | 15 |
| 1200 | 2 | 10½ | 3700 | 8 | 2½ |
| 1300 | 2 | 14 | 3800 | 8 | 6 |
| 1400 | 3 | 1½ | 3900 | 8 | 9 |
| 1500 | 3 | 5 | 4000 | 8 | 13 |
| 1600 | 3 | 8½ | 4100 | 9 | 0½ |
| 1700 | 3 | 12 | 4200 | 9 | 4 |
| 1800 | 3 | 15½ | 4300 | 9 | 7½ |
| 1900 | 4 | 3 | 4400 | 9 | 11 |
| 2000 | 4 | 6½ | 4500 | 9 | 14½ |
| 2100 | 4 | 10 | 4600 | 10 | 2 |
| 2200 | 4 | 13½ | 4700 | 10 | 6½ |
| 2300 | 5 | 1 | 4800 | 10 | 9½ |

# Appendixes

Conversion tables

| g | lbs | oz | g | lbs | oz |
|---|---|---|---|---|---|
| 2400 | 5 | 4½ | 4900 | 10 | 13 |
| 2500 | 5 | 8 | 5000 | 11 | 0½ |
| 2600 | 5 | 11½ | 5100 | 11 | 4 |
| 2700 | 5 | 15 | 5200 | 11 | 7½ |
| 2800 | 6 | 3 | 5300 | 11 | 11 |
| 2900 | 6 | 6½ | 5400 | 11 | 14½ |

# Appendixes

Useful addresses

## Multiples of SI units

| name | symbol | factor |
|---|---|---|
| kilo- | k | $10^3$ |
| centi- | c | $10^{-2}$ |
| mili- | m | $10^{-3}$ |
| micro- | $\mu$ | $10^{-6}$ |
| nano- | n | $10^{-9}$ |
| pico- | p | $10^{-12}$ |
| fento- | f | $10^{-15}$ |

## Useful Addresses

Assocition for all Speech
 Impaired Children
347 Central Market
London EC1A 9NH
01-236 6487

Birth centres (see local
 directories)

Cleft Lip and Palate
 Association (CLAPA)
Dental Department
Hospital for Sick Children
Great Ormond Street
London WC1N 3JH
01-405 9200 (Ext. 316)

MAMA—Meet a Mum
 Association (National postnatal support)
26A Cumnor Hill
Oxford OX2 9HA

National Association for
 Maternal and Child Welfare
1 South Audley Street
London W1Y 6JS
01-491 1315

National Association for Spina
 Bifida and Hydrocephalus
Tavistock House North
Tavistock Square
London WC1H 9HJ
01-388 1382

# Appendixes

Useful addresses

Family Planning Association
27 Mortimer Street
London W1N 7RU
01-636 7866

Foundation for the Study of
　Infant Deaths (Cot Deaths)
5th Floor
4–5 Grosvenor Place
London SW1X 7HD
01-235 1721

The Haemophilia Society
P.O. Box 9
16 Trinity Street
London SE1 1DE
01-407 1010

La Lèche League
P.O. Box 3424
London WC1V 6XX
01-406 5011

National Childbirth Trust
9 Queensborough Terrace
London W2 3TB
01-221 3833

National Marriage Guidance
　Council
Little Church Street
Rugby
Warwickshire CV21 3AP
0788 73241

Parents Anonymous (see local
　directories or telephone
　01-688 4805: 24-hour service)

Stillbirth and Perinatal Death
　Association
15A Christchurch Hill
London NW3 1JY
01-794 4601

# Index

Abortion, late missed 163–4
Abscess, breast 282
Acquired immune deficiency
    syndrome (AIDS) 137
Adrenal function 18
Age, maternal, and infant
    mortality 248
Albumin 12
Alcohol 114–15
Aldosterone 18
Alimentary function 20
Alimentary tract diseases 108–9
Alkaline phosphatase 14–15
Alpha-feto protein 40
  screening for neural tube
    defects 71–3
Aminoglycosides 291
Amniocentesis 75–6
  Rhesus iso-immunization 124
α-methyldopa 86–7
Amniotic fluid 35, 37–40
  analysis, Rhesus
    iso-immunization 123–4
  assessment of lung
    maturity 158–9
  embolism 235–6
  meconium staining 222–3
Amnionitis 180
Anaemia
  aplastic 82
  haemolytic 82
  prophylaxis 77
  severe, management 79
Anaesthetics, local 295
Analgesia
  epidural 186–90
  in labour 184–90
  instrumental delivery 208–10
Analgesics 291–2
Anencephaly 70
Angiotensin-converting enzyme
    inhibitors 88
Ankle dorsiflexion 263
Antacid therapy 210
Antenatal care 47
  provision of 49–57
  routine examinations and
    investigations 57
Antenatal classes 169
Antenatal clinic procedures 49–51
Antepartum haemorrhage 151–3
Anticoagulants 293
Anticonvulsants 293
  effect on fetus 105–6
Antidiabetic agents 295
Anti-D immunoglobulin 121–2

Anti-emetics 290
Anti-hypertensive drugs 86–8,
    294–5
Anti-infective agents 290
Apgar score 257
Aplastic anaemia 82
Apt's test 153
Arm recoil 267
Arrhythmias, management 100
Asthma, bronchial 107
Atenolol 87
Australia antigen 51

Bacteriuria 144
Barbiturates 114, 293
Basal metabolic rate 18
BCG vaccination, neonate 272–3
Beta-adrenergic blocking
    agents 87–8
β-haemolytic streptococcus 141–2
Beta-sympathomimetic drugs 203
  contra-indications 205
Bilirubin 20
Biophysical profile 155–7
Birthweight 25–8
  low 31–2
  mortality and 246
Bishop score of cervical state 181
Blastocyst, stages of formation 3
Blood
  coagulation 15–17
  composition 9–15
  fetal, sampling 220–2
  pressure 7–8
    measurement 83
  routine tests 51
Bottle feeding 281
Breast
  abscess 282
  cancer 116–17
Breast-feeding 55, 279–80
Breech presentation 160–2
  external cephalic version 160–2
  labour 192–5
Broad ligament haematoma 238
Brow presentation 195–6

Caesarean section 212–15
  breech presentation 193–4
  death rate from 254
  epidural analgesia 190
  general anaesthesia 210
  multiple pregnancy 196–7
  pre-term labour 206–7
Calcium 11
Candidiasis 129–30

308

# Index

Carbohydrate metabolism 20–1
Carbon dioxide 9
Cardiac arrest, neonate 260
Cardiac disease 97–101
Cardiac failure 98–9
Cardiac surgery 100
Cardiotocograph 216
Cardiovascular dynamics 7
Cephalometry 28–9
Cervix
  cancer 115–16
  dilation 172
  ripeness 181–2
Chest X-ray 54
Chloramphenicol 290
Chlordiazepoxide 292
Chlormethiazole 232
Chloroquine 291
Chlorpromazine 292
Cholelithiasis 109–10
Cholesterol 13
Chorionic villus sampling 76
Chromosomal disorders 63–6
Cleft palate/lip 74, 271
Clot observation test 234
Coagulation defects 234–5
Coeliac disease 111
Coitus 55
Confinement
  GP unit 48–9
  home 49
  hospital 48
Congenital malformations 63–76
Contractions 172–4
Convulsions, in eclampsia 231–2
Copper 12
Cord prolapse 229–30
Corticosteroids 293
Cortisol 18
Co-trimoxazole 291
Creatinine
  clearance 17
  pre-eclampsia 89
Crohn's disease 111
Cystic fibrosis 67–70
  detection of 274–5
Cytomegalovirus 140
Cytotoxic drugs 296

Death
  intra-uterine 163–4
  neonatal, dealing with 164–5
Deep vein thrombosis 147
Delivery, expected date of 3–4
Dental care 55
Depressive illness 112

Desoxycorticosterone 18
Diabetes mellitus 90–7
  antenatal screening 91
  beta-sympathomimetic drugs 205
  delivery 95–6
  gestational 95
  management 93–7
  risks associated with 92–3
Diazepam 231–2, 292
Diet 57–9
Diuretics 88
Down's syndrome 65–6
Drug abuse 113–14
Drugs 289–98
  best avoided 297
  specialist supervision 298
Dubowitz scoring system 263–5

Eclampsia 231–4
  management 233–4
Electrolytes, serum 11–12
Embolism
  amniotic fluid 235–6
  pulmonary 147
Emergencies 227–39
Endocarditis, infective 100
Entonox 186
Enzymes, serum 14–15
Epidural analgesia 186–90
  caesarean section 214
  hazards 187–8
  instrumental delivery 209
  management 189–90
Epilepsy 105–6
Episiotomy 198–9
Ergotamine 296
Erythrocytes 9–10
Erythropoiesis 11
External cephalic version 160–2

Face presentation 195
Family planning advice 284
Fertilization 3
Fetal alcohol syndrome 114–15
Fetal distress 215
Fetal heart rate
  first stage of labour,
    interpretation 217–20
  recording 174–5
    continuous 216–17
    programme for 154
    stethoscope 216
Fetal monitoring,
  intrapartum 215–23
  methods 215–23
Fetal skull, moulding 176

309

# Index

Fetal welfare, assessment 153–5
Feto-placental synthetic
    function 85–7
Fetus
  anomalies, detection 53–4
  growth and development 25
  movements, count of 154
  normal, average measurements 25
*Fetus papyraceous* 162
Fibrinogen 15
Fibrinolytic system 15–17
Flying Squad 227–9
  equipment 228
Folate 11
Forceps
  conditions for proper use 207–8
  trial of 212
  use of 211

Gastric aspiration 236
General anaesthesia, instrumental
    delivery 209–10
General practitioner unit
    confinement 48–9
Genetic counselling 55
Genital warts 135
Gestational age 3
  assessment 4, 28–31
    accurate 53
    neonate 263–9
Glucocorticoid therapy, respiratory
    distress syndrome 206
Glucose tolerance, impaired 91
Glucose tolerance test 91–2
Glucose-6-phosphate 82
Glycosuria 21
Gonorrhoea 130–1
Gravidity 4

Haematological disorders 77–82
Haematological indices 9–10
Haematoma, broad ligament 238
Haemoglobin, falling, causes 77–8
Haemoglobinopathies 79–82
  diagnosis and screening 81
Haemolytic anaemia 82
Haemorrhage
  antepartum 151–3
  primary postpartum 200–1
  secondary postpartum 283
Head
  descent of 172–3
  lag 269
Health education and advice 55–6
Heart
  congenital lesions 73–4
  defects, in pregnancy 97, 101
Heartburn 110
Heel to ear manoeuvre 268
Heparin 150–2
Hepatitis 51, 109
Herpes simplex virus 134–5
Hips, congenital dislocation 270
Hodgkin's disease 82, 117
Hodgkin's lymphoma 82
Home confinement 49
Hospital
  confinement, criteria for 48
  discharge from 285
Hydatidiform mole 19
Hydralazine 87
Hypertension
  antenatal monitoring 88–9
  causes 83–5
  control 233
  mild, management 85–6
  severe, management 86
Hypertensive disorders 82–90
Hyperthyroidism 102
Hypnotics 293
Hypotension, epidural analgesia 187
Hypothalamo-pituitary
    function 19–20
Hypothyroidism 102–3
  congenital, screening for 273
Hypoxia
  effects of 215
  management 223

Impacted shoulders 230
Implantation 3
Infant feeding 279–82
Inhalational agents 186
Instrumental delivery 207–12
  analgesia for 208–10
  indications for 210–11
Insulin 21
  in pregnancy 94
Intra-uterine death 163–4
Intra-uterine growth retardation 29, 155–8
  special care 261
Intra-uterine transfusion 124–5
Iodides 295
Iodine, protein bound 18
Iron 11
  parenteral 77, 79
Irradiation 75

Jaundice 108–10
  neonate 271
    induction of labour 180

# Index

Ketoconazole 291
Kleihauer test 76

Labetalol 87–8
Labour
  analgesia in 184–90
  augmentation 177–8
  bony pelvis and 190–2
  diagnosis 171
  first stage 170–1
  induction 179–83
    failed 180–1
    hazards 180–1
    indications for 179–80
    methods of 182–3
    post-term pregnancy 163
  malpresentation 195–6
  monitoring progress 172–6
  multiple pregnancy 197–8
  normal 170–1
    management 171–6
    progress in 177
  onset 170
  posture during 177
  preparation for 169
  pre-term 201–7
    mode of delivery 206–7
    multiple pregnancy 162
    treatment 203–5
  second stage 178
  third stage 199–200
Lactate, measurement in fetal scalp sample 222
Lactation
  and contraception 284
  enhancement 281
  prescribing during 289
  suppression 281
Lactogen, human placental 43
Leg recoil 268
Legitimacy, and mortality 246–8
Leucocytes 10
Leukaemia
  acute 117
  chronic myeloid 82
Lipids, serum 13–14
Listeriosis 143
Lithium carbonate 292
Live birth, definition 243
Liver 20
  acute fatty degeneration of 109
  diseases 108–11
Lung maturity 158–9
Lupus anticoagulant 104

Magnesium 12
Magnesium sulphate 232
Malaria 142–3
Malignancy 115–17
Mastitis 281–2
Maternity benefit 55–6
Meconium, staining in liquor 222–3
Melanoma 117
Membranes
  premature rupture 207
  spontaneous rupture 183–4
  state of 175–6
Mendelson's syndrome 236
Metronidazole 291
Mortality
  maternal 251–4
    causes 252–3
  perinatal and infant 243–8
    causes 244–6
    factors influencing 246–8
Mosaicism 63, 65
Multiple pregnancy 162
  diagnosis 53
  labour 196–7
  mortality 248
Myasthenia gravis 104–5

*Neisseria gonorrhoea* 272
Neonate 257–75
  death 164–5
  examination
    at birth 262–3
    routine discharge 269
  exchange transfusion 126
  febrile 262
  resuscitation 258–60
  'special care' 261–2
  temperature, maintenance 259–60
Neural tube defects 70–3
Nifedipine 88
Nitrogen 12

Obstetric emergencies 227–39
Oestradiol 35
Oestriol 35
Oestrogen/creatinine ratio 42–3
Oestrogens 35–6
  lactation 281
  urinary 41–2
Oestrone 35
Ophthalmia neonatorum 272
Opiates 113–14, 292
  in labour 185–6
Ossification centres 31
Ovarian tumours 116

311

# Index

Oxprenolol 87
Oxygen, consumption 9
Oxytocin 19
  induction of labour 182–3
  intra-uterine death 164
  lactation 281

Paediatrician, presence at delivery 260
Pain relief, methods for 184–5
Pancreatitis 110
Paracervical block 190
Paralysis, epidural analgesia 187
Parity 4
  and infant mortality 248
Partogram 172
Pediculosis pubis 136
Pelvimetry, X-ray 191–2
Pelvis
  bony, and labour 190–2
  ideal 191
Peptic ulceration 111
Perineal infiltration 208
Pethidine 185
Phenindione 293
Phenothiazines 186
Phenylketonuria 67
  screening for 273
Phenytoin 106
  eclampsia 232
Phosphatidyl-glycerol 158
Phospholipids 13
Phototherapy, jaundice 271
Pituitary tumours 107
Placenta 35–7
  accreta 239
  expulsion 199–200
  functions, tests 40–3
  localization 53
  morbid adherence 239
  postpartum haemorrhage 200–1
  praevia 53, 152
  proteins 36–9
Placental abruption 152
Plasma volume 7
Plasmaphoresis, maternal 125–6
Platelets 10
Pneumonia 108
Polyhydramnios 159–60
Popliteal angle 268
Postnatal exercises 284
Postnatal visit 285
Postpartum 'blues' 122
Post-term
  definition 32
  pregnancy 163

Potassium 11
Pre-eclampsia 84–5
  jaundice complicating 109
  optimum delivery time 90
Pregnancy
  early diagnosis 47–8
  length of 3
  physiological changes in 7–22
  prescribing during 289
  tests 47–8
Pre-term
  definition 32
  labour 201–7
Progesterone 36
Propranolol 87, 295
Prostacyclin 14
Prostaglandins 13–14
  induction of labour 182–3
  intra-uterine death 164
Prostaglandin-synthetase inhibitors 205
Proteins
  placental 36–9
  serum 12–13
Psychiatric disorders 111–15
Psychotropic drugs 113, 292
Pudendal nerve block 208–9
Puerperal psychosis 113
Puerperium 279
  pyrexia 282–3
Pulmonary embolism 147
Pyelonephritis 144–5
Pyloric stenosis 74–5
Pyrexia, puerperal 282–3

Relaxin 15
Renal function 17
Renin 17
Reserpine 294
Respiratory diseases 107–8
Respiratory distress syndrome 206
Respiratory function 8–9
Resuscitation 258–60
Rh factor 121–2
Rhesus iso-immunization 121–6
  prediction of severity 122–4
  timing of intervention 124
Rhesus sensitization, prevention 283
Rheumatic heart disease 97
Rifampicin 291
Ritodrine hydrochloride 204–5
Rubella 138–40
  vaccination 284

Salbutamol 204
Salicylates 291

# Index

Scabies 136
Scarf sign 268
Seat belts 55
Sedatives, hypertension 88
Sex steroids 294
Sexually transmitted
 diseases 129−37
Shake test 158−9
Shoulders, impacted 230
Sickle-cell disease 80−1
Sickling crises 80−1
Single gene disorders 66−70
Smoking 27, 55
 and mortality 248
Social class, and mortality 246−8
Sodium 11
Spalding's sign 163
Special care baby unit 261−2
Spina bifida 70
Square window 263
Status asthmaticus 107
Status eclampticus 233
Status epilepticus 106
Steroids 293
 sex 294
Stethoscope 216
Stillbirth 164−5
Sulphonamides 290
Syntometrine 199
Syphilis 132−3
 congenital 134
Systemic lupus erythematosus 104

Talipes equinovarus 270
Tears, third degree 198−9
Term, definition 32
Tetracyclines 290
Thalassaemias 70, 79−80
Thrombocytopaenic purpura,
 idiopathic 81−2
Thrombo-embolism 147−51
 management 148−50
 prophylaxis 150−1
Thrombosis, deep vein 147
Thromboxane 14
Thyroid disorders 102−3
Thyroid drugs 295
Thyroid function 18
Thyroid stimulating hormone 19
Thyroidectomy, subtotal 102
Thyroiditis, post-partum 103
Thyroxine 18
 free index 19
Toxoplasmosis 142
Tranquillizers, hypertension 88

Transfusion
 intra-uterine 124−5
 neonatal exchange 126
Transverse lie 196
Travel during pregnancy 55
Treponemal infections 131−4
TRIC agent 272
Trichomoniasis 130
Tri-iodothyronine 18
 resin uptake test 19
Trisomy 65
Trypsin testing, cystic fibrosis 275
Tubal ligation 284
Tuberculosis, pulmonary 107−8
 neonate 272−3
Twin labour, management 197
Twin pregnancy, presentations 196

Ulcerative colitis 111
Ulcers, peptic 111
Ultrasound 51−4
 cephalometry 28−9
 diagnostic, use of 52−4
 multiple pregnancy 162
 safety 51−2
Unstable lie 162−3
Urea, pre-eclampsia 89
Urethritis, non-specific 135−6
Uric acid 12
 pre-eclampsia 89
Urinary tract infections 144−5
Uterus
 fundus, height 31
 inversion 238−9
 rupture 236−7

Vaccination 55
 BCG 272−3
 rubella 139−40, 284
Vaccines 291
Venography 147
Ventouse 208
 use of 212
Ventral suspension 269
Viral infections 141
Vitamin $B_{12}$ 11

Warfarin therapy 150, 293
Water intoxication 183
Weight gain in pregnancy 21−2

X-linked disorders 67
X-ray pelvimetry 191−2

Yaws 132

# When Grandad Went Train Spotting

## Maxwell Jackson

Published in the UK in 2023 by M & H Press,

Email: jacksonhms@gmail.com

ISBN: 978-1-3999-5989-6

Copyright © 2023 Maxwell J B Jackson

The right of Maxwell J B Jackson to be identified as the Author of this book has been asserted in accordance with the Copyrights, Designs and Patents Act 1988.

All rights reserved. No part of this book may be reproduced in any form or by any means without prior written permission from the publisher.

A CIP record for this book is available from the British Library.

Set in 12 Pt Times New Roman

Printed and bound by Ashley House Printing, Exeter, EX2 8QF

**For my wife, Héloïse,**

who deserves some explanation for my ongoing fascination with the steam railway and to thank her for all the work she put into the preparation of this book.

# CONTENTS

| Chapter | | Page |
|---|---|---|
| 1 | Awakening the Interest | 1 |
| 2 | Holidays with Steam | 24 |
| 3 | Like Minds | 35 |
| 4 | Intrepid Pursuits | 52 |
| 5 | Memorable Places | 74 |
| 6 | Rambling Around | 103 |
| 7 | Digging Deeper | 117 |
| 8 | Collecting the Memories | 134 |
| 9 | A Scottish Diversion | 152 |
| 10 | Timetables, Guides and other Distractions | 157 |
| 11 | Questions of Colour and other Reflections | 167 |
| 12 | Somewhat off the Rails | 185 |
| 13 | Legacy | 201 |
| | POSTSCRIPT | 212 |

# ACKNOWLEDGEMENTS

Thanks are due to all those shed masters and works managers who so willingly facilitated visits to their premises; also to all those well-disposed railwaymen, present and departed, who understood our enthusiasm.

Thanks to:

Crécy Publishing for permission to include pictures of early Ian Allan ABCs.

Samuel Jackson (www.jxnfilms.com) film maker and all round digital whizz, for help with layout.

James Mutton for his valued guidance on the cover design.

All photographs are by the author. Those taken at the National Railway Museum are published with permission from the Science Museum Group.

# PREFACE

Trainspotting, or more accurately loco spotting, was a minor social phenomenon in Britain, especially between about 1947 and 1967.

Its participants were mostly teenage boys. That said, many older men took a keen but less conspicuous interest in all aspects of railways, especially the locomotives.

The activity has always attracted good natured ridicule. It was never a surprise when utter incomprehension evoked jokes about anoraks, nerds and watching puff-puffs. It took more than that to stop us. After all, it was not all idyllic summer days; we could suffer for our hobby in rain, wind and cold! Any attempt to explain or rationalise loco-spotting is bound to be inadequate, simply because every spotter's experience could be so different. Maybe there was a little more to it than was apparent at first sight.

For all its shortcomings, here is an attempt to look beyond mere number collecting and the comradeship which that might have engendered. Why did they bother and more interestingly, what made such a pastime so engaging?

In the following pages I invite you to share some personal recollections and reflections and, if you were ever a spotter, I suspect they might evoke some memories of your own. Alternatively, they may explain what grandad got up to.

From the social historian to the merely curious, I beg your indulgence for any technical or other references which I have included for the benefit of those 'in the know'.

M.J.

# EXPLANATORY NOTES

Steam locomotives fell into two principal types. Tender engines carried their coal and water supplies in a following tender, typically up to 5,000 gallons of water and 5 tons of coal. Tank engines usually carried their coal in a rear bunker and their water in side tanks, a saddle tank sitting astride the boiler, pannier tanks either side of the boiler or well tanks, a rare arrangement with the tanks within the loco frames.

Names like Bullied, Robinson, Wainwright and others occur in the text. They refer to the Chief Mechanical Engineers of pre-Nationalisation companies and they were responsible for specific locomotive designs.

Loco wheel arrangements were described using the Whyte notation; e.g. 4-6-2 denoted 4 leading wheels, 6 driving wheels and 2 trailing wheels. Each notation had a corresponding name; thus 4-6-2 was *Pacific*. In the case of tank engines, the suffix would indicate the type of tanks; e.g. 0-6-0 PT (Pannier).

Named classes of locomotives had official class designations but spotters often adopted unofficial names. The nickname chosen varied in different parts of the country.

When many more stations operated, terms like Express, Semi-fast and Slow, (affectionately called 'Stoppers'), generally reflected the duration of a journey. The pace of acceleration and average line speeds to-day have rendered those distinctions largely meaningless.

# CHAPTER ONE — Awakening the Interest

The constant passage of trains, not 200 yards from my bedroom window, was the noisy backdrop to my early years. It was not any railway line, but the main line from London to the West Country.

So normal was the background sound of trains that if ever I was away from home, I did not exactly worry about the relative silence, but I would enquire whether there was a railway somewhere in the vicinity. In that case, I remained curious until an indulgent parent took me to see it.

At home, the trains ran along the top of an embankment, separated from my home by nothing more than a single house and an expanse of allotment gardens, so I enjoyed a good view of all the comings and goings.

By the age of five or six I was wondering where exactly all these trains were going to and where did they stop on the way? Why did most of the engines follow one of two or three basic shapes? Why did they mostly head trains of twelve carriages but sometimes only eight? Almost everything was green, and that included the frequent electric trains. The local ones slipped quietly by, but those bound for Portsmouth, as I later learned, were faster and made much more noise.

For sheer drama though, nothing could beat the steam-hauled expresses, either accelerating westwards or easing off as they approached the final nine miles of suburbs into Waterloo. They usually announced their approach by a distant whistle and, after a moment's delay, were seen pounding along the embankment top. A brief change of note followed as they crossed a steel road bridge, before disappearing behind distant trees or houses and then they were gone.

Sometimes, a slight purple haze hung in the air for a few moments, but otherwise they left no trace. It never much mattered. There would soon be another one and meanwhile those electrics provided some distraction. That is how it all started, a long-standing interest in railways generally and steam trains in particular.

Meanwhile, I cannot have been alone. In 1942, Ian Allan, a 20 year old employee of the then Southern Railway at Waterloo, published a booklet listing the different classes of locomotives and their identifying numbers. That edition of just 2000 copies was a success and ultimately represented the foundation of the extensive publishing company bearing his name. Similar booklets, ABCs as they were titled, soon became available for the remaining three pre-nationalisation companies, the Great Western, the London Midland and Scottish and the London and North Eastern Railways, companies known collectively as the Big Four. Thus a hobby was born and train spotting, from the late 1940s to the end of steam in the late 1960s, came to acquire a huge following.

That was not quite the full story because men, and boys in particular, had been fascinated by trains from their earliest appearance. The National Railway Museum holds a letter from a fourteen year old boy, describing Stephenson's Locomotion No.1 and its train, on the occasion of the opening of the Stockton and Darlington railway in 1825. The Berkshire Records Office has a diary of a John Treacher of Sonning, noting the names of locomotives passing Reading during 1840. This is probably the earliest evidence of loco spotting as we know it to-day. That early dependence on names alone to distinguish locomotives was clearly not sustainable. By that year there were, for example, already no less than ten engines named 'Liver' or 'Liverpool'. Another 14 year old, this time in 1861, a girl named Fanny Johnson, from Westbourne Park, listed the names and numbers of Great Western engines. That was another early example of noting what had been observed and no doubt many other train watchers were recording their own observations.

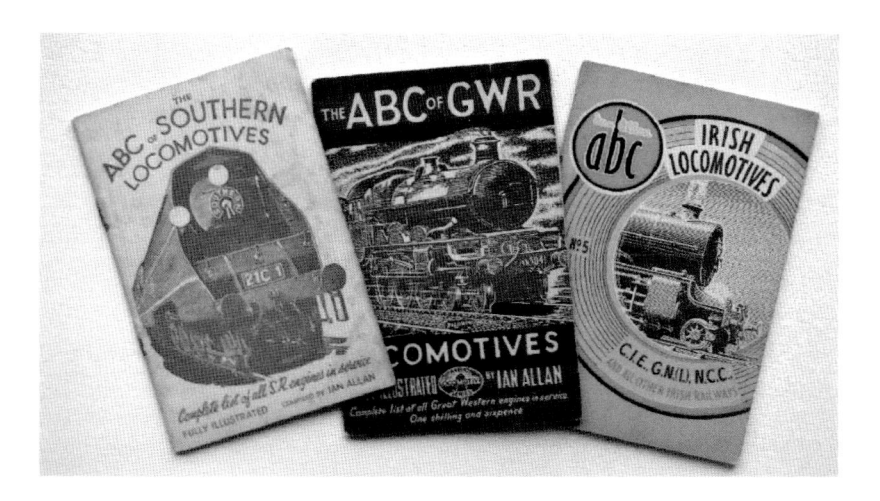

*Some early ABCs: The Southern 5th edition, dated October 1943, is noteworthy, considering the first edition had appeared only ten months previously. The Great Western example dates from October 1945, whilst the 1949 Irish edition follows a slightly different format. It includes a lot of fascinating historical information regarding the constituent companies*

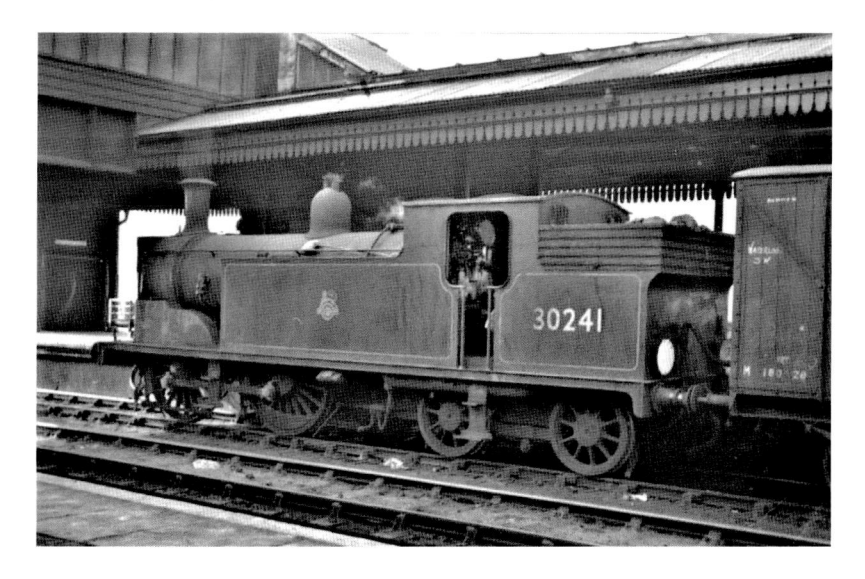

*Pictures of specific engines can still evoke vivid memories all these years later. To the casual observer, this is just another M7 class tank. For the writer it recalls a Sunday afternoon riding on the footplate whilst shunting empty carriages in the yard at Clapham Junction.*

Some railway publicity departments encouraged the publication of postcards illustrating their trains and these became collectable, much in the way people collect postage stamps. Clearly the band of enthusiasts was on the increase, giving rise to the appearance of the Railway Magazine in 1897. It came to review new locomotive types, new routes and services, improvements in stations, developments in freight handling, signalling, railway catering and just about every other aspect of railway history and operation.

By 1899 several lists of engine names and numbers had been published. Nevertheless, it was the eventual arrival of the ABC's which enabled enthusiasts to put their sightings into some sort of coherent order and context. It was no longer just names and numbers for their own sake, but it offered an element of challenge, the search to see every example of each class of locomotive. That in turn encouraged close observation of detail variations between engines, whilst some numbers acquired an almost mythical status when they represented a unique locomotive or a type identified with a very particular location. Those examples often had a fascinating history of their own which was of wider engineering or geographical interest.

Until 1923, something approaching 150 separate railway companies had operated in the UK. Although it made economic and operating sense to group them into the Big Four, a good deal of regional character was lost in doing so, not least in the appearance of locomotives and trains.

The individual companies adopted different colour liveries, lettering styles, approaches to locomotive and rolling stock design and for the paying passenger, different levels of speed and comfort. Some enthusiasts concentrated their energies on railway photography and it is remarkable just how many railway related photographs were taken prior to the 1923 grouping, bearing in mind that photography as a widespread popular interest, really took off only during the 1920s. Others concentrated on locomotive performance. The privileged few with footplate access, minutely recorded train loads, journey times and speeds, coal consumption, gradients and how the driver was handling his engine at every stage along the route, and these records were published in magazines.

All this, together with the considerable physical legacy from those days, was shared by all railway enthusiasts. Nevertheless, despite the diversity of interests, it was the steam locomotive itself which provided the common thread between the great majority of them and it was therefore no surprise that Ian Allan's ABCs met with such immediate success.

Because my grand-parents lived in London, my mother frequently took me by train to Waterloo, when I would be puzzled by ticket barriers where it was frequently announced that 'All tickets must be shewn'. The quaint spelling did not seem to bother either of my parents and I never encountered it elsewhere. If my father joined us after his work I knew the journey home would be fun. Dad and I would leave the bus at Bank station and Mum would continue to Waterloo. Meanwhile, we would take the 'Shooter', as City workers nicknamed the Waterloo and City underground train. The line itself was less glamorously named 'The Drain'. Both titles amused me.

At that time there was a late evening service every few minutes, though scarcely anyone used it at that hour. Dad threw off any sense of City suited propriety and like two liberated school boys we would hurtle down the endless short flights of steps in the tunnel which led down to the train. It was always waiting for us and we would tumble in giggling and breathless.

There was no confusing these trains with the red London Transport variety. These were instead a rather mysterious shade of metallic malachite green. In spite of their very modern appearance, internally they were both cramped and very noisy. There were fretwork metal ventilator grilles either side of the carriage ends, reading 'SOUTHERN' and 'RAILWAY', and it was a long time into British Railways days before the

'RAILWAY' grilles were replaced by rather shaky hand-cut aluminium versions of 'REGION'. Surely, that was one of the very last references to the pre-nationalisation company.

Arriving at Waterloo we met Mum and a quick conference decided if the fun could continue. The formula was for her to take the 8:25pm stopping train to Raynes Park and meanwhile Dad and I took the 8:30pm to Guildford, first stop Wimbledon. This produced the slightly nail-biting uncertainty of whether or not we would overhaul Mum's train just before she reached Wimbledon. Sometimes it was a close run thing but we always managed to scurry across the platform in time to join her for the last couple of miles home.

Sometimes Dad took me to work with him on a Saturday morning, after which we might visit the Science Museum, with its locomotive related display. The annual Model Railway Engineers' Exhibition at Central hall, Westminster, was a favourite, and for a couple of years, a close up inspection of a Romney Hythe and Dymchurch Railway engine, displayed on the concourse of Waterloo station, was another treat. In 1947, the 15 inch gauge RH & D Railway was re-opened to the public after its war-time years of coastal defence service.

Displaying one of its locomotives in London was good publicity for the revived railway and presumably the main line railway saw it as a means of encouraging excursion traffic to the Kent coast. Not too many families had cars in those days and holiday traffic on the railways in the summer months was intense, especially on Saturdays. It was not long before my parents treated me to such a trip, including a ride on the RH & D Railway behind No.1, Green Goddess, which left a big impression.

My grandfather never showed any particular interest in locomotives. What was noticeable however, was his apparent knowledge of routes, scenery and journey times to destinations within a large radius of London. He would express them in pre-grouping terms. For example, if a journey to Exeter was contemplated, he would ask if it was to be by Great Western or the South Western. I later came to see that this sort of detailed knowledge would be common currency amongst business and tradespeople who had grown up before almost universal car use.

As he introduced me to London bus travel, I noticed in some central areas there were bold printed cards, displayed in the windows of certain commercial premises. They might display letters like NWR, GE or LTS. Grandfather was immediately able to explain that these were messages to railway carters on their regular rounds, to stop by for a collection, in these cases for the ex-London and North Western Railway route from Euston, the ex-Great Eastern from Liverpool Street or the London Tilbury and Southend from Fenchurch Street. Such was the intimate role the railways played in commercial life, even until the early years immediately after nationalisation.

At that time, my grandfather would occasionally take me on a Saturday trip from Liverpool Street to Southend, which was still before I became a committed spotter. Nevertheless, the fact it was steam and not electric travel was sufficient to attract my interest. To arrive at Southend Victoria behind a Sandringham 4-6-0 and see it at close quarters was, for me, a pleasing introduction to the town. There followed a regular pattern involving ice-cream, whelks, a walk to the end of the 1 and 1/3 mile long pier and a ride back on the pier railway.

On one of these occasions the return journey was undertaken in some decidedly elderly carriages, unusually painted in an overall somewhat bilious shade of brown, presumably reserved for excursion traffic. They were noticeably uncomfortable too. On the other hand I was quite excited by the fact that after passing Stratford we took a left turn to end up at Fenchurch Street station. What particularly caught my attention were the rather ghostly and obviously closed stations of Bow Road and Burdett Road which we passed through on the way. The impression they left stayed with me and was to re-surface some years later when stations were fast closing and steam was in rapid decline.

My regular trips up to Waterloo had made me aware of the peculiarities of the suburban electric trains, as well as the detail interest along the route, in particular the best places to see locomotives. We usually boarded the train at Raynes Park station where there was a likelihood of seeing steam hauled expresses at close quarters. They would busy themselves through on the up and down fast lines, which ran between the suburban tracks. The thunderous noise as they crossed the bridge above Approach Road added to the drama.

Just occasionally the routine would be broken by the passing of, for example, a train of nothing but parcels vans, or at ten minutes past seven of an evening, a short loose-coupled freight train from the local goods yard would come bustling up the steep gradient from the underpass loop off the Epsom branch, on its way to Wimbledon yard, behind an 1880's vintage London & South Western '0395' freight locomotive.

On one occasion a King Arthur class loco, obviously struggling on its way to London, struck me how differently individual members of a class could appear. The King Arthurs usually went about their work in a business-like way and drew no particular attention, but on this occasion this two-cylinder engine was oscillating alarmingly from side to side, the tender whipping violently. It looked not unlike a car driver losing control of an unstable caravan. The whole thing was so disconcerting that it occurred to me to identify the engine for future reference but by then it was too late to read its name or number.

Sometimes, we took the train from Wimbledon, which I associated with two things; first was Wimbledon Nell, a stuffed dog in a display case, which had once progressed around the station collecting coins for the railway orphanage, and secondly, the noise. The sound of express trains passing through was deafening, especially since drivers seemed to delight in sounding their whistles for several seconds at a time. I liked both these features but found each, in its way, slightly uncomfortable.

After Wimbledon, it was worth looking out for the electric shunter, which spent most of its life on the coaling ramp at Durnsford Road power station. Built in 1899 and carrying the departmental service number of DS74, this was already an ageing electric pioneer and something of a curiosity, which eventually survived until 1965. Equally predictable was the greater activity found at Clapham Junction, where shunting engines worked the carriage sidings. I soon got to remember some of their numbers and realised they were regulars on these duties. These same engines often appeared at Waterloo, where they had delivered an empty train, cleaned and prepared for perhaps a west of England express, or maybe for a Southampton boat train.

From Clapham Junction, the next stretch was interesting because it took us past Nine Elms loco sheds. These were set back, effectively out of view. However, there was a spot where engines stood before entering or leaving the depot area. On one occasion our local train made a signal stop and we found ourselves alongside a row of three of these engines. In such proximity, simmering gently, their appearance contrasted sharply with their appearance when in full cry.

These were the same engines which came screeching past in view from my bedroom window, throughout the day and into the night. Then, the orange glow from open firebox doors reflected off the underside of the plume of exhaust steam, as it traced above the cab and which then gave way to the blurred yellow glow of the carriage lights, following in its wake. Now, much pacified, as they waited to return to the shed, it took a bit of mental adjustment to recognise them in such different circumstances.

Next was Vauxhall, which had two features which caught my eye. On the up side, platform No.1 was almost always occupied by a milk train, apparently in the process of being discharged via the pipe work permanently installed on the platform.

Almost without exception it was headed by an M7 0-4-4 tank which had brought it up from Clapham Junction, following its arrival from Torrington, as I was later to learn. The six-wheeled milk tank wagons employed were introduced in the 1920s and continued to operate until 1981. They mostly looked very grubby. Although they might have born announcements that they were glass or stainless steel lined, they never looked very savoury.

By all accounts, the footplate crews, who had to stand-by during this lengthy process, were inclined to make the most of it by catching up on reading or grabbing a nap, especially on the night shift, and who could blame them?

The wall flanking the down slow line on the opposite side of the station also caught my attention, not for any loco interest but for its repetitious insistent advertising. Each panel in the wall construction bore a prominent enamelled advertisement. These alternated between a sign for the food supplement, Virol, and one for Stephen's Ink, extending the greater length of the platform. Eventually, the Virol signs expired and gave way to repeated ink advertisements. Both these signs had been widely displayed both on the railways and elsewhere and were very much of their time, i.e. pre-grouping days, some lingering on until the 1970s. Both products faded from popular memory in the years following the end of steam, so, by the time the signs were removed from Vauxhall, they were simply providing no more than a familiar decorative feature to the station.

Waterloo at that time had 21 platforms. Although electric trains dominated, there was nevertheless nearly always a number of steam engines to be seen close up, at the buffer

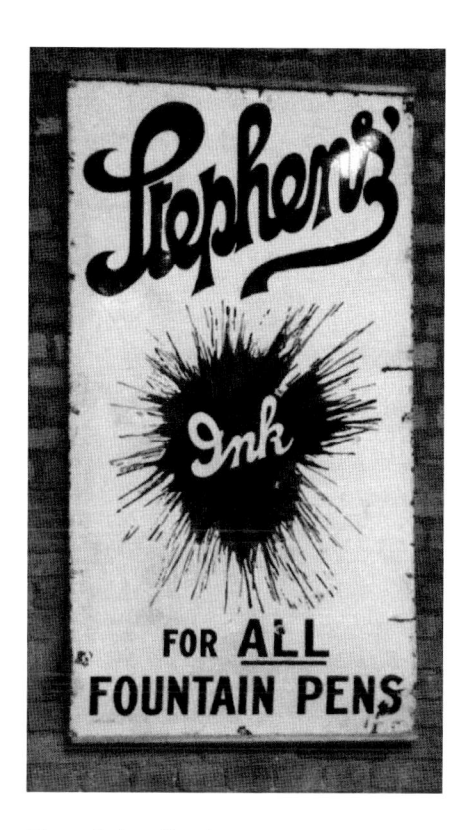

*Enamel signs like these appeared widely on stations in the first half of the 20th century. They had been a common form of advertising since the late 1800s, covering anything from bicycles and motor oil to paint and patent medicines. Stephens' Ink and VIROL were particularly prominent on railway stations. The VIROL food supplement signs employed a number of strap lines which themselves were almost worth collecting. They included 'Nervous people need it', 'Anaemic girls need it' and 'Delicate children need it'. The oddest of all was 'Wonderful flesh former'!*

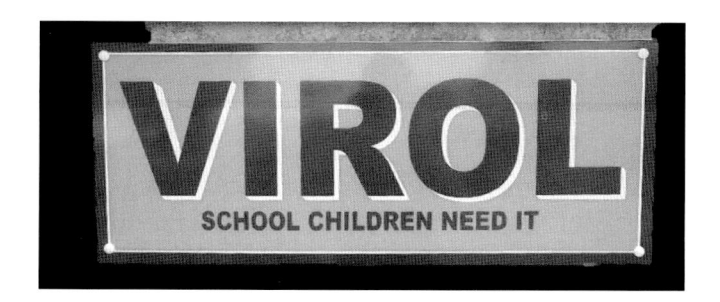

stops. These were in total contrast to the tantalising glimpses of distant clusters of engines at Stewarts Lane shed, or rather closer examples when we passed Nine Elms depot, all seen from our local trains to Waterloo.

These regular visits to Waterloo produced some vivid memories, not all directly concerned with the railway. For example, for many weeks in 1948 there were film sets to be seen for the making of the Ealing comedy, 'Passport to Pimlico'. These were off to the right, on flattened bomb sites, just before the approach to the terminus.

Then, before entering the station, we often paused at a signal check. If we were travelling outside the rush hour, there would be three or four sidings occupied by empty electric trains, but at busier times, when these were pressed into service, there was an intriguing view of two rather mysterious platforms, lying a little way off to the right. I puzzled over these for some time and then gradually, over a year or two, they were tidied up, shortened one after the other, and finally they disappeared, before a series of cabins and temporary buildings began to appear. It was many years later when I discovered these platforms had been the track-side remains of the London Necropolis Company's funeral station, much of which had been laid to ruin by bombing in April 1941.

With a bit of luck I would sometimes catch sight of a departing express, just as our electric pulled in. In fact it was often the journey back home from Waterloo which I enjoyed the most. Waiting for our train to leave, I might watch a wheel tapper with his long shafted hammer, working along the train opposite. When it was explained to me that a dull clunk would indicate a cracked wheel, I would listen intently. One day the clunk actually came but to my disappointment the wheel tapper just moved on nonchalantly.

A more engrossing distraction was provided by the guards who would switch their hand oil lamps from white to

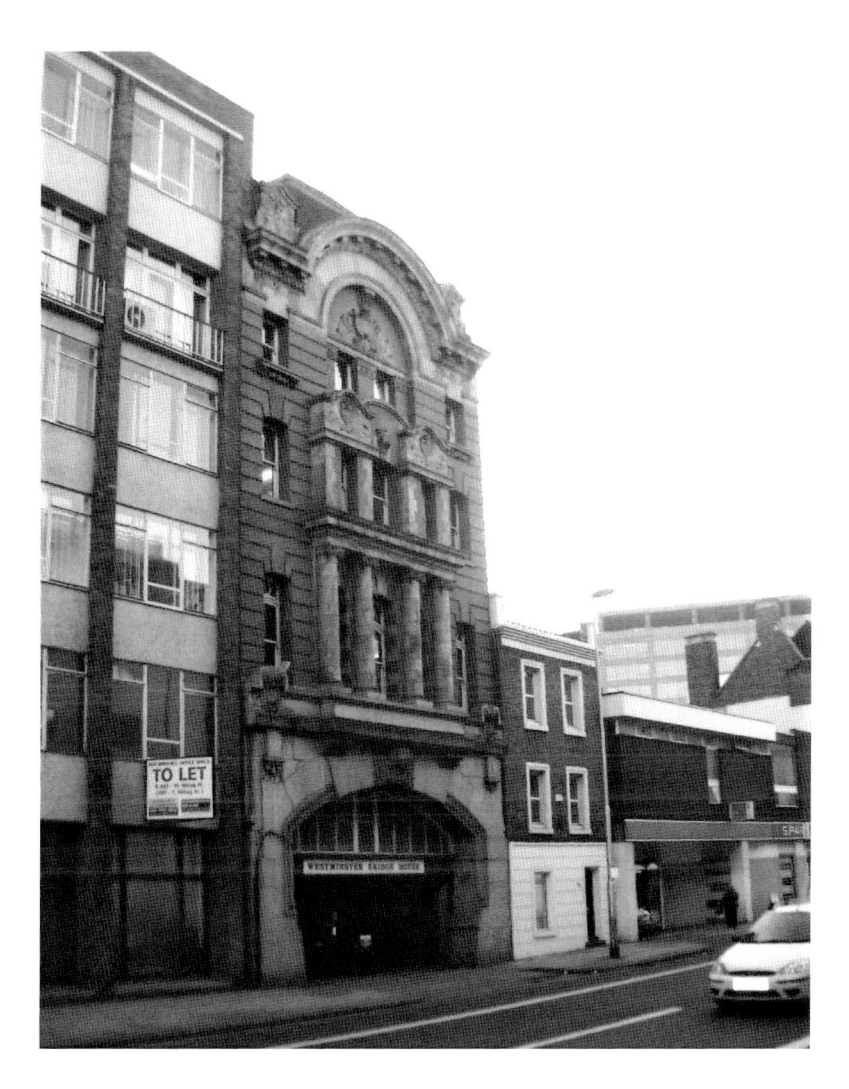

*An interest in the loco spotting environment could lead in all manner of unexpected directions. Although the track level buildings of Waterloo Necropolis station were obliterated during a Second World War bombing raid, the 1902 office building of the London Necropolis Co. survived intact, along with the two platforms at track level above. Funeral trains to Brookwood continued briefly from the main station after the bombing but soon ceased and in due course, the old Necropolis platforms were removed. A little research revealed that M7 0-4-4 tank engines, more familiar on empty carriage workings between Clapham Junction and Waterloo, had regularly worked the funeral trains. Is it imagination that the building seems to project an appropriate doom laden quality? After all, the arched entrance off the street is not everyone's idea of the Pearly Gates.*

green to give the driver the all-clear, but swing themselves aboard the train only once it was in motion. To my secret disappointment I never saw a guard get left behind as a result of this practiced bravado.

The best moments came when our departure time corresponded with that of a main line train, preferably hauled by a Lord Nelson. Sometimes we would run alongside the locomotive for a few seconds when I would watch the tender springs flexing as it worked its way towards the down fast line. A second or two later I would glimpse the fireman already at work and the driver getting his eye in for the road ahead.

That, though, was just the beginning. Our suburban electric would surge forward towards our first stop at Vauxhall. Only as we moved off again might we get a rearward glimpse of the express we had left behind. We were usually leaving Clapham Junction before it overtook us, accelerating purposefully, if not yet very fast. Then we would overhaul it again, this time rather slowly, getting the full sensation of pent up power as we drew alongside and passed the locomotive which, by now, was getting into a rhythm. It had not yet hit the pace of those trains seen from my bedroom window but it undoubtedly meant business.

The repetitive motion of valve gear and connecting rods, along with the staccato huff of the four cylinder exhaust, momentarily blocked out other impressions. If we were yet to get ahead of the express we knew it would not be for long. From almost rubbing shoulders with this 83 ton engine, it was now bearing down upon us, the driver giving it its head, no time to watch it now as it thumped past, carriages clickety clacking, nine, ten, eleven, twelve and gone, our upstart electric put firmly in its place.

These regular observations increasingly engaged my curiosity. I wanted to know where various branch-lines led to, what sort of trains served the numerous destinations on the Waterloo departure indicator and just where those places were.

Then, there were the little motor tractors which sped around the station concourse diving around groups of waiting passengers and hauling their own trains of trolleys, frequently stacked high with mail bags. Occasionally the groups of passengers would include some oddly dressed boys who, it was explained to me, were Blue Coat School boys wearing their traditional Tudor style uniforms. More correctly, they were pupils of Christ's Hospital School, probably returning to school at Horsham for the beginning of term.

More frequently observed obstacles on the station concourse were stacked up wicker baskets of racing pigeons, with their destination labels clearly attached. The birds always seemed happy enough but were, no doubt, seen as priority traffic to be transported in the guard's compartment and released at, for the pigeons, some bewildering unfamiliar location. In short, I wanted to understand everything about the working environment in which the locomotives operated. So far, I had noticed that locomotive depots and large stations always promised plenty of activity.

The Nine Elms goods yard by contrast, in spite of its extent, seemed very unpromising, with nothing to see apart from one or two pre-War, ex-Southern Railway, diesel electric shunters, of classic English Electric type. Not once do I recall seeing a freight train on the move in that area. I did occasionally see a main line train of parcels vans but that did not seem to be anything special since it was common practice to add one or two vans to the tail of West of England expresses. No, what was missing was the sight of an out and out freight engine at work on the main line.

I was aware of the shunting that went on in Wimbledon west yard but I had not appreciated that the Southern Region was essentially passenger orientated. There was no reason I would be taken to Feltham, where 'proper' freights were marshalled and in any case they would have headed south-west or northwards on inter-regional traffic. Dad suggested goods trains to and from Nine Elms probably moved at night, so I rather stopped looking out for them.

Some while later, I was taken to see family members living in Chiswick. In the evening, misjudging the time it took to walk to Chiswick station, we arrived there to see our Clapham Junction bound electric train just departing. That meant half an hour to sit on a platform bench in the dark, quite a demand on a six or seven year old.

Boredom set in quickly when suddenly, out of the darkness appeared a train of twenty to thirty empty loose coupled mineral wagons. The 0-6-0 tender engine, puffed gently past without remark, but what followed was much more attention-grabbing. Firstly the wagons started to concertina together, gently at first but then the rapid series of compressions which followed progressively down the length of the train, set in motion a corresponding series of staccato metallic rings, as buffers met buffers, like hammers on anvils.

Before that sequence was complete the driver opened the regulator so the engine and the first few wagons surged forwards, inducing a cacophony of echoing booms, groans, squeaks and clangs in the following wagons, as their three-link couplings protested against being snatched one by one, in quick succession, as the train visibly accelerated away.

As quickly as the engine had appeared, so too did the guard's brake van disappear into the night. I was impressed by the proximity of all this theatre and became aware of just how massive were those 16 ton wagons which looked small and insignificant when seen sitting idle in sidings. From that point forward I became even more on the look-out for freight trains but had to be content with the odd glimpse of one until my spotting days started seriously.

Until the late 1950s coal remained a major commodity transported by rail. Large quantities were still carried for domestic use, to say nothing of some twelve million or so tons consumed as loco coal and another two million tons for generating electricity for railway use, which, taking an example, was the case in 1957. Little wonder the long coal train was perhaps the archetypal freight train of the 1950s and where there were coal trains, there were empty wagon trains. The train seen at Chiswick that night had probably come from Willesden or Brent, bound for Nine Elms, but why were the wagons empty when it was heading towards Clapham Junction and Nine Elms?

I cannot answer that question but what I do know is the importance of sounds as much as imagery in creating a mood and sense of place. Much as the sounds of that train of empties impressed me, it was no accident that films and plays used similar background noises of wagon-shunting to set the scene. There was something about those sounds which was meaningful to a wide audience. I wonder if it would still have the same resonance with a modern film or theatre audience.

Something a little less usual happened at Waterloo one Saturday morning when my father took me through an open ticket barrier for a close up look at a rather smart, moderately sized engine, standing at the buffers. I was admiring its olive green paintwork and polished brass fittings in the cab, when the driver stepped down with an oil can and rag in his hand. As he walked forward, he paused to say something to my father, nodding towards the engine. Dad bent down to relay the message that this was the Royal Engine. He seemed to say it with a sort of hushed respect as if he was in the privileged presence of the King himself. I must have been about 6 years old at the time but it was enough to impress upon me that some engines were indeed special. I now realise this must have been T9 class no. 119.

From the frequency of my journeys to and from Waterloo, I had already come to remember those engines I saw regularly. From then on I started to look at the numbers even more carefully, with no real purpose other than knowing that a number conferred a certain individuality on an engine. I also became aware of just how many engines carried name plates, which was a further confirmation of their uniqueness.

After nationalisation, which had occurred on the 1$^{st}$ January 1948, the Southern Railway had become the Southern Region of British Railways, and all its steam locomotives were renumbered in the 30,000 series. I never had occasion to remark on this at the time and continued my wider railway observations, albeit mostly over the same route to Waterloo and always by electric train.

The electrics moved in sets; that is to say in fixed formations of carriages, mostly in twos or fours. They carried their identification numbers on each end of the set, in the corresponding number plate position found at the front of a steam engine. Historically, most locomotives had carried painted numbers on their front buffer beams. Only at nationalisation did the other companies fall in line with LMS practice, displaying a cast iron number plate on the smoke box door.

Electric trains did not compare with steam locomotives. Nevertheless, they were not devoid of interest. Some of the older ones dated from pre-grouping days and might consist of carriages of quite different shapes. A common variation occurred when a three-carriage set had been lengthened by the insertion of an extra carriage, but of very different provenance, leading to a rather ad hoc appearance. Continuous running boards and rows of bulky brass grab handles along their sides could add to their period character, whilst creaking bodywork and loudly ticking electric motors further betrayed their age.

The interiors too could produce some strange arrangements. Just occasionally, one could find oneself not in a compartment at all but in a family saloon, complete with a fixed central black varnished table and bench seats along the sides. How was it ever used? Did families of twenty hire them for the day? Another odd experience was the half compartment, where a row of passengers sat facing a blank 'wall'. Presumably it had been an attempt to carry a few more passengers in the train. Then, there were the compartments with generous armrests between the seats, which had been sewn up in the closed upright position, again in order to seat an extra couple of passengers in each compartment. I gathered this was done during the Second World War.

One of my favourites had a rather low gently curving ceiling. Each compartment had a circular brass ventilator and a cornice moulding around the perimeter of what looked like a heavily embossed lincrusta lined ceiling. Below were correspondingly low bench seats on either side of the compartment. Covered with deep horse hair filled mattress-like cushions, these completed the impression of a tiny Edwardian sitting-room.

Another characteristic of the electric trains was a letter displayed on the front, which indicated the route it was taking. That could help passengers when they decoded it by reference to departure indicators on station platforms. On the other hand, steam locomotives carried white painted discs in an assortment of positions. On the Southern Region, these gave similar indications and also whether they were light engines or hauling freight trains. This was informative to signalmen but remained a bit esoteric to the casual observer.

One Saturday, I was invited to join my father and a friend of his who was planning to buy a cottage in north Buckinghamshire. We were to travel from Baker Street to Aylesbury by train. When I understood this to be a London Transport route I was not over enthusiastic. That changed when it was explained we would change from electric to steam traction at Rickmansworth.

On that basis, it was hard to resist. What I had not appreciated was that the journey was to start in brown painted former Metropolitan Railway carriages, known as 'Dreadnoughts', pulled by an ageing electric locomotive. This was painted a dismal grey colour which had been adopted as a

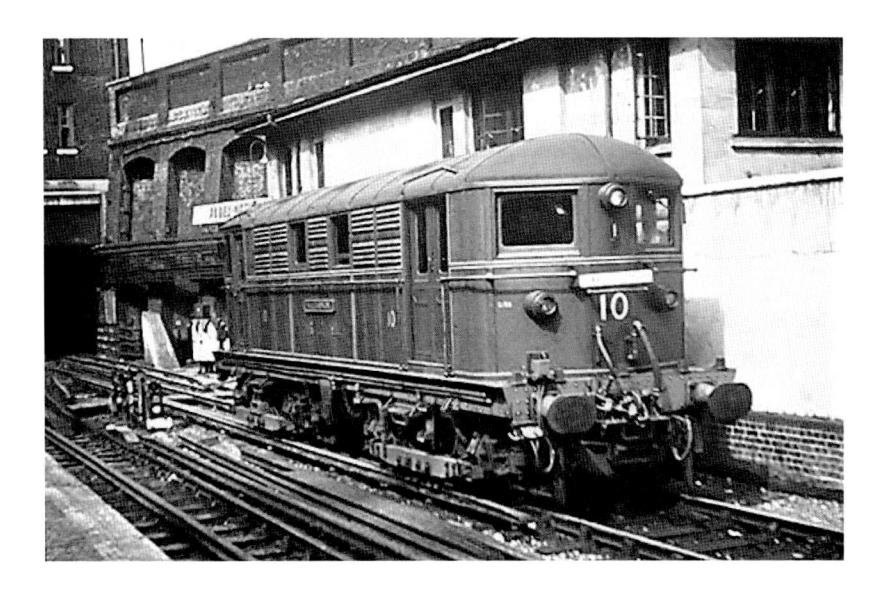

A 'Growler'; Metropolitan Railway electric locomotive No. 10, W E Gladstone, at Baker Street in April 1960. It had been built in 1923 and named William Ewart Gladstone. During the Second World War, all members of the class were painted a drab light grey, without their nameplates. From 1953 they retrieved their Metropolitan red livery and their nameplates, but this example had its name abbreviated. Had one of the plates been lost or damaged during the War? No.10 and its colleagues were withdrawn in 1962, a year after electrification to Amersham was completed.

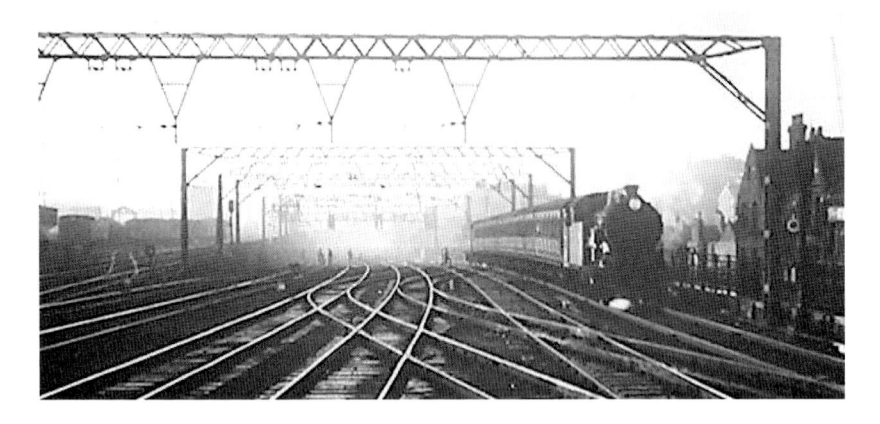

An N7 class tank, with its 'Quint-Art' group of five articulated carriages, crests the top of the bank as it approaches Bethnal Green station in 1960. The tracks on the extreme left, cross through the haze above Bethnal Green bank, towards Bishopsgate goods station off to the right. All is set for imminent electrification.

20

wartime economy and which was not to be replaced for a few more years yet.

The enduring memory of that journey was the noise the engine emitted on the long climb up from Baker Street to Finchley Road. We passed the still evident remains of the closed Lords and Marlborough Road stations, as it groaned and scraped and whined through the tunnels like a beast in pain. No wonder they were nicknamed 'Growlers'.

At Finchley Road, I spotted a pair of parallel wires running the length of the platform, a little above head height. Later, I saw Metropolitan guards using a brass ferule on their flags which they used to touch these wires together to sound a starting bell, positioned near the standing loco. It was an interesting practice when compared with the hand oil lamps and the waving of flags and arms, which the national network relied on.

Further examples of Growlers were seen on passing the extensive London Transport railway depot at Neasden, but there was very little else of interest until we reached Rickmansworth, where an ex-LNER L1 2-6-4 tank made a very smart change over with our Growler. At Chalfont and Latimer there was a glimpse of the Chesham branch train behind a former Great Central tank engine and my eye caught its number, beginning with a '6'. The carriages, some of the oldest I had seen in use, can still be seen to-day, working on the Bluebell Railway in Sussex. Then it was on to Aylesbury, where I had a distant glimpse of a Great Western engine and a Marylebone bound express made a stop, again with a number in the 60,000s.

Overall, it has to be admitted that I found much of that day excruciatingly boring, which was perhaps why the few items of railway interest lingered in my memory. On the return journey, my eye followed the route map displayed beneath the luggage rack, gradually ticking off the stations, and this time there was a second similar tank engine at Chalfont and Latimer, to catch my attention.

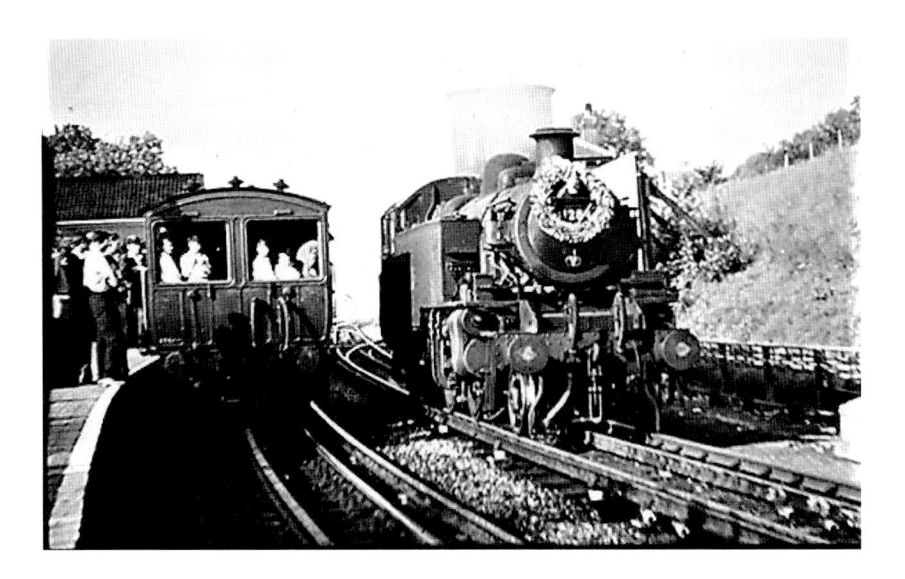

The last full day of steam operation at Chesham. London Midland Region 2-6-2T 41284, runs round its shuttle branch train on 11 September 1960. The smokebox door wreath was a typical marker of such occasions.

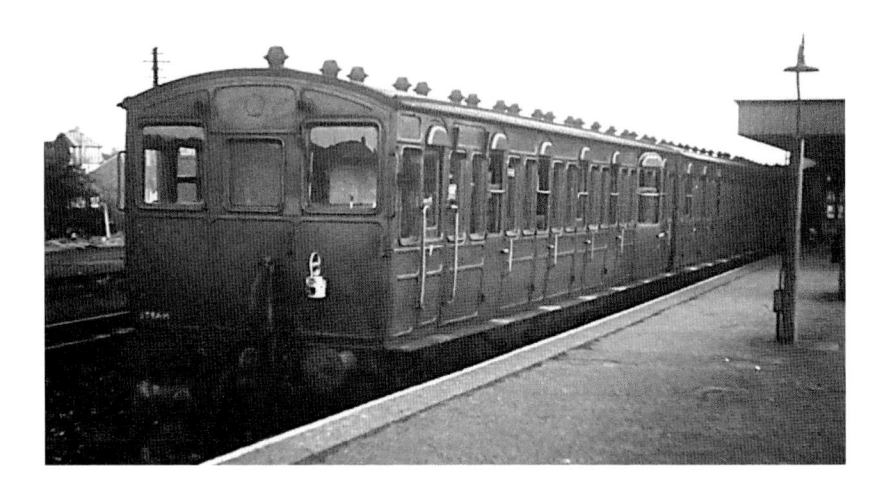

The Chesham branch train, dating from the turn of the last century, seen at Chalfont and Latimer. I always thought the brown livery, adopted for locomotive hauled Metropolitan trains, gave them a rather agricultural look. I also wondered why carriages of that vintage sported a grab handle to every door. Did people find it that difficult to step up into a compartment? The prominent roof ventilators too were very much of their period.

22

Eventually, as we approached the Neasden depot again, I was surprised to glimpse a dark red London Transport tank engine which I must have missed on the way out. At that tender age, I failed to make the connection with one of my favourite possessions, a set of cigarette cards. Before World War II, cigarette manufacturers included cards in their packets. They covered many different subjects and could be collected or pasted into specially printed albums. They could be hot currency in early post war school playgrounds where duplicates, or 'swaps', regularly changed hands or were won or lost in card flicking contests. I had no intention of losing my well fingered set, based on railway locomotives and equipment, not least because they included pictures of Metropolitan passenger engines.

I was particularly intrigued by their deep red livery and unusual wheel arrangements. Even as quite a small boy I had looked out for but never seen a 4-4-4 or 0-6-4 tank engine of any kind. I did not realise it at the time, but the last of them had been scrapped shortly before that visit to Metroland, and indeed, we had been travelling on their very own home ground. It was another decade or so before I was able to search for the outlying vestiges of that Metropolitan territory, at Brill and Verney Junction.

# CHAPTER TWO                    Holidays with Steam

I longed to travel behind an express steam locomotive and when the opportunity came, it was not on the Southern Region at all. We were to visit Mundesley-on-Sea, on the Norfolk coast, for our family holiday. This time, in my impatience to see Liverpool Street station, I took little notice of the usual crowd of holiday-makers as we passed through Waterloo, nor of the stacked-up wicker baskets of racing pigeons, nor of those tractor-hauled trains of mail bag trolleys, weaving across the concourse. This was the summer of 1950, and Liverpool Street was undergoing repairs and maintenance, presumably resulting from war damage and neglect. The station proved a disappointment. The crowds were dense and we had to jostle our way to the departure platform, dodging scaffolding and baggage, under a low hanging tarpaulin. I imagine glass was being replaced overhead and any sense of it being a special place was lost in the gloom. My father disappeared for a few minutes with a view to confirming this was indeed our train. Meanwhile, remembering the sweeping concourse at Waterloo, I formed such a dim view of Liverpool Street that I took little interest in the train we were boarding and did not even think of looking for locomotives.

The carriage was packed and I was offered a seat on my father's knee. My spirits were quickly raised when I realised I could spend the journey standing in the corridor, an arrangement which suited us both. Things looked up from the very moment the train gave a jolt and slowly got under way. Within a minute or so the driver was getting to grips with the climb up Bethnal Green bank. The bark of the locomotive exhaust echoing off the line-side retaining walls, was something I had never heard before and a far cry from my previous experience, limited to electric travel.

As we passed the long closed Bishopsgate low-level platforms, I caught the sound of another train and was taken by surprise by the volumes of steam and sound issuing from the cavernous gloom below Bishopsgate goods station. A tank engine was busily blustering through the darkness, trailing a string of plum red carriages. Dull yellow light glowed from their compartments. This was primitive stuff compared with Southern Electrics. What was more, that upstart of a local train was overtaking *our* express! By the time we passed Bethnal Green we were again in the lead and with honour restored I resumed my concentration on this line, which was so new to me.

Extensive carriage sidings near Stratford impressed me though I was disappointed to see so few steam engines. There was passing interest in the still new electric trains, especially seeing a group of them on display at their Ilford depot. They carried the familiar green colour of those back home and offered the novelty of using overhead wires rather than a third rail for their electricity supply. With their sliding doors and open plan interiors, they were reminiscent of the London Underground, rather than the Southern's slam doors. I was even aware of the modernised suburban stations with their LNER blue and white tiling – the basis, I suppose, of what we would now describe as a corporate image. Looking back, I am surprised just how much detail I took in, but nevertheless it all added up to a disappointment after Waterloo and the West of England main line.

Much of the journey was eventless, with boring spells of watching the rise and fall of the telegraph wires between poles and listening to the clickety-clack of wheels on rail joints. Eventually corridor travel lost its appeal and I returned to the compartment. Wriggling on my father's knee and frequently bombarding him with, 'How much longer Dad?', we at last pulled into Norwich Thorpe, when I belatedly realised we had just passed the engine shed, just off the platform end. Another test of patience was to follow. Apparently we had to stay in the train which would be hauled in reverse, bound for North Walsham and Cromer.  This sounded like an interesting manoeuvre but it was only after an interminable wait, we set off behind a Sandringham 4-6-0 on what proved to be a dull journey for an 8 year old who had seen enough countryside for one day.

Getting out at North Walsham, I noticed each carriage end of the departing train bore the legend 'Norfolkman', presumably allocated to the rolling stock of the named train we had arrived in. As it cleared the platform I spotted the lower level ex-Midland and Great Northern station a short way off and realised that even in such relatively remote railway outposts, there was exploration to be undertaken.

Meanwhile, I had not seen any more engines and I was about to learn that we would be continuing our journey to Mundesley by taxi.  I ask you; what is it about adults? Nevertheless, in spite of everything, I had noticed the few engines I did manage to see all had numbers beginning with a '6', like those I had spotted on the Metropolitan and Great Central line to Aylesbury. This bore further examination.

We were to stay for a couple of weeks with a great-aunt. Within the first day, I was making enquiries as to the whereabouts of the station. Although I quite enjoyed the daily trip to the beach, it took until the end of the first week before I was allowed to walk alone to the station itself.  I was getting on towards 9 years old at the time and in 1950, nobody took any notice of small boys going about their business alone.

In the station yard, I stood watching two coalmen unloading coal from a railway wagon into hefty black sacks, which were weighed on heavy cast-iron scales and stacked on the back of their Austin lorry.  It caused a moment's bewilderment when I later got home and asked what a 'cwt' was. Yes, I had definitely seen this written on the side of the weights they were using.  After that, I knew what a hundredweight of coal looked like!

The station itself was impressive for a small village, looking a bit like a grand cricket pavilion topped by a small cupola. Strangely there were no railway staff in sight. I ventured onto the station platform, through the entrance hall with its heavy black wooden central table, past the shuttered ticket window and now, there I was, ready to explore. Emboldened by the absence of authority, I took a good look at a horse box parked in the bay platform, crossed the footbridge, from which I could see the men in the yard still loading their lorry, and then walked the length of the opposite platform until it terminated at a road over-bridge. I had worked out that beyond that led to Cromer but apart from looking at the dripping water crane, there was nothing else of interest. Happily this was remedied the following day when it was explained to me that if I wanted to see a train, it might be better to visit when people were coming home from work in the evening.

This proved to be my very first unaccompanied spotting expedition. Sure enough, I was duly rewarded by the sight of quite an important looking engine, at least for these parts. It was a tender type which came bustling in with what looked like a sizeable train of perhaps four or five coaches. A dozen or so people seemed to tumble out and equally quickly make their way towards the footbridge. With an abrupt whistle, the train was away again and by the time the last carriage had disappeared round the bend under the road bridge, there was not a passenger left to be seen. I had scarcely had time to savour the activity but one thing did stand out and that was the fact that the engine number had begun with a '4'. This was my first sighting of a London Midland Region engine whose locos all fell in the 40 and 50,000 series. It was quite a time later when I concluded it had probably been an Ivatt class 2, 2-6-0. These latter figures indicated two wheels in front of six larger driving wheels and none behind. The different wheel arrangements were a major distinguishing characteristic between loco types or classes. In fact, at that time, about a third of all engines were 0-6-0s, either tank or tender types, in turn divided into many classes. It was probably no more than ten minutes later when I was delighted by a second arrival. Fewer people disembarked and this time the fireman came down to uncouple the engine. Now this was more like it and the driver must have sensed my interest. "Do you want a ride?" he asked. It was all so unexpected. I was overwhelmed by the idea. Where would we be going? Would he bring me back? "No thank you", I heard myself saying, and settled back to watch what was going to happen next. The engine duly ran round its train, which then headed off back towards North Walsham, so I need not have worried after all. There was not a passenger in sight and the station had returned to its more familiar state of slumber.

When my mother decided to come along the next evening, to put in a word for me with the driver, the holidays were definitely livening up. Sure enough, he thrust a handful of cotton waste into my hand and told me where to stand safely in the cab. Every second on that little trip was magical. As we pulled forward under the road bridge I sensed the solidity of everything around me, the steel on steel and lack of resilience as we clicked over the rail joints. The cab was a surprisingly quiet and cosy place to be, a warm, private world. I watched the reversing lever being operated and its locking mechanism engaged in its quadrant of square cut teeth and then it was back through the station to run round the empty train. The exhaust note was now more staccato, echoing underneath the platform canopy on one side and against the parked carriages on the other. The odd thing was just how far away the sound seemed to be coming from. I would like to have been able to wave proudly to passengers along the platform, but there was not a soul to be seen as we rumbled past the horse box, still in the bay platform, and as far as the cross-over.

Reversing once more, we were all too soon back at the other end of the train. I was lost for words and my smiling mother had to remind me to say thank you and hand back the

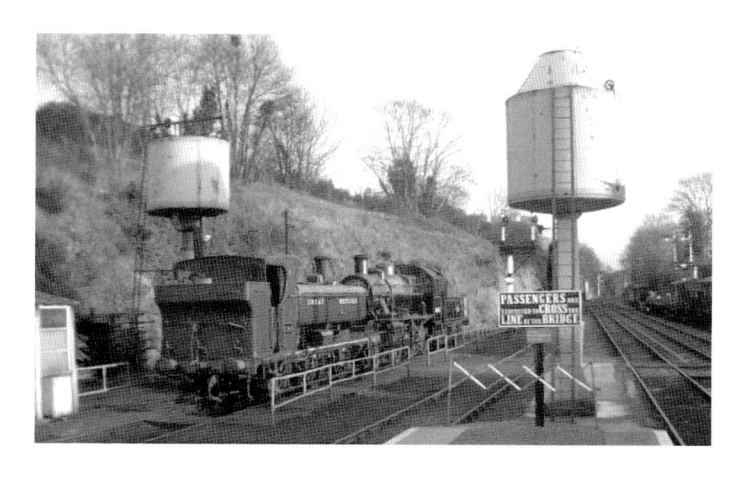

*Seen here, at the preserved Severn Valley Railway's Bewdley station, is a pair of characteristic Great Western water towers, framing a 5700 class 0-6-0PT in Great Western livery, together with an LMS designed class 2 mixed traffic 2-6-0. The 5700s had numbered 863 examples and were the most prolific class of British steam loco. The 2 MTs were still being built until 1953 and some of these were allocated to secondary routes in East Anglia. It would have been one of these which impressed the writer at Mundesley, on his very first lone spotting trip in 1950.*

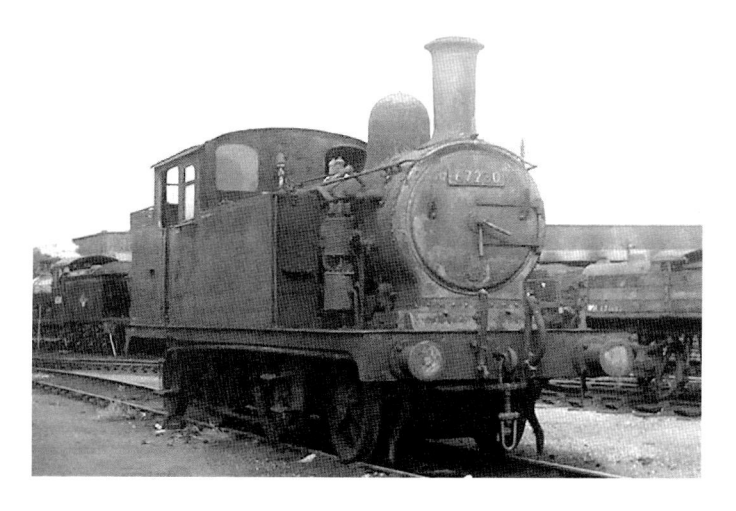

*67230 was the last surviving class F6 2-4-2T and was the type of engine which gave the writer his first footplate ride. It had already been withdrawn during May 1958 and was seen here on 3 August 1958, on the dump west of Stratford shed. It was finally scrapped the following December. The sound of Westinghouse brake pumps, as seen here mounted in front of the side tank, is forever reminiscent of the former west side suburban concourse at Liverpool Street.*

wodge of cotton waste. My excitement must have impressed my parents because, at the end of the holiday, it was not too hard to convince them to start the journey home by train to North Walsham, rather than the bus previously planned. Now that could have been the limit to my exploration of locomotives and railways. After all, apart from that engine ride, train travel in East Anglia had not been exceptionally exciting. Meanwhile, I had plenty of railway distractions at home, and that was how it stayed for the next two or three years.

The year following the Mundesley adventure, our family holiday was to be at Lyme Regis. For the first time I was to travel on a steam hauled express from Waterloo and that meant more to me than the destination itself. This time, the early Saturday morning start saw us arriving at a crowded Waterloo station. Even in the winter months there were a couple of dozen daily expresses to Exeter and Bournemouth whilst a summer Saturday saw this number exceeding sixty. That was without counting the steam-hauled semi-fasts to Basingstoke and beyond and the Southampton boat trains which sometimes reached double figures on exceptional days.

Many people arriving from the suburbs still worked on Saturday mornings at that time. Their movements were in direct conflict with the intending holiday makers who hovered around the ticket barriers to their respective departure platforms. Little wonder there was confusion, which was mostly overcome by the simple introduction of blackboards opposite the main line departure platform gates. These were set well back so as not to impede pedestrian flow along the length of the concourse. By indicating the destination, the platform and the departure times, some semblance of order was introduced to the holiday crowds. With so many departures at these peak times the blackboard expedient probably solved many a 'right platform, wrong train' mishap, making it easier for both ticket collectors and luggage burdened families.

As we waited in the appropriate queue, we were serenaded by recordings of what Dad later jokingly recalled as 'military marching melodies'. For some years after the Second World War, that kind of music was played over the loud speakers and perhaps it was a natural choice given the number of armed forces personnel who had passed through – sailors for Portsmouth, soldiers for Aldershot, airmen for airfields across southern England.

On week days, bowler hats, briefcases and rolled umbrellas were much in evidence and characterised a large proportion of arriving commuters who, sometimes a bit out of step, would purposefully stride along in time to the music towards the Waterloo and City line entrance.

Now, from our queue, the musical effect was somewhat marred by frequent interruptions from the station announcer, mostly no doubt, repeating information clearly visible on the large Suburban and Main Line departure indicators. These indicators had fascinated me since I had grasped the basics of reading, and was able to interpret them. At frequent intervals, after a few trains had left, they would rattle into life and a different set of destinations would appear. Should one of the rotating name panels get stuck, the man in charge would reach up with a long pole and poke the offending panel into its correct position. Hence, an erroneous 'Woking' might be made to give way to a 'Basingstoke', whilst an interloping 'Byfleet' might be made to disappear.

Before long, the queue ahead started shuffling forward, suitcases, raincoats, children and all. Repeating some of the experience of the previous year, I again opted to spend most of the journey standing in the corridor. As for the journey itself, there was some novelty to be enjoyed from running on the down fast line and travelling non-stop through all the familiar suburban stations, but there were not many engines to be seen and once again, the overall journey remained relatively uninteresting. There had been a passing view of the pre-war

Brooklands motor racing circuit, with the Vickers aircraft sheds in the background, but not a lot else to catch my attention. Somewhere along the way I did manage to glimpse our engine and identify the 'air-smoothed' outline of a Bullied Pacific, but I did not record any numbers at that time. It must still have been in the balance as to whether loco spotting would attract me further or not.

As we traversed Somerset, I became intrigued by lineside signs announcing that we were approaching the 'Strong Country', so that as we arrived at Axminster I was able to ask Dad if that was the Strong Country. He remained as puzzled as I was, or perhaps he was just preoccupied in getting us safely off the train with our luggage. I was not to know at the time, the 'Strong Country' in question related to Strong's brewery in Romsey. With the signs visible from both eastbound and westbound trains, passengers could have been forgiven for wondering if they were coming or going.

Meanwhile, back at Axminster, there was a huge flurry of activity as passengers and luggage filled the platform for a few hesitant moments before surging en-masse towards the pedestrian over-bridge.

My parents had been caught off guard and we found ourselves as stragglers as we watched the fast disappearing crowd. It seemed to be all suitcases, jumpers and raincoats, the standard precautionary impedimenta for holidaying in England – and not a bucket and spade in sight. I was more interested in the departing train. I could scarcely hear the engine, only the slow rhythmic ker-dunk-ker-dunk, as carriages passed over the rail joints, finishing with a fading 'kerdak' from the last bogie as it grew further away.

Arriving on the opposite platform, most families had already packed into the waiting train for Lyme Regis. The elderly compartment carriages were all but full by the time I was bundled aboard. We were soon climbing to cross over above the main line. The engine was pulling hard and I looked forward to seeing it at close quarters when we arrived. Meanwhile, the compartment was hot and crowded and I was aware of the creaking carriage and scraping wheel flanges. We stopped at Combpyne for no obvious reason since nobody displayed any signs of movement. Even if they had wished to alight, it might have proved difficult, with every square inch of the floor space seemingly packed tight with feet and luggage. The universal destination was clearly the seaside and twenty minutes of modest discomfort was a small price to pay. Nevertheless, for me it seemed an age.

      Beautiful countryside was all very well but what about some trains to see? There was a brief interruption to this growing ennui when the ground dropped away dramatically as we crossed what I later learned was Cannington viaduct. This was some 600 feet long and 90 feet high and had been opened in 1903, not long after the Glenfinnan viaduct of Harry Potter film fame. Both viaducts were pioneers of mass concrete construction and are now listed for preservation. Otherwise nothing of note happened until we arrived at Lyme Regis station, high above the town. This time my parents were better prepared and I found myself swept past the engine into the crowd which was making its way out of the station. The abiding memory was the convoy of suitcase-carrying holiday makers stretching out ahead towards the town, along with my unsatisfied wish to properly inspect the branch line engine. It is odd to recall now that there was not a wheel to be seen on any of those suitcases, to lighten the load. Today little remains of the station area, transformed like many a country terminus into a light industrial area, whilst the station building itself has been re-erected on the Watercress Line station at Alresford. Such has become the raw material of nostalgia.

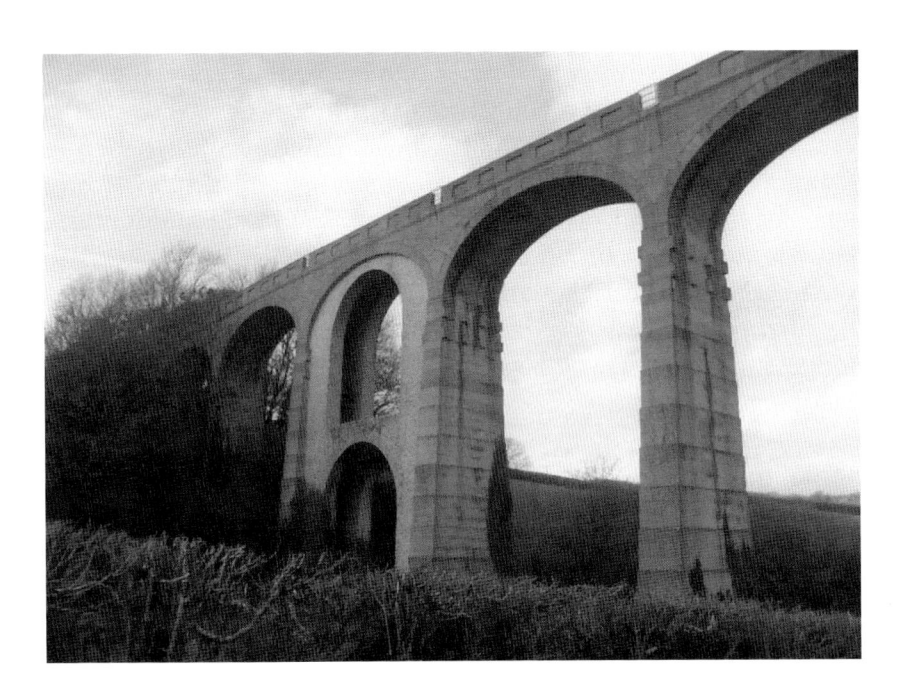

*Cannington viaduct once served the Axminster-Lyme Regis branch. Only when spotters became car drivers did they discover many aspects of railway history not apparent from a train. This ten arch viaduct was some 600 ft wide and 90 ft high. During construction in 1901-03 the westernmost abutment and adjacent pier slipped, which accounts for the brick infill stiffening arch. The viaduct's claim to fame is that it employed pioneering mass concrete construction, as did the Glenfinnan viaduct, which featured in the Harry Potter films. The construction technique is clearly expressed in the slightly stepped piers. A wooden box formwork was filled with concrete. Once set, a slightly smaller form was placed upon it and the process repeated. The projecting nibs at the top of the piers were to support the temporary wooden centering upon which the arches were formed.*

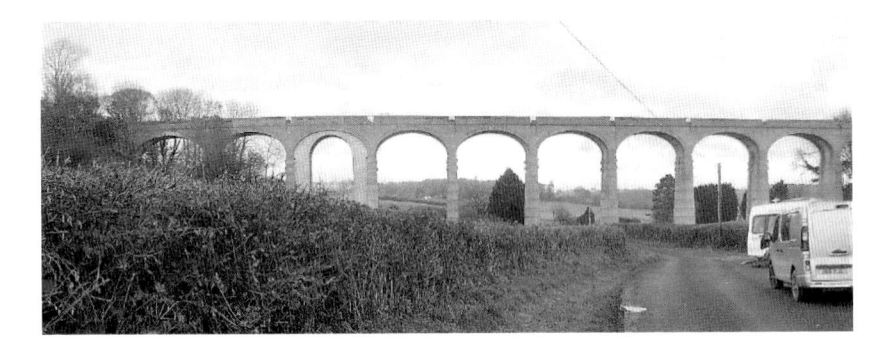

# CHAPTER THREE                           Like Minds

When I changed school, I encountered a whole range of hobbies amongst my classmates. There was coin and stamp collecting, a boy who could talk only about Ford cars and another enthusiastic about motor racing. One boy bred pet mice and yet another filled his head with tennis statistics. My immediate neighbour in class was fascinated by magic tricks and had a talent for drawing cartoons of both the teachers and pupils. Included in all this diversity was Roger, a lad who was clever in class and rather mysteriously seemed to know about other things too. He knew how long and how far it was to travel between different towns. He seemingly knew where to change trains for any journey and he knew the London Underground map by heart. Sometimes he would stop the apparent doodle he was drawing on any scrap of paper to hand, saying things like, 'That is the down slow and that is the up relief line', and then he would further elaborate it until the complete detailed track diagram emerged of perhaps the entire Norwood Junction area or the maze of tracks around Battersea.

I saw all this as a bit of a party trick until he started to point out, very precisely, the best vantage points to see railway engines. Why he thought I would be interested I cannot imagine. Maybe he was just talking at me like our Ford fanatic did to anyone who would listen. It turned out he was one of these 'loco spotters' I had heard about and his unselfconscious enquiries soon revealed two or three others in our class.

Feeling I might be missing out on something interesting, I resolved to buy the Southern Region ABC which he told me about, in order to record my sightings. My first impression was that there was an awful lot of engines to see, yet it was a challenge and it would involve seeking them out. I liked the idea of hunting them down and resolved to make a start locally by cycling to a footbridge at the approach to Wimbledon goods yard. A whole Saturday morning spent there yielded what seemed like a lot of numbers, but when they were ruled off in the ABC they made little impression.

Nevertheless, I had been accompanied by another lad who lived near home and we had enjoyed ourselves enough for this to become a regular haunt for several Saturdays. There was usually enough train activity to keep us interested though I do recall once becoming fascinated by a 'Black Motor'. That was an early nickname, unused by my generation of spotters, for the LSWR 700 class of freight 0-6-0s. It was shuffling back and forth in the western goods yard at Wimbledon, puffing clouds of steam up through the gaps in the wooden footbridge decking. The obvious distraction was to place ourselves strategically so as to be engulfed in the temporary fog. That led to giggles at the sensation of being momentarily disorientated until the mist cleared. Once the novelty wore off the next challenge was to drop a couple of toffee wrappers, screwed-up in a blank page from my note-book, into the loco chimney, just as it passed below. This felt a bit naughty but it was a harmless challenge. Nothing was left to chance. We estimated the time between exhaust beats and made a guess how long it would take for the paper ball to drop. Most surprisingly, we got it right first time, immediately followed by a mighty puff of exhaust which sent our paper missile sky high. After the whoops of joy, it was time to get back to serious business since an approaching London bound express had been spotted.

The many scarcely marked pages of my ABC were either to remain intimidating or would become an on-going challenge, to say nothing of the competitive element with class-mates. To help things along a bit, I delved into various corners to retrieve a few numbers I had previously noted down, mostly in a booklet given with a short lived publication called, 'Every Spotters Weekly'. I even looked into my mother's holiday snaps to discover her picture of me at Mundesley on the footplate of 67228. Alas, as an Eastern Region engine, that particular one began with a '6' and had to be noted in the cover of my Southern ABC until I could afford to buy the appropriate Eastern Region edition and to travel further afield.

Something similar occurred in the spring of 1953 when a Bullied Pacific had an axle failure at high speed, resulting in similar locos being withdrawn for examination. When their temporary ex-LNER V2, B1, or ex-LMS Black Five replacements were spotted, their numbers too had to go on my reserve list.

The great benefit of living in the London suburbs was the relatively easy access to stations representing all the former Big Four railway companies. I knew about the existence of the pre-nationalisation companies from those cigarette cards, together with books which I was starting to receive as birthday or Christmas presents. Consequently, when school friend Roger suggested a trip to Kings Cross would give us a sporting chance of seeing world steam record holder, 'Mallard', yes, *the* 'Mallard' and no, 'Cock o'the North' was no longer a 2-8-2 but you could still see it in rebuilt form and the suburban trains were all steam worked, yes, steam, and with articulated coaches too – what were they? Well, a visit was irresistible.

Climbing the steps from the Underground, I was struck by the heavy sulphurous mustiness of the air. We slipped into the station between the old cab road across the station front and the collection of wooden sheds and outbuildings which then occupied the forecourt, serving various railway and postal activities.

The first engine we encountered was a grubby N2 0-6-2 tank which had brought in the empty carriages for a northbound express. Then, simultaneously, we heard each other saying: ' Hey, look', as our attention was drawn to a pair of streamlined A4 Pacifics standing at the buffers on the arrival side of the narrow concourse. Neither of them was Mallard, but never mind, they made a handsome pair and a memorable introduction to spotting on the Eastern Region.

It was not long before we extended our range. We made several trips on the South London line between Victoria and London Bridge and we devised a way between us of recording as many engine numbers as possible. In the brief time it took to travel on the elevated line above Stewarts Lane engine shed, one of us would scribble a number down but just call out the next one, and so on. The other one would take down the dictation. We collected the electric unit numbers too. Because these trains came in so many forms they provided a marginal interest in their own right.

Soon Roger came up with more ambitious trips in mind, starting with an electric train to Guildford, followed by the little steam hauled cross-country to Horsham and then back home on a suburban electric. A visit to Guildford gave us access to a new range of locomotives. The wider hunt was on! Interestingly, most engines spent their working lives in the territory of their originating company. In the case of older examples, and there were many of these, that meant along the routes of the 150 or so private railways which had been grouped into the Big Four in 1923.

The South Eastern and Chatham Railway for example, extended a tentacle as far west as Reading, via a section of the London and South Western, which included Guildford. Consequently we were able to see some unfamiliar engine types at Guildford. I well remember 31737, a black and grimy object which still moved with a certain grace. It was one of Wainwright's SECR designs dating back to 1901 and I was later delighted to see it had been preserved at the National Railway Museum. Restored to its former glory, in lined out green and polished brass, it reveals the underlying elegance of design for which Wainwright was noted.

In many people's eyes, the other end of the scale was represented by Bullied's wartime austerity Q1 class, examples

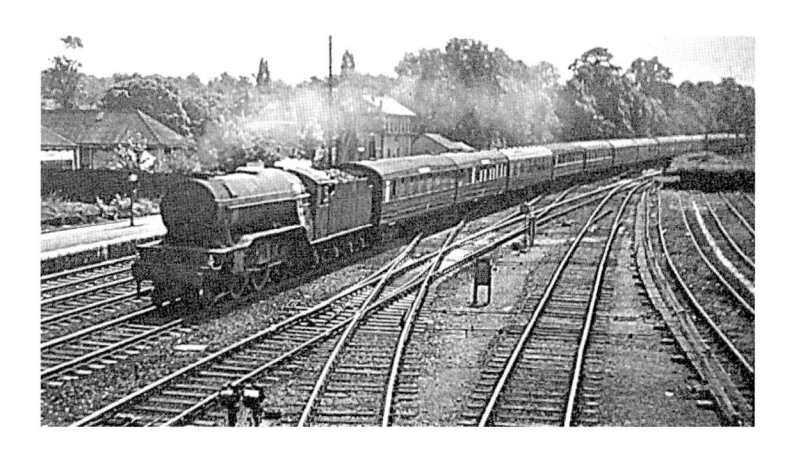

A down express passing Hatfield behind a V2 class 2-6-2, in the late fifties. They were handsome engines, equally at home on passenger or freight trains. It was a pity they were so dirty, as often as not, like the example seen here. Had they all been painted green they may have attracted more interest. When the Bullied pacifics were temporarily withdrawn following the 1953 axle failure incident at Crewekerne, they certainly impressed my young neighbours more than the B1s and Black Fives which had also been drafted in. What is more, Nine Elms kept them clean!

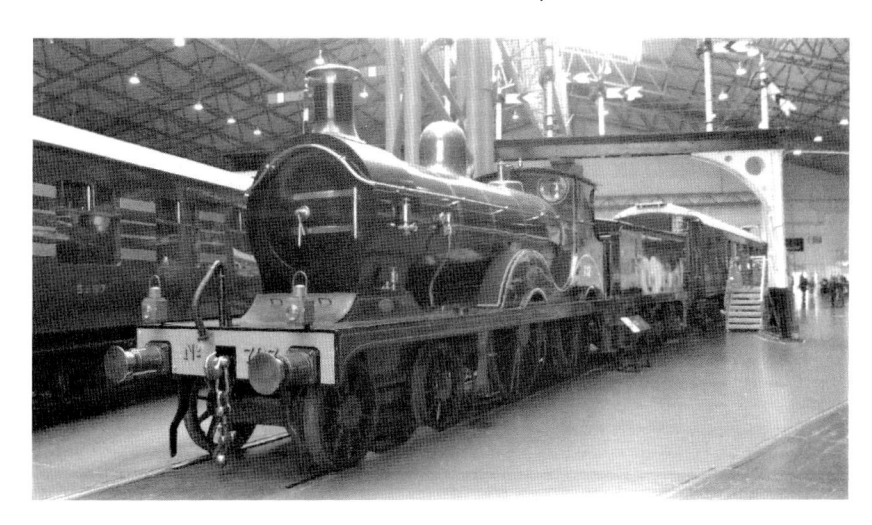

Wainwright's engines for the South Eastern and Chatham Railway were notable for their pleasing lines and handsome liveries, right down to the skill and care taken over lettering and lining out. No.737, displayed here at the National Railway Museum, is unrecognisable as the grubby black apparition once seen gliding gently through Guildford station, in the guise of Southern Region No.31737.

of which were also usually found at Guildford. These 6-wheeled tender engines were paired down to a box-like profile, lacking such refinements as splashers or running plates over the fully exposed wheels. I liked them for their originality and their simplicity and saw no reason to judge them by historic aesthetic standards. One of these too has survived into the National Collection.

Guildford's loco shed was built on the roundhouse principle; that is to say, the tracks radiated as a crescent from a central turntable. It nestled up against a retaining wall at the south-west corner of the station site and was just a bit too obscured from the platforms to provide an immediate view of the engines stabled there. For the spotter who just collected numbers, this was a frustration. For those of us who enjoyed the chase and enjoyed savouring the whole environment, then patience brought its rewards.

Roger, being the informed young fellow he was, had advised me that 'Ironside' could be seen at Guildford. This, it transpired, was a rare sighting. I had checked my ABC to discover that it was indeed a unique locomotive, built in 1890 as a four-wheeled dock shunter for Southampton docks, and was now the shed pilot for Guildford. This effectively meant it spent its days pottering around the shed area. Providing it was in steam that day, there was a good chance of seeing it. Sure enough it briefly appeared from behind the coaling stage, hauling a single wagon, before returning out of view. That made the day and plans were immediately laid for further exploration.

Roger's choice of returning via Horsham introduced me to the wider pleasures of railway exploration and discovery. At the time, Horsham or Guildford based E5X and E6X tank engines regularly served this route. In the late afternoon sunshine, the train's outline was sharply silhouetted against the track-side, when I got a nudge on the arm. "Look, that's cute, isn't it?" "Cute" struck me as fashionably American but I saw the point he was making. These particular engines unusually

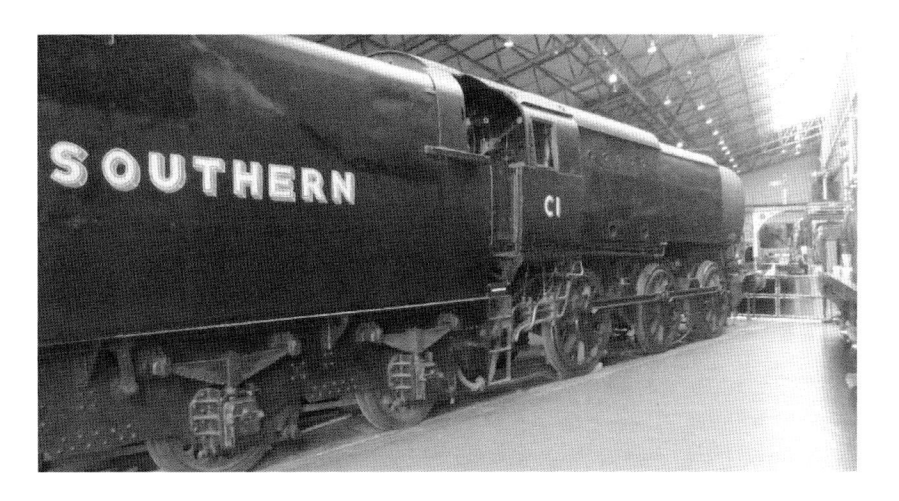

Bullied's wartime 1942 Austerity 0-6-0 freight engines were a radical departure from tradition with their boxy shape and lack of running plates above the wheels, contrasting fiercely with elegant machines like Wainwright's No. 737. Commentators usually decry them as ugly but would we choose a 40 or 50 year old style for a car or caravan when times move on? Spotters, however, never seemed to complain about them. Wartime austerity or not, the Southern Railway still took the trouble to use 3-dimentional lettering on the tender sides.     The cabside number indicates 'C' for six coupled wheels and '1' as the serial number.  Had the complexities of Bullied's numbering system endured, it would likely have deterred many a spotter.  For example, a 4-6-2 loco would have carried a 2 1 C prefix, indicating two leading axles, one trailing axle and six-coupled wheels, all before a possible 3 digit serial number. Unsurprisingly the system was abandoned upon nationalisation.

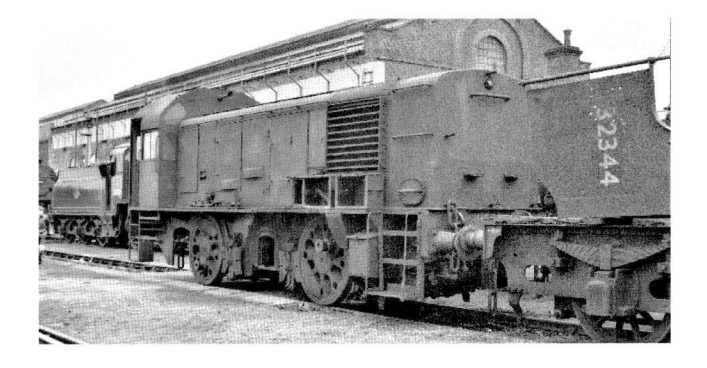

Diesel locomotives had a certain novelty interest in the 1950s. This Bullied freight prototype from 1950, seen at Ashford in April 1958, continued the use of Bullied/Firth Brown wheels,  favoured for his steam locos.  It was displayed at the International Railway Congress at Willesdon motive power depot in May 1954 but officially withdrawn in 1959.  It would appear ex LBSCR K class, 32344 was already beyond saving.

carried a thin handrail around their boiler domes and even this detail was clearly visible in the bobbing silhouette. This, along with the sounds of creaking carriages, exhausting steam, the rhythmic clicking of rail joints and the occasional waft of sulphurous smoke, combined into a kind of reassuring timelessness. There I was, a 12 year old budding romantic.

It was not long before I came across copies of Trains Illustrated magazines. These circulated at school, not exactly clandestinely, but rather like precious artefacts to be poured over by the cognoscenti. I do not think many of us had sufficient pocket money to pay for these, as well as for train travel, and I suspect there were a few interested dads out there who provided them.

When funds did permit, I would treat myself to a magazine. Trains Illustrated and The Railway Magazine were the most accessible and there used to exist one or two other titles which I enjoyed, like Railway World. Deciding which to buy would be a struggle. Browsing through these magazines, I noticed regular photo credits to Lens of Sutton. Living within cycling distance, it was not long before I determined its exact whereabouts and became an occasional Saturday morning visitor. His advertisement used to say 'Anything of a railway nature, bought, sold or exchanged'. Others have described John Smith's emporium at length. Suffice to say it offered a veritable cornucopia of railway photographs and publications. More of a shed than a shop in the conventional sense, it hung precariously on the side of a deep excavated pit, a short way along Carshalton Road. There had not been so many railway books published in those days. What was available included relatively rare publications, some quite old, along with printed ephemera, time-tables and so on. Lens of Sutton was a major source of back numbers of railway periodicals and I remember references indicating the ready availability of copies of Trains Illustrated from issue no.4 onwards. There was a waiting list kept for customers wanting issues 1 to 3 and no doubt those early issues are like gold dust to-day.

The other great attraction was the boxes of postcards which lined the walls. These offered photographs of seemingly every imaginable type of locomotive, past and present. The only problem was that none of these photographs were in any fathomable order, let alone an index. Enthusiasts of all ages poured over the racks, shoulder to shoulder, rather like librarians sifting through card indexes. Sometimes, one had to join a short queue to wait for John Smith to reappear behind the counter, to pay for one's purchase. Seeing as the shop had room for only four or five standing customers, that 'queue' was rarely more than two people long. The proprietor would eventually emerge from a trap-door in the floor, having retrieved either a mug of tea or some item from his store room, which apparently hung below the shop. The effect was somewhat like that of the old time theatre organist rising from the orchestra pit and filling the auditorium with his presence. Only then could we pay for our postcards at 6 old pennies a time. During one of these visits, I bought an unmarked copy of the 1948 edition of the ABC, recording as it did, all the engines inherited by British Railways. It brought home just how many classes I had missed by just four or five years.

This did not seem to matter so much at the time. There were still many thousands of engines to be seen. Nevertheless, it struck home a few years later. As one became familiar with the different loco types encountered, there was no doubt that watching some of them offered the enthusiast more interest and engagement than did others. It is difficult to put a finger on why that should have been. For example, the N2 0-6-2 tanks from Kings Cross and their N7 opposite numbers from Liverpool Street, both exuded a character of dependable machines regularly going about their local business. We tended to take them for granted but they were providing a backdrop to the activities of more glamorous express types which were more likely to catch our attention. The latter seemed to depart from their city terminus with purpose and optimism. Conversely though, they arrived looking hot and tired as they cruised to a halt at the buffer stops. Perhaps those impressions could be likened to the mechanical equivalents of how their crews felt.

Certainly it was quite usual to see a driver relaxing for a moment upon arrival. Whilst his fireman uncoupled, changed lamps and headcodes and tidied up the footplate, the driver might be seen at the cab window or standing at the open tender gate, watching the alighting crowds stream past. Sometimes he would be exchanging a few words with an appreciative passenger, invariably a middle aged man.

When Roger read about a loco spotters' special excursion to Rugby, I jumped at it. If I remember correctly, the last two carriages of a train from Euston had been reserved for us and this was to be my first serious introduction to ex-LMS locomotives on the Midland Region. Not only did it mean a notebook full of engines in the 40,000 series but also a sprinkling numbered in the 50,000 series too. That raised a comment or two since the latter were quite rare around London. Most were allocated to Scotland, Lancashire and Yorkshire and with others scattered across the Midlands.

On the way to Rugby we passed the Wolverton carriage and wagon works where we spotted some of the elderly saddle tanks bearing numbers in their own service-loco series. That was a bit special too, as was what greeted us at Rugby. After being coaxed into a long line, we threaded our way in schoolboy crocodile fashion towards the shed. Quickly the word went round to look out for an ex-LNWR tank. It was the last of its class and I only wish I still had a note of its number now. A flickering memory tells me it was 46601.

I have the impression that although there were lads who kept meticulous records, most of us were pretty casual about retaining note books. Although I still have one or two, they do not always indicate dates or locations of engines seen. Some spotters underlined numbers directly into well-thumbed ABCs. Most, like me, carried soot-smudged note books which could be carefully scanned through back home, whilst a few spotters seemed to make do with any scruffy bit of paper to hand.

Having finished the formal visit, many of us explored Rugby station for the best vantage points. I remember a friendly fireman of a 4-4-0 Midland compound, which was waiting at the platform, asking us why there were so many spotters around and I recall making my way to the south end of the platforms. From there could be seen the massive Great Central viaduct in the distance, which then crossed the former London and North Western main line. Not many trains seemed to use the viaduct but there was a sighting of a northbound express behind an unidentified A3 class, the same class to which Flying Scotsman itself belonged.

Somebody pointed out the celebrated Rugby locomotive testing station and there were general mumbles of regret that the excursion had not been extended to include it. A final treat was provided by the passing of a southbound express making rapid progress behind Duchess of Athol, 46231. In those days when many young boys aspired to model railway ownership, the Hornby model of that very engine was known to us all, so there was a fluster of excitement as it roared past on its way to London. I cannot recall much more from that day beyond a personal resolution to explore the London Midland Region further and to equip myself with a combined volume of the separate regional ABCs.

I was lucky enough to have sympathetic grand-parents who approved of my pastime and what they saw in me as a spirit of adventure. Consequently they would slip me a few shillings which always seemed to be just sufficient for my next jaunt. I remember my first tentative visit alone to St Pancras. Approaching it from the Underground platforms involved a pedestrian subway, not at all up to the usual standard of London Transport pedestrian tunnels. Instead it consisted of gloomily lit, rather grubby tiled walls, free of the usual colourful posters and, as one grew nearer to the main line station, the malodorous air took on the distinctive sulphurous tang of steam locomotives.

A choice of stairs enabled one to pop up into the station above at alternative points on the concourse. There was indeed a feeling of 'popping up' since, after the claustrophobic passage approach, one felt almost projected into the huge volume of space contained within the overall roof of St Pancras. Later, one came to realise that the quality of the environment outshone the quality of the loco spotting; it was not a hugely busy station. I decided to take a train to St Albans because I fancied the idea of travelling behind a double header; that is a train with two engines. These regularly left St Pancras behind a class 2P 4-4-0 of Midland Railway origin, leading an ex-LMS Class 5MT. The Black Fives, as they were popularly known, were a class of 842 engines, the most numerous class of tender engines in fact. They were versatile machines, liked by enginemen, but so prolific as to hardly attract a second glance. Double heading had been a Midland Railway practice at the beginning of the 20th century, as trains were growing heavier, and the company had been a bit slow to develop more powerful engines. It surprised me to see the practice continuing, even with trains which I would have thought were well within a Black Five's capacity.

When my grandparents asked me if I had visited the town of St Albans I had to admit that I had stayed at the station. They agreed it was a bit of a walk to the town centre and were apparently not disappointed. At least my travel allowance was not affected. Most spotters travelled with the sole intention of observing trains and engine movements, so one might have travelled a hundred miles or more and not left the station, before taking the train home. I still think my grand-parents might have remained puzzled at that extravagance.

Clearly, my grandmother had been impressed by my loco spotting endeavours and it so happened she had a long-standing friend whose husband was in a responsible post at Waterloo.

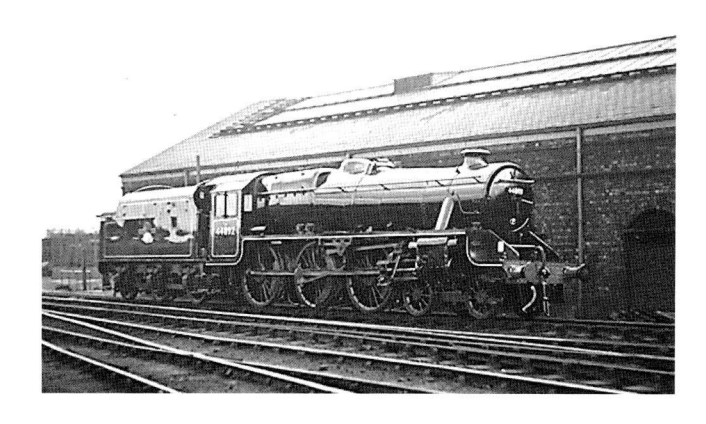

*5MT or Black Five, 44892, seen on 21 June 1961, newly outshopped in lined black at Crewe works. This mixed traffic class was the most prolific type of tender loco in Britain. There were variations but most of them carried a straight running plate just clear of the driving wheels, as seen here. Like most black painted engines, they attracted less attention to their appearance than did a green painted passenger design. That did not prevent them being well respected, if a little unexciting.*

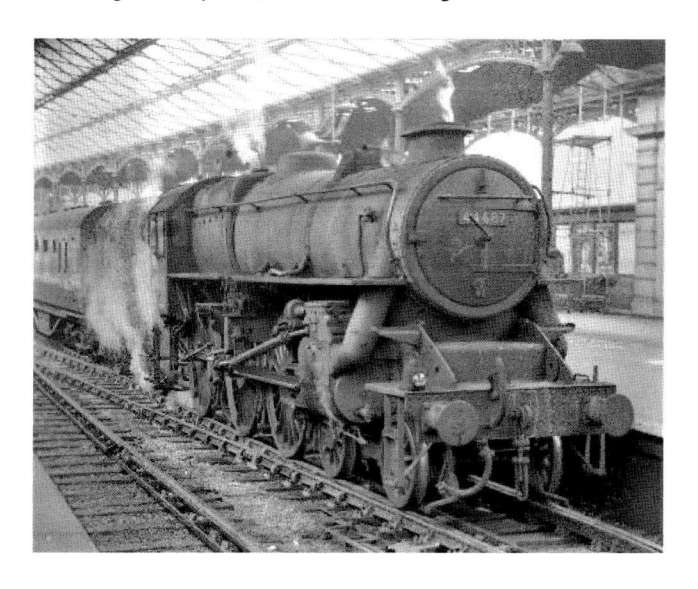

*Amongst the slightly monotonous class of Black Fives were a number of examples worth looking out for. For example, there were just four which bore names and a group of twenty-two which were equipped with Caprotti valve gear. Seen here at Euston is a British Railways variation of one of these, 44687, with double chimney and very high running plate. The appearance was slightly awkward and certainly distinctive when seen against the rest of the class.*

When asked if I would like a visit to Nine Elms loco shed, it took but a couple of days to arrange. A Saturday morning saw me reporting to the offices at Waterloo, where I was introduced to a kindly locomotive inspector who whisked me off to ... a BUS stop! Oh, what disappointment! I had so hoped a footplate ride might have been planned. Nevertheless, enthusiasm only slightly dented, I started to ply my host with questions, historical, organisational and technical. My eagerness to learn must have encouraged his generous response to my questions. Only once did he seem a little reticent and that was when I enquired about Bullied's largely experimental and ill-fated 'Leader' class. He seemed to know more than he was prepared to divulge. Although it was over three years since the project had been abandoned, a delayed storm of adverse press publicity concerning huge sums of wasted money had broken out only a year or so before. Subsequently I wondered if the subject was embargoed or if he was just manifesting old company loyalty, regarding that embarrassing episode. Even six years after nationalisation, it was not unusual to hear railwaymen still referring to 'the Company', so it may have been no more than that.

By the time we alighted from the bus along Wandsworth Road, I had already learned a great deal. I noticed the short walk to the shed gates was along Brookland Road. The association with the pre-war Brooklands motor racing circuit did seem inappropriate, if not distasteful in the circumstances, but that quickly evaporated as I caught my first sight of the expanse of tracks, both left and right.

My guide recounted how, in London and South Western Railway days, drivers were frequently allocated their own engine, which they expected the cleaners to keep spick and span. They might call in on the shed of a Sunday morning to give 'their' engine the once over and would then wipe the copper work with half a lemon to bring out the rainbow reflections.

Then I learned about the operating sequence of locomotives coming off the main line. Two or three would wait at the back-shunt next to the main line and then couple up together before moving into the shed area where they uncoupled and took their turn to refuel under the coaling tower. We watched the operation in progress and my guide pointed out the concrete stumps which remained as vestiges of the former hand coaling stage. He explained the original layout of the depot and how it had evolved and he pointed to a building which had been part of the original loco works. It had been superseded by the new works at Eastleigh, after 1909.

Seeing so many engines in close proximity from ground level for the first time, I started to appreciate their true scale. As we penetrated deeper into the shed, the gentle hiss of steam, the smell of hot oil and the acrid wafting smoke of the engines we had already passed, gave way to sounds of dripping water, metallic clunks and occasional muffled voices. These were the sounds of dead engines awaiting or receiving attention from the fitters.

Seeing engines off-duty revealed them in a very different light. Once out of steam, locos seemed to me to lose much of the individual personality which belonged to each class. They assumed instead an almost morose shared anonymity. Even the 'namers', with their polished name plates, had something of the air of imposters about them. I noted their numbers almost automatically until I was startled by the sight of a shadowy face at ankle level, seen through the spokes of an engine's driving wheels. Fitters were working under an engine in the inspection pit between the rails. They were operating by the sooty light of open flame oil lamps, so the theatrical effect of a disembodied head had awoken me abruptly from my musings.

Eventually, lurking at the back of the shed, I spotted the distinctive number, 30777, a King Arthur class engine which filled a conspicuous gap in the blocks of numbers I had previously collected. Years later, it remained the only engine I

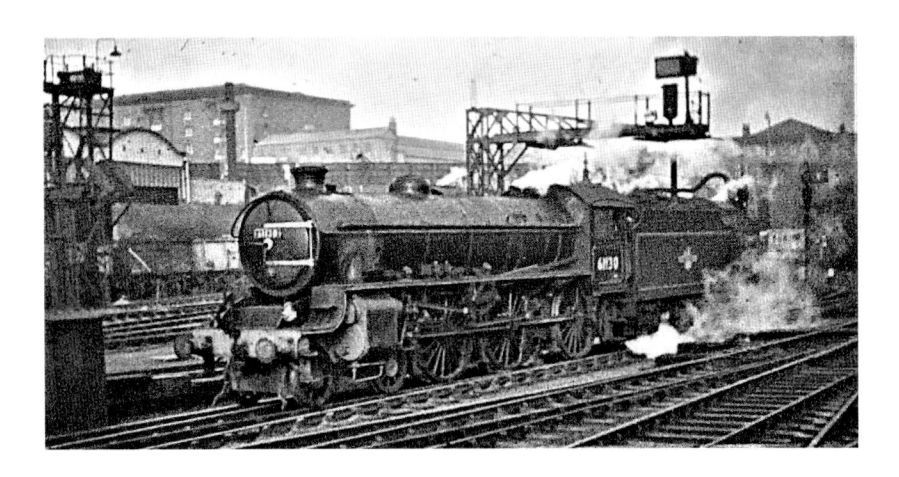

B1 class, 61130, displaying a little unofficial decoration in its white painted smokebox door hinges, as it passes in front of the Kings Cross loco servicing area on 27 December 1958. The B1s appeared in 1942, gradually replacing pre-grouping 4-4-0s and 4-4-2s along with Great Central 4-6-0s. New B1s were still appearing into the British Railways era in 1950. As a class they seemed to go about their work in a business like way but as a spotter I never felt they matched the self-confidence and swagger of the LMS Black Fives. It was strange how one could attribute human characteristics to distinguish locomotives, yet the moment they were out of steam all classes resorted to being just 'things'.

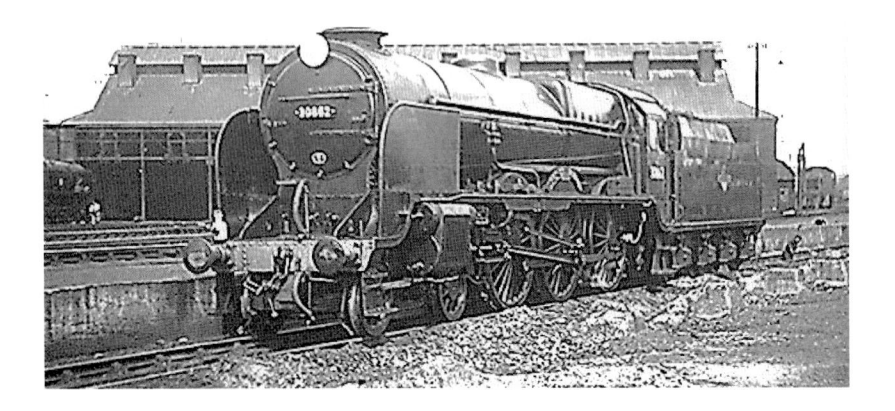

Lord Nelson class 30862, 'Lord Collingwood', at Nine Elms, standing next to the site of the former hand-coaling stage, marked by its crumbling concrete foundation bases, on 6 August 1961. There were just sixteen of these handsome engines built. They were not the best steamers until Bullied made some modifications. By the 1950s they were particularly identified with the South Western section east of Salisbury, when they regularly hauled heavily loaded Southampton boat trains. The building in the background is the 10 road 'New Shed' of 1910.

remembered from that visit, and as chance would have it, it survives to-day in the National Collection.

We visited just about every corner of the running sheds and finally it ended with the same disappointment with which it had begun. There were apparently no engines due to go to Waterloo and so it was back to the bus. There was still a minor treat to come though, when I was shown behind platform 21 at Waterloo to inspect the hoist which served the Waterloo and City underground line. I heard the story of how, six years previously, an M7 tank had fallen into the hoist shaft and had had to be cut up in situ.

After that excellent morning's spotting, I made my way towards my train home, still reflecting on the whole experience and overlooking the fact that it was from that very station that Ian Allan had effectively launched the whole business of loco spotting.

# CHAPTER FOUR                           Intrepid Pursuits

Initially, most of my spotting was undertaken in good weather. As I became increasingly keen, I was not to be deterred by poorer conditions. Without thinking much about it at the time, I adopted what became the archetypal spotters' uniform – the anorak.

School caps were common garb – nothing so vulgar as a baseball cap in sight, along with shorts, long socks and knobbly knees, at least up to the age of about 12 or 13. In the winter months, belted gabardine raincoats appeared. Then, in the late fifties, duffle coats sold from army surplus stores, led to a widespread fashion which, in turn, became the standard cold weather choice of spotters.

The virtue of anoraks and duffle coats lay in their generous pockets. These were appreciated for carrying pencils, notebooks, ABCs and perhaps the odd Mars bar. Spotters making a long day of it, or maybe those with big appetites, were likely to carry an old school satchel or perhaps an army surplus gas mask bag, slung over their shoulder. I have seen time-tables, marmalade sandwiches, buttered Weetabix, bottles of pop, warm gloves and cameras, emerge from these.

Generally speaking, few of us regularly patronised station buffets. We preferred to reserve our money for travel. As often as not, it might be no more than a couple of stations along the line, so as to pass an engine shed or a busy shunting yard, or just to see trains passing at speed. Budgeting for travel was simple enough, with fares based on a flat rate per mile, together with an additional fifty per cent for first class, an option we never considered. Half fares applied up to the age of fourteen, at which point small, or baby-faced boys, were able to push it for another year or so.

Gradually one got to chat with other enthusiasts who were also idling away time until the next train came along. One soon picked up the jargon. An engine seen for the first time was a 'cop'. Some lads boasted of 'cabbing' an engine, though I never saw much merit in that, unless a ride was involved. 'Bunking', was the term applied to an unofficial visit to a loco shed or works, without formal permission.

I was nervous about that and, not wanting to get into trouble, I had to find out whom to ask for permission. Opinion varied between approaching the appropriate regional Public Relations and Publicity Department and writing directly to the shed-master concerned. I received some useful tips regarding whether permission might be granted for just a couple of people, whether a small group had a better chance of acceptance and whether mention should be made, on the application, of an accompanying adult. What was more, the regular bunkers were more pragmatic and dismissed the automatic need for official permission. They were though, quick to warn of sheds which were hard to penetrate, and again, where the best unofficial entry points were to be found to avoid ejection.

It all sounded a bit naughty and a bit intimidating to me. I hit on the idea of a compromise approach, getting my Dad to join me as the responsible adult and to try for The Big One. Stratford shed had the biggest loco allocation in the UK, said to be between 300 and 400 engines. It also had a reputation for being difficult to bunk and needing an organised party if a permit were to be granted. I later appreciated the reasons because the sheds and some of the works areas were intermixed in a tangle of lines over a huge area.

Putting theory into practice, Dad and I emerged from Stratford station on the chosen Sunday afternoon, turned left and entered the claustrophobic pedestrian tunnel which led to the motive power depot and works – a route strictly reserved for authorised personnel. Some way along in the gloom a sign indicated a branch tunnel off to the right, leading to the works, immediately before negotiating an S-bend which led towards daylight.

There, was located the gatekeeper's lodge. Dad tapped on the window to attract the attention of the man on duty. He raised no objections at all, pointing vaguely in the right direction and, I dare say, returning directly to his Sunday newspaper. I know we saw a host of engines though I am not sure we winkled out everything present. On the other hand, my one abiding memory was of the first engine we saw which was 69060, one of the very last L3 class former Great Central 2-6-4 tanks. Its bunker was empty and its coupling rods had been removed and it was clearly awaiting scrapping. That 97 ton monster really was a special cop.

In school term time we had only week-ends for spotting sorties, and more especially, Saturdays. Sundays saw reduced time tables and very little activity, although we came to realise that Sundays would be the best time to bunk around sheds, when they were full of engines and there was little likelihood of being thrown off the premises. For seeing engines at work, Saturdays, and especially summer Saturdays, suited us very well. There were often holiday relief trains, and sometimes visiting excursion specials up from the country could bring rare sightings, in addition to the regular services.

So far I had not sampled the Western Region, so Roger and I decided to start with Paddington. It was an eye opener in every respect. I had made a tentative visit to St Pancras and I was, of course, already familiar with the sweeping concourse of Waterloo station. I was always impressed by its size and apparently efficient layout, but otherwise I do not recall being particularly moved by it. Back to Paddington, though. It was certainly a good deal smaller than Waterloo, though its magnificent train shed made up for that. It had a much greater sense of place. The trains were immediately present, not obscured by ticket barriers, screens, bookstalls and so on. What was more, everything was steam hauled. Meanwhile, the space within had a mixture of both transparency and enclosure. As a twelve or thirteen year old, I am sure I would not have described it quite in those terms, but looking back, those were indeed some of the qualities that impressed me.

The engines were the first things that attracted us. I had already seen photographs of GWR locos, but the reality was something special. The Southern had its share of well turned out engines, whilst at Paddington, they possessed an extra sparkle. They all had copper rimmed chimneys and brass safety valve covers, often along with polished brass name plates. Instead of the usual five digit painted cab-side number I was used to, all these engines flaunted a four digit brass number plate. I was aware too that one might encounter two or three digit numbers, but not at Paddington itself. One historically famous example was a Castle class engine, No.111. This was the rebuilt version of the celebrated 'Great Bear', the only GWR example of a 4-6-2 locomotive, dating from 1908, and converted to a 4-6-0 in 1924, when it was re-named 'Viscount Churchill'. Roger drew my attention to this in his 1952 edition of the ABC. He had been lucky enough to have seen it but it was withdrawn later the following year, shortly before this, my first visit to Paddington. He also pointed out the last remaining Saint and Star class members so these became quarries for my early forays on the Western Region. The Stars I did see but the last Saint was to elude me. One became aware that the last of many loco classes were about to disappear and it was frustrating not to have the time or resources to hunt them down.

Later, there was to be particular interest in discovering examples of just one, two or three digit numbers. The numbers themselves were not the only unusual things. These Western Region engines smelled differently, no doubt a product of the South Wales coal they burned.

The first two GW engines I ever recorded were 1008 and 1011, both members of the 4-6-0 County class. I did not realise at the time that Counties were not a common sight at Paddington, so to find two of them together was indeed a bit special. Both then and on subsequent visits, we always ended up at the end of platform 8, which was the spotters' favourite viewing point.

It was here that I once witnessed a rare example of spotters misbehaving. A little group was taking it in turns to walk down the sloping platform end to place pennies on the rails. These were squashed by the next engine to pass over them. I read later that spotters had been banned for bad behaviour, at Preston in 1951, and again at Willesden Junction in 1954. As early as 1944 the press had reported incidents at Tamworth, but this event at Paddington was the only case of bad behaviour I ever encountered. In fact, platform end observers had always struck me as pretty docile groups. About the most rowdy thing we might sometimes have encountered was the first lad to identify an approaching locomotive by its plate frame bogie and elbow steam pipes, when he might shout out, 'King!' Not exactly a breach of the peace!

Between the comings and goings of the main line trains, we would catch sight of the suburban ones, which slipped in and out of the platforms they shared with the Hammersmith line of London Transport. These lay just off the country end of the main platforms. The engines were almost exclusively 2-6-2 tank engines in the number series starting with 6100, being nicknamed, somewhat labouriously, 'tanner-oners'. Remembering the old pre-metric six-pence coin was popularly called a 'tanner', I suppose it just about made sense. Generally though, nicknames were reserved for more impressive engines. Some otherwise modest locos could be attractive just for the character they exuded. The 1400s were a class of little 0-4-2 tanks, sometimes seen on empty carriage workings. Their tall chimneys and steam domes gave them a quaint appearance which made me think of little old men in top hats. Where that association came from, I really do not know. Similarly, the 1500s, a small class of 0-6-0 tanks, echoed the Southern Q1s, (the wartime utility freight engines) in so far as they too were

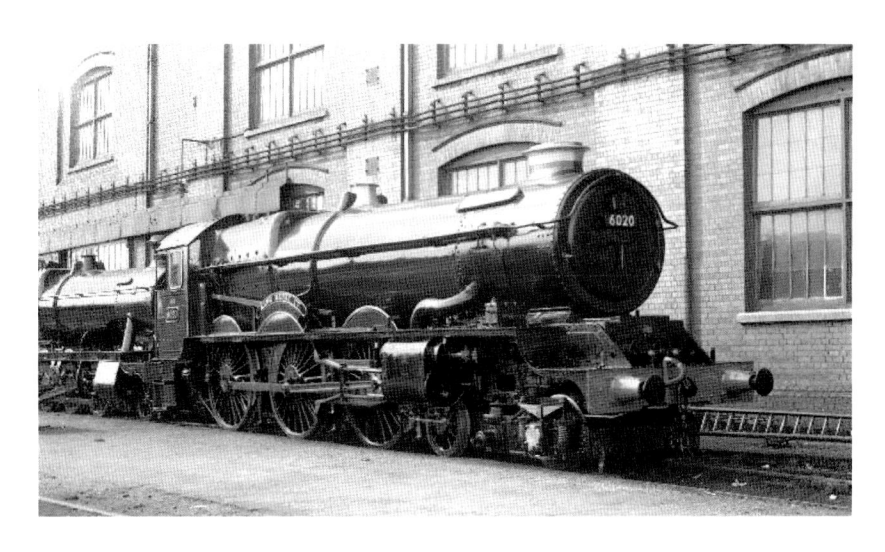

6020, King Henry IV, ex-works at Swindon in Sept 1957, waits to be reunited with its tender. The Kings were the Western Region's most glamorous class which spotters quickly identified from their elbow steam pipes and their unique plate frame bogies with outside bearings to their leading axles.

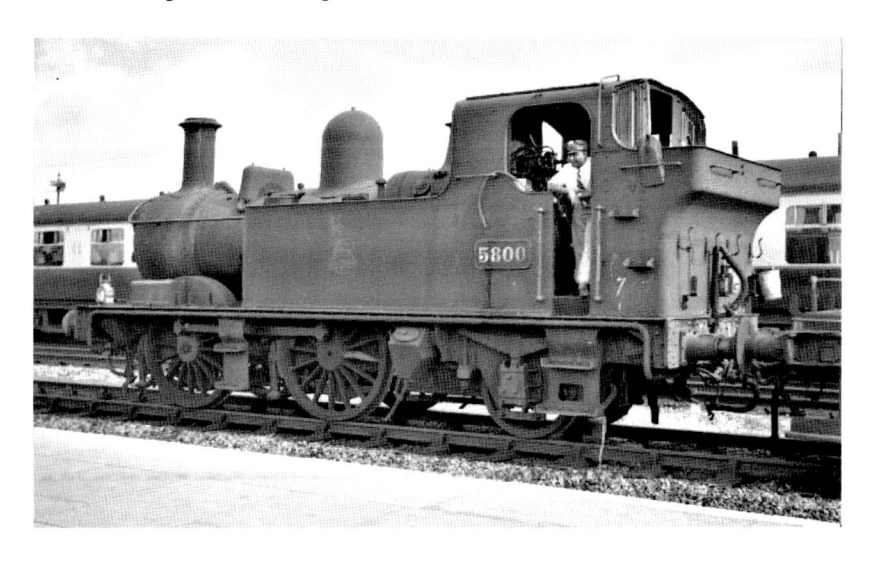

At the other extreme, the diminutive 1400/5800s were designed for light passenger work. Notice the fireman wears a tie in this 1958 photograph; something which could still be seen in some quarters until the end of steam. In the London area they operated the Ealing Broadway to Greenford services and were not unknown pottering around Paddington.

without running plates above their wheels and which, to my mind, gave them a tough pugnacious look.

Soon after those initial sorties, our school announced plans for a summer camp in Brittany, travelling first from Southampton to St Malo. That sounded like an interesting but unknown venture. What was known was that rather odd looking USA class 0-6-0 tank engines were to be seen in Southampton docks. That much my young mentor, Roger, had informed me when we had first seen Ironside at Guildford. He also mentioned B4s, another unusual type of small locomotive, once particularly associated with the docks. That was enough for me to sign up for the trip.

Probably noticing my enthusiasm for this venture, another lad in our class, who had no interest in trains, kindly gave me an unwanted copy of a 'Bradshaw's Continental Railway Guide, 1853, 3/6d'. Aimed at a rather more prosperous clientele than school boy campers, it had no immediate relevance to our planned adventure. 1853 was a century ago, but I could not help noticing some of the guidance offered for foreign travel.

'**Hotels** – It is not necessary, in travelling on the continent, for a gentleman and his wife … to take a sitting room as well as a bedroom, as is the custom in British Holels' – no difficulty there since our sitting room was to be a grassy field and our bedroom was a tent.

'**Knapsacks** – may be purchased much cheaper abroad, and much better than in England' – our government-surplus kit bags did the job for us.

'**Portemanteaus** – are better purchased in England than anywhere else.' – I could see no immediate need for one of these.

The outward journey with thirty excitable youngsters was hardly conducive to spotting. Even so, I was still surprised just how few engines I did glimpse, especially in the Eastleigh or Southampton areas, so I just hoped for better luck in a couple of weeks time on the way home. When we eventually reached our destination in Brittany, I immediately detected a railway line in a cutting which flanked our campsite and where an ungainly and asthmatic sounding steam train, passed a few times a day. The engine, covered in external plumbing, leaked steam from every available joint and seemed to struggle against its three or four all but empty carriages, lumbering reluctantly behind it. Enquiries at the local station revealed that this was the service to Morlaix, which I duly noted, should the opportunity arise to visit that town.

   Meanwhile, things looked up when a couple of us were allowed to go off to explore the next village. There, next to the main street, I discovered just the sort of scenery I enjoyed, in the form of a complete station yard. What made it special was that everything was in miniature, for this was on the extensive one metre gauge regional network which used to serve many a small Breton community. The centre piece of the scene was a rather narrow and upright 0-6-0 tank engine whose tall chimney emitted lazy black whirls of smoke which formed a dense canopy above it and which only began to disperse at its extremities. The driver was tinkering about, oil can and hammer to hand, and the fireman was raking out ashes from under the engine and shovelling them into miniature tub wagons. He hardly needed to have bothered because the entire yard was covered in black cinders to the extent that no sleepers were visible at all in the loco sidings, only the rails themselves shining against the greasy black background. The engine was black, the sky was black and the ground was black. At first sight one would not have noticed the modest pile of loco coal strategically placed to supply the engines. What had first caught my eye was a small heap of coal briquettes, distinguishable only by their shape, but otherwise as black as everything else.

   Just beyond this scene stood a second engine of the same type which had been taking water. It was at least a bit cleaner, with a smear of red indicating the buffer beam and no more than a black haze emanating from the chimney. Fire irons and shovels seemed to lie around indiscriminately and there was no sign of life beyond the two engine crews. A short train of ancient once varnished wooden carriages, sat disconsolately off to one side. Passing the same spot two days later, nothing much had changed and even at my tender age of twelve, I sensed that could not go on for many more years. There were too many shiny new Simcas, Panhards, and Renaults around, and still no train passengers in sight.

During the second week of our stay, a coach excursion to Morlaix was announced. It was agreed two of us could go by train rather than the coach, if we preferred, and so it was we made our way to catch the 'puffer', as it had been christened. The ticket collector seemed surprised and puzzled that two English boys should want to travel by train. Although we dutifully presented our tickets to be clipped before boarding, he just waved us through onto the platform and was still watching us with some curiosity as we boarded near the engine. We found ourselves alone in the corridor carriage and the journey was uneventful. In due course, we were impressed by the lofty railway viaduct which crossed the town of Morlaix but the highlight of the day for me was watching the engines stabled next to the station platform, when we were waiting for our train home. Two of them were large express engines, one painted green, which looked impressive by their size alone.

These modern looking machines were probably amongst those supplied by the USA in the years after the War. They were definitely in a different category from the USA shunters I was to spot at Southampton docks during our journey home. The boat train awaiting the arrival of our former Southern Railway ferry, 'Falaise', was headed by a King Arthur 4-6-0. This time, I was better prepared so that, having copped three or four USA tanks, I was able to make a log of the journey to Waterloo. As we passed Winchester, I was disappointed that the shed was so small. At least it gave me my first B4 cop. It also taught me that if cops were not to be missed some preparatory research was useful for any journey. By that time, I was resigned to the fact it was not going to be a scintillating run to London. In fact the average speed turned out to be a rather modest 46 mph.

Of the few French engines I had seen during those two weeks, the enduring memory was of those metre gauge examples. We had little quite like them at home but we did have the British Railways Vale of Rheidol line with its three engines Nos. 7, 8 and 9 on their 1foot 11½ inch gauge track. Also in Wales, there was the Welshpool and Llanfair 2 foot 6½ inch gauge line with its two engines, 822 The Earl and 823, later named Countess.

The novelty value of narrow gauge within the British national railway system was enough to mark out those five numbers, so there was a particular satisfaction to be had in spotting them. When, therefore, the Welshpool and Llanfair, which had been a freight only line since 1931, was closed in 1956, it was a relief to learn its locomotives had been put in store. That made them feel even more inaccessible but there was always hope. So it proved when a group of enthusiasts partially reopened the route in 1963. Meanwhile, it fell to the Vale of Rheidol trio to fly the flag for narrow gauge on British Rail and to supply the very last steam engine to run on British Rail tracks in 1989, at which time the V of R was privatised, twenty-one years after the end of main line steam.

There was novelty value too in other low number locos, all of which fell within the purlieu of the Western Region. These were types, generally of South Wales origins, which had been inherited by the GWR from sources like the Rhymney Railway, the Taff Vale Railway, the Swansea Harbour Trust and from elsewhere. Many of them acquired Great Western boilers but others betrayed their obvious 'foreign' origins to the end. Many of them were cut up in 1953 and 1954, so for spotters from the eastern end of the region, a visit to Swindon in those years was rewarded with a last chance to cop some unusually low numbers.

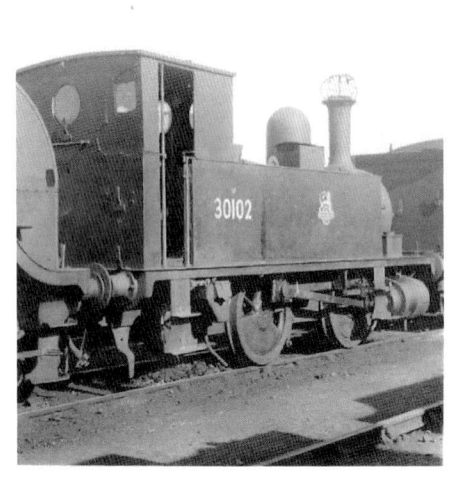

B4 class 30102 is seen at Eastleigh in 1958. Built in 1893, it was to bear the painted name 'Granville' when it spent time working in the Southern Railway's Southampton docks. One wonders just how effective was the primitive wire cage spark arrester perched on the chimney top. It spent its last years shunting at Winchester. Withdrawn in 1963, it was sold to Butlins for holiday camp display and then moved to the Bressingham Steam Museum, Norfolk, in 1971. Looking carefully, one can make out the original profile of the cab rear screen. It originally had only the central circular spectacle, flanked by curved cut-outs. Later the missing corners of the cab were made up, each with its rectangular spectacle.

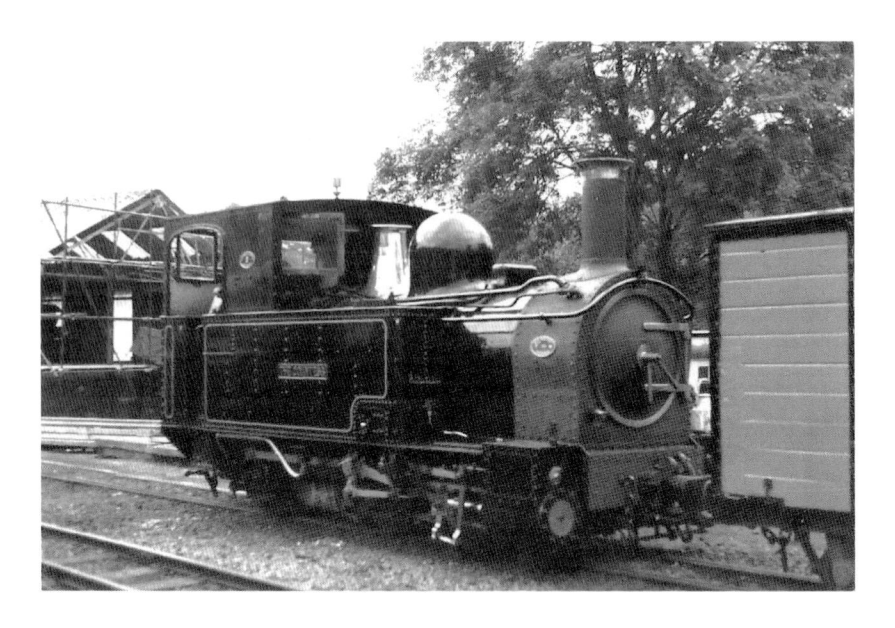

The charm of narrow gauge could attract diehards to remote locations. Formerly 823 'Countess', is seen here after enthusiasts succeeded in progressively reopening the Welshpool and Llanfair line from 1963 onwards. By this time she was running as 'The Countess', presumably to match her partner, formerly.822, 'The Earl'. No longer part of British Railways, neither carried its former Great Western number. Nevertheless, they made acceptable belated cops.

Gradually our spotting range increased. The rest of that South Eastern and Chatham stretch from Tonbridge to Redhill to Guildford was completed, and again, with a satisfying mix of locomotive activity and stretches of cross-country tranquillity. That particular run was accomplished behind one of the 2-6-0 classes which had their design origins in the SE & CR and, unexpectedly, the carriage we had to ourselves was an elderly open saloon, with seating along the sides and facing a central table. There were tantalising glimpses of unfamiliar engine types at Redhill but it was not possible to identify them. My regular companion on these excursions notified me we would have to go to Brighton to see these properly. That was often how future trips were agreed upon, with no need for further discussion.

Over a few months we visited not only most of the London terminal stations but we started to venture further afield from them. An interesting circuit was to take a train to Basingstoke, then a cross country link to Reading, and finally a fast train back to Paddington. This was a journey of contrasts which we were subsequently to undertake several times. Some of what we were to see was predictable and some things varied according to the time of year or the time of day. At that time, we still talked of expresses and semi-fast trains for longer journeys. A semi-fast might stop at Woking, beyond which the West of England main line was almost solely steam hauled, allowing for the regular appearance of diesels, 10201 and 10203. Our train was typically pulled by one of the green painted 'King Arthur' class 4-6-0s, all sporting names from Arthurian legends, but equally we might have been hauled by one of the less glamourous black unnamed freight variations of the Arthurs. These were not particularly attractive to watch, but in terms of loco spotting, they kept us on our toes.

Through quirks of history, the number series of Southern Region classes of engines, in particular, were frequently scrambled together. Consequently it was not always immediately obvious whether or not we had seen all the members of a particular class. This made one look harder at loco details in order to identify their type. It could be more difficult when a class contained a range of variations, or sometimes included details cobbled together from parts of long defunct classes.

What decided the train we took was the price of travel, as much as anything. Although fares were generally based on a flat rate of 1 3/4d per mile (or 73p/100 miles), it was possible to keep an eye open for cheaper excursion tickets, which usually specified particular travel times. This worked better for an out and return trip but did not help for a circular trip like our Waterloo, Basingstoke, Reading, Paddington route. Summer Saturday mornings tended to be very crowded with holiday makers. They also yielded sightings of rare and elderly passenger engines, pressed into service at these peak times. These included 4-4-0s of the S11, L12 and D15 classes. I suspect they were doing little more than working out their time, shuffling back and forth to Basingstoke. Strangely enough, the more numerous T9s, or 'Greyhounds', put in fewer appearances. Once famous for their turn of speed on the West of England main line, they were by then largely confined to the south-west of England.

During school holidays of course, it did not matter which day we chose to travel. In fact weekday journeys were likely to give us a corridor or compartment to ourselves, which enabled us to dive from one side of the train to the other, according to whatever caught our eye. It has to be remembered we spent a lot of time hanging out of open windows, anticipating what was coming and, incidentally, collecting in the process our fair share of ash and smuts from the engine. It was easy enough to arrive home, after a long day, our hair full of grit and our faces one or two shades darker than when we set out. Perhaps surprisingly, only once did I catch a piece of grit in my eye, whereupon I was steered towards a first aid post on the concourse of Waterloo

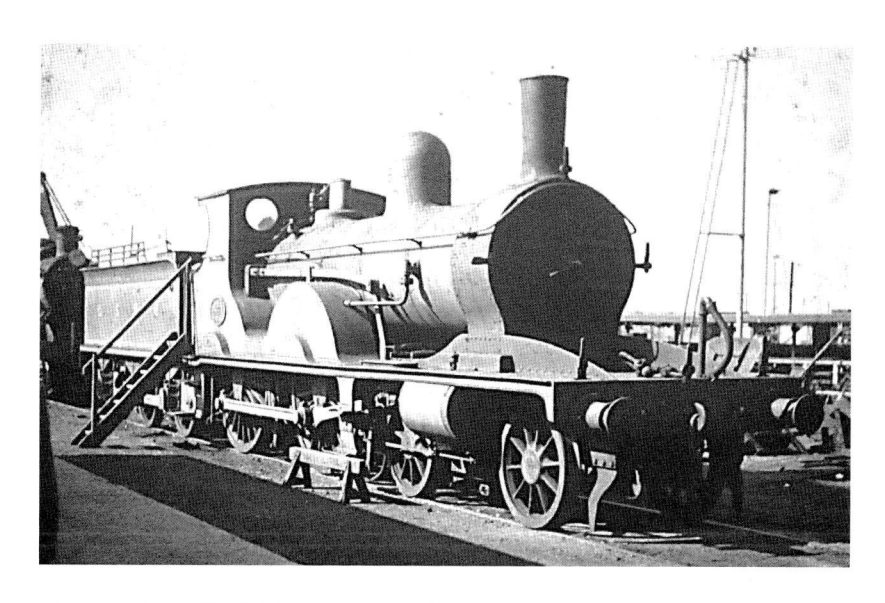

*The open day at Eastleigh on 3 August 1960, warranted bringing out of storage Adams class T3, 563. Built in 1893 and withdrawn in 1945, the Southern Railway displayed it at Waterloo in 1948, along with an M7 tank and preserved Bodmin and Wadebridge Railway vehicles. Waterloo station had undergone a complete transformation in its rebuilding between 1901 and 1922 and 1948 marked the station's centenary. From 1963, No.563 was displayed at the Clapham Transport Museum, moving to York when the National Railway Museum opened in 1975. Demoted to the reserve collection at Shildon in 2010, it was eventually passed to the Swanage Railway Trust in 2017. Not a cop in the usual sense but a joy to see.*

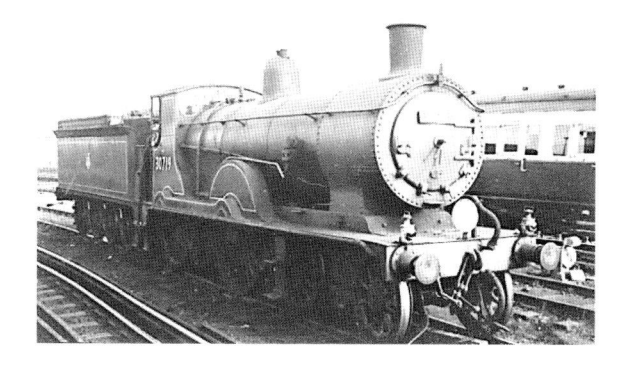

*Former LSWR loco, class T9 30719 at Clapham Junction in the late 1950s. Their turn of speed in their heyday earned them the name of Greyhound. They remained more active west of Salisbury. Not all examples carried the original pattern 'water cart' eight wheel tender seen here. Built in 1899, 30719 lasted until March 1961.*

station to have it quickly flushed out. One imagines it was a routine procedure for the nurse in attendance. The irony was that I had been travelling in an electric train at the time.

There was always a moment or two of excited anticipation before departure. Our preference was to be in the very first carriage directly behind the engine, where we could see it, hear it and smell it. A little before departure time, Roger would announce, "We've got the flash," though I never knew how authentic this expression was amongst railwaymen. He had told me his grandfather was on the railway, so I tended to accept this way of announcing the green colour light signal was showing all clear. There would be a distant whistle from the guard; the last carriage door would thump shut; there would be a brief warning whistle from the engine and we were underway.

What we really hoped for was a fast non-stop run to Basingstoke behind a Merchant Navy or West Country class, something we did manage on one occasion. These unconventional, rather boxy looking engines, could really fly, even if they were popularly known in some quarters as 'spam cans'. They were notoriously light footed. If a train was well loaded or the rails were wet or greasy, there was every chance the wheels would lose their grip upon starting. You could almost sense it coming. First there would be a slight clunk as the coupling slack was taken up and then almost a hesitation as the driver judged just how much further he dared open the regulator. If he got it wrong, there could be an almighty explosion of exhaust through the chimney, as the driving wheels struggled for adhesion. The driver would instantaneously shut off steam and try again. If he were lucky, the second time around, it might be no more than a momentary slip and then the train would be coaxed into movement, as it threaded its way across the complicated point-work, towards the down fast main line.

That was exactly the scenario we witnessed. The tentative start gave no indication of what was to follow, so by the time we reached Wimbledon, we were in full cry, whistle

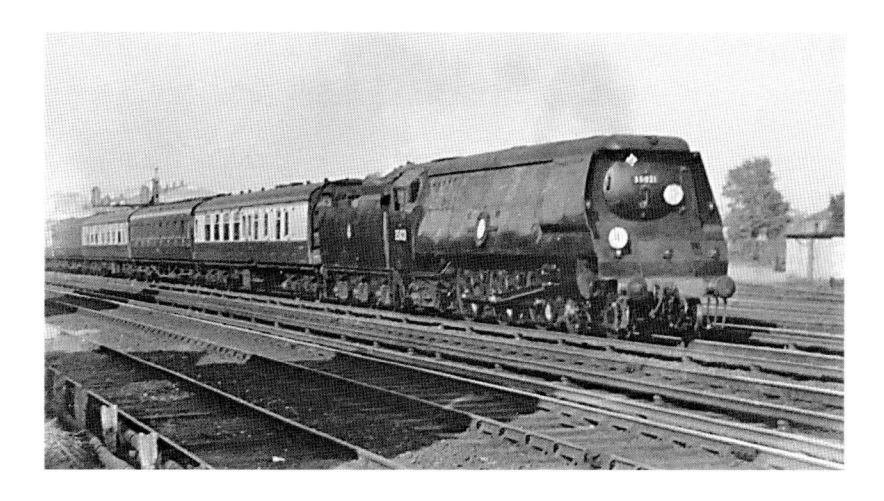

*Un-rebuilt Merchant Navy class, No.35021, New Zealand Line, accelerating westwards past Wimbledon in 1955, sporting a Bournemouth West headcode. The rag-bag effect of mixed carriage liveries is evident. The Merchants were nearly two and a half feet longer than the West Countries – a perceptible difference which was enough to make them that bit more impressive. There has been talk of re-streamlining one of the surviving rebuilt Merchant Navies and that would certainly lead to an interesting comparison to-day.*

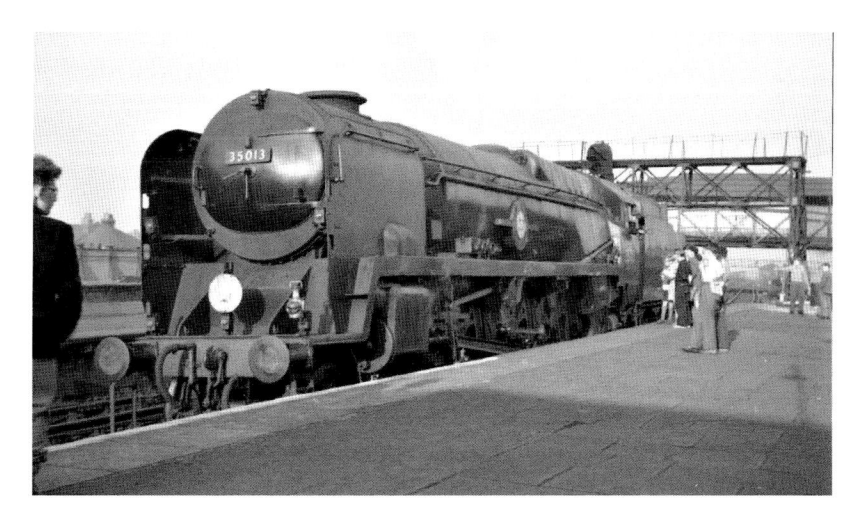

The first Merchant Navy rebuilds appeared in February 1956. This is 35013, only the 3rd example, seen at Waterloo shortly after its conversion in May of that year. Waterloo rarely witnessed more than two or three spotters. However, the novelty of these new arrivals brought out the newly curious throughout that summer.

67

screaming as we rushed through that particularly reverberative station, bursting out from below the road over-bridge and accelerating westwards.

Having arrived at Basingstoke, we might pause long enough to watch a couple of London bound expresses passing through, but the truth was we were unlikely to see many Southern engines we could not have seen nearer home. This applied equally to the semi-fasts and to freight trains. Sometimes on these trips we made the effort to leave the station, taking the road which passed under the tracks towards the small loco shed. It took only a minute to see what was inside but there was, after all, the possibility of spotting something unusual which had perhaps failed or was temporarily in store. Disappointingly, as far as I recall, our visits to the shed never actually yielded much more than a panoramic view back towards passing expresses.

We forewent this little deviation on the occasions when our connecting train to Reading was shortly due. This marked a change in tempo. It was almost always hauled by a Remembrance class loco. This would be one of a small group of seven 4-6-0s which had originated on the London, Brighton & South Coast Railway in 1914, as 4-6-4 tank engines. Rebuilt from 1934, they perpetuated the names of pioneer locomotive engineers, with the exception of 32333 which was named "Remembrance", as a form of mobile war memorial to fallen railway staff. They were equally to be seen on semi-fasts to London. Painted black, they were denied the glamour of other named engines and seemed to go largely unnoticed, despite their interesting background.

The journey to Reading was leisurely and the train was usually all but devoid of passengers. With nothing better to do during this part of our circuit, we would wander up and down the corridor, daring to stand in the corridor connections between carriages. The carriages themselves had seen better days and jolted disconcertingly as the overlapping floor plates crunched

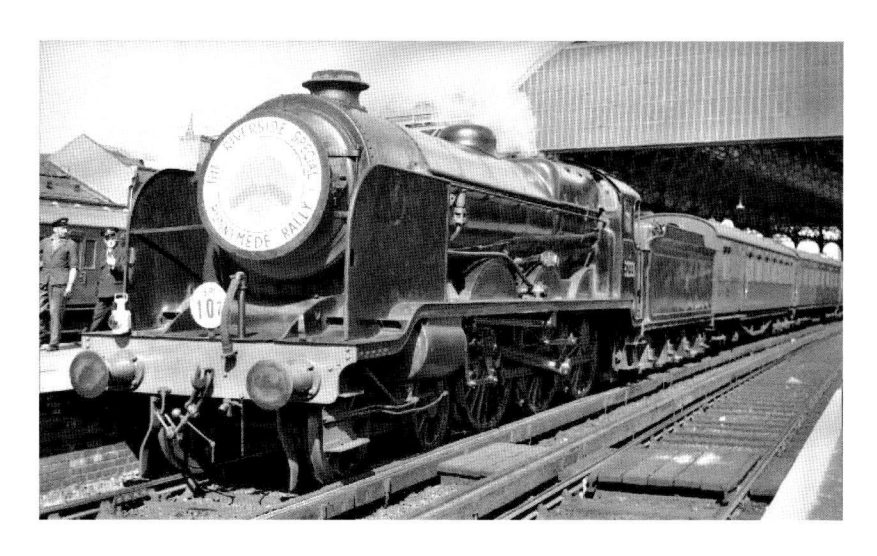

*The last of the Remembrances, 32331 Beattie, on the 'Riverside Special', waiting to leave London Bridge on 23 June 1957. They had been a regular sight on Waterloo – Basingstoke – Reading services for many years. Large disc headboards like the one displayed here were associated with private excursion specials.*

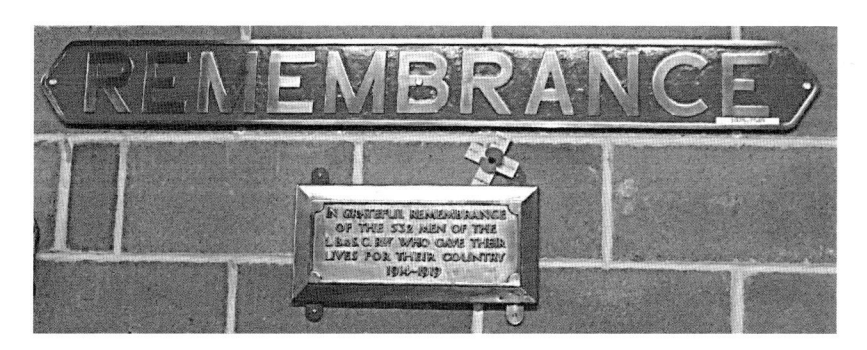

Locomotive nameplates can hide fascinating histories which lift them above being mere souvenirs. Those of British Railways No. 32333 are displayed at the National Railway Museum. The initial London Brighton and South Coast Railway 'L' class locomotives appeared as 4-6-4 tanks in 1914, painted black. The last one was adopted as a mobile war memorial. They were changed to SR olive green from 1924 and their boldly painted names were replaced with straight name plates in 1927. In 1934 they were all rebuilt as tender engines as the N15X class. They then acquired curved name plates and the cab-side memorial plaques of engine No.333 Remembrance were affixed to the splashers below its new nameplates. The N15X s were painted black during the 1939 – 45 War, then malachite green until 1949, when British Railways took them almost full circle, back to mixed traffic lined black. 'Remembrance' itself had been built in 1922 and was withdrawn in 1956.

69

and scraped against each other. We knew it was safe enough, but it still felt that the gap between carriages might open up at any second.

Only on the approach to Reading would we resume the serious business of spotting. Watching the working patterns of locomotives and observing the details which distinguished one class from another, was a major part of it. Recording numbers came to be an extension of this. I realised that for some enthusiasts, number collecting was an end in itself. Subsequently I met one or two people who displayed an almost obsessive desire to hunt down every locomotive in the land, to the exclusion of any wider interest. One of these I recall vividly. Rather seriously, this sixteen or seventeen year old asked if I had seen any of the three London Midland engine numbers he quoted. These were the very last cops he needed to have seen every British Railways steam locomotive, or so he said. He was not going to find them where we stood, at the end of platform 10 at Kings Cross, but perhaps he could just not resist the appeal of Eastern Region express passenger engines.

I came to see it as something of a chicken and egg situation. Collecting numbers necessitated travel and observation. Observation widened interest and awareness. Recording numbers gave a sort of validity to the time and effort expended. Inevitably one saw numerous engines time and again if one frequented the same territory. In that case, it became something of an event to return home with a few 'cops'.

Watching familiar engines at work may not have raised much excitement but they still represented an animated part of an engaging landscape. It is tempting to draw comparisons with bird watching, with its parallels of species and their variations of behaviour, colouring and sound, along with location, time of day, frequency of occurrence, occasional visitors, long distance flyers or local residents.

It is surprising how close these similarities are. Alright, the comparison can break down. In one pursuit the quarry is animal and alive, in the other it is material and inert, yet even then the latter takes on an elemental and metaphorical form of life where earth, fire, air and water combine to produce lifelike motion.  Nothing highlighted that more than the contrast with those dead engines seen in locomotive sheds and yards.

None of these considerations would have bothered us as we left Reading West and looked across towards Reading motive power depot.  The small size of the brass number plates in the distance made it tricky to record many Western Region numbers from the moving train, but we usually bagged a few cops. Then, there could still be a surprise or two to come.  As we drew into the bay platform we would perhaps see a 'Flying Banana', the nickname for the streamlined ex-GWR rail cars which had been introduced in the mid-1930s.  They were something of a curiosity.  Diesel powered, they sounded more like buses and, as one-carriage 'trains', they discreetly slipped in and out of stations almost unnoticed.

Once, here at Reading, and waiting for our London bound train, we stood back safely from the platform edge as a non-stop express rushed through.  There was nothing odd about that except, some seconds later, we were surprised by the spectacle of an unpowered single carriage rolling into the platform and a group of passengers alighting.  As it happened, we had witnessed one of the few slip coach services still in operation, whereby a guard detached one or two carriages from a fast moving train, which therefore avoided the need to stop for relatively few passengers to alight.  The GWR had been the last railway to retain slip working by 1939, so it was a surprise to see it re-introduced on the Western Region in 1950.  It was to last for another ten years.

Another attraction of Reading for loco spotters was the almost adjacent Southern Region terminus, Reading South.  It may have been less busy than Reading General but it did attract engines from as far afield as Tonbridge, so a cop or two were quite possible.   It also had its own engine shed where it was

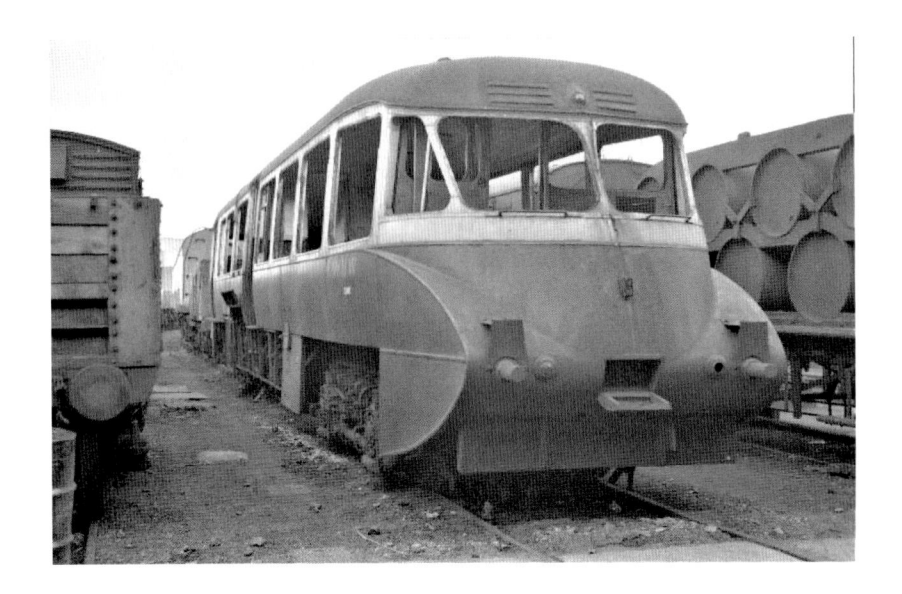

In 1932, Bugatti designed a railcar capable of speeds exceeding 100 mph, which entered service from Paris the following year. It was 1934 when the GWR introduced their own rather more modest railcar design. It was perhaps no coincidence that they took a design cue from Bugatti in dispensing with the conventional disc-like face to the buffers.

Ex-GWR diesel railcar No.11 was built by Gloucester Railway Carriage & Wagon Co. in 1936. It is seen here in April 1958 in the Swindon carriage works yard having been withdrawn some months previously. Unlike the missing glass windows, the side valances had been removed early in its career. The original streamlined design looked very slick but appearance gave way to practicality when the valances impeded access to the running gear.

This particular 'Flying Banana' had 63 seats and toilet facilities. Others in the class had variations covering seating capacity, engine type and buffet facilities. In service, they operated at speeds up to 60-70mph.

possible to see ex-South Eastern and Chatham designs, of the kinds which looked more at home around Tonbridge.

A station like Reading General was always something of a hot spot for spotters. A main line, a junction bringing trains from several directions, a loco shed or busy goods yard – all these things meant enough activity to attract the spotter's interest. Indeed, such was the interest that in the late 50s and into the 60s, a sunny summer's day could draw three or four dozen spotters to the west end of the platforms. They must have been generally well behaved since after the demise of steam and into the 1970s, Reading station was probably unique in encouraging loco spotters by issuing a special ten pence 'Train Spotter Ticket', available from 9am to 5pm. It is not clear what the advantage was over an ordinary platform ticket or indeed what function it served if the spotter had arrived by train anyway.

By the time we reached Paddington it was usually enough to make a quick check on what was standing at the buffer stops, maybe a brief examination of the glass case tucked away in the corner of the concourse, which housed a superb large scale model of a King class locomotive and a carriage, and then off to the Underground for our journey homewards, with the lure of Swindon in our minds.

# CHAPTER FIVE                    **Memorable Places**

I learnt on the grapevine that Swindon works held regular open days, so it was easy enough to get permission to visit. On reflection, visits were all remarkably casual, with little formal supervision. Consequently we tended to follow our nose rather than any specific directions.

The works yard contained several very low number engines from the former South Wales valley companies, like the Taff Vale and Rhymney Railways. Some of these were probably about to be scrapped but alongside them, in complete contrast, were glamorous express passenger engines in shiny freshly painted ex-works condition, one or two awaiting their tenders to be attached.

The spotters' Mecca was 'A-shop', the principal works building which housed row upon row of locomotives in varying states of assembly. None of the men working on them ever gave more than a passing glance in our direction, as we made our way up and down the rows. Sometimes a slight deviation was necessary to ascertain the identity of a particular engine, which was in such a state of undress as to be anonymous at first glance. Usually its cab, and therefore its number plate, was close to hand and the number would again appear, chalked on the major components as if against any risk of parts being mistakenly separated.

This could pose a minor ethical problem for spotters. What component identified a locomotive? Was it enough just to record a number? Was the running number on the front of a boiler sufficient, especially as boilers could be interchanged or replaced? The works yard contained a number of boilers, sometimes from rare or otherwise extinct engines. The temptation to record them as cops was considerable. There were no rules, but if pushed, the consensus seemed to be that you had to see the frames. Even then, there were cases mentioned of

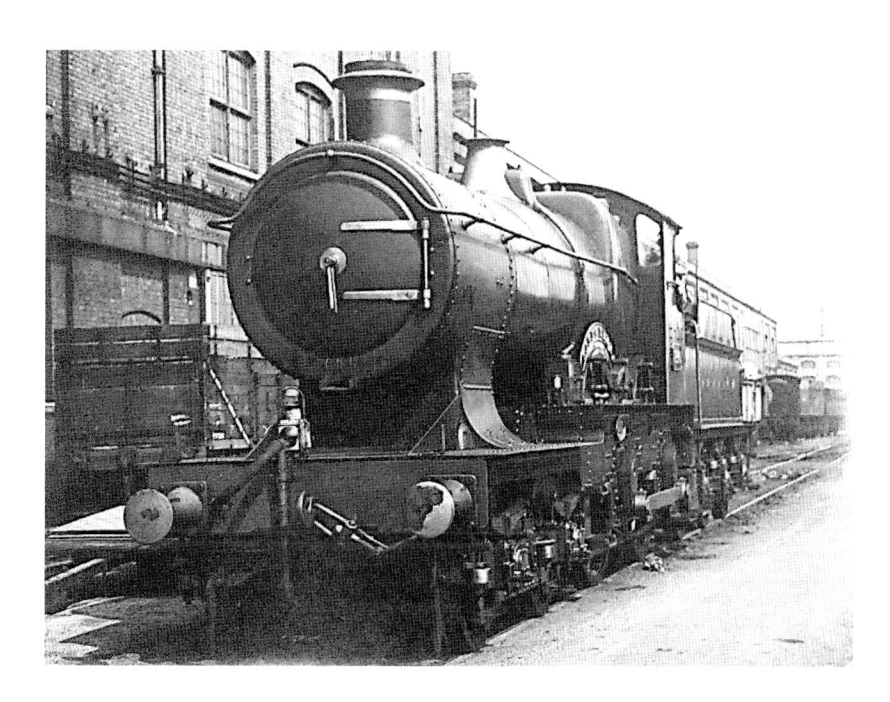

*Built in 1903, outside frame GWR No.3440 City of Truro, is seen at Swindon works on13 April, 1958. In 1904, it was probably the first locomotive to have reached a speed of 100mph. Withdrawn in 1931 and after many years in the LNER's Queen Street collection at York, it was restored to revenue earning service and worked regularly on the Didcot, Newbury & Southampton line from 1957 to 1961.*

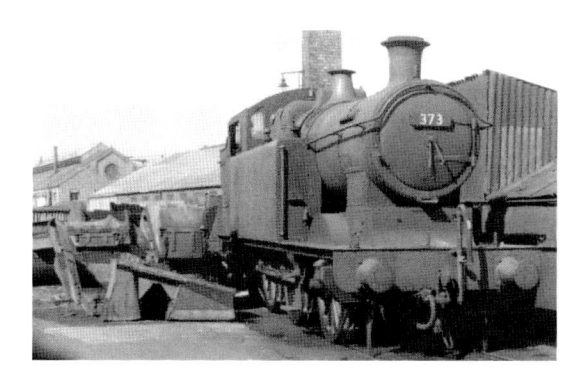

*Low number cops were somewhat prized by home-county spotters. This 0-6-2 tank had been given a Great Western boiler and details, which disguised its former Taff Vale Railway origins. It was seen here in Swindon works yard on 29 September 1957, having been withdrawn the previous month from Abercynon shed.*

frames and identities being exchanged, but I think most of us drew the line at sorting out such niceties.

A little further west came a sizeable yard, containing a motley collection of bedraggled wagons and locomotives. One hoped some of them were waiting their turn in A-shop. However, if they carried a daubed on cab-side symbol in the form of a cross within a circle, or the abbreviation, 'CON', then they were certainly heading for the cutter's torch. They might be demolished outside or within 'C'- shop, which had been built to facilitate the process. Along with its lifting equipment, it allowed the workmen to operate in sheltered conditions. One might also have seen it as a discreet veil over their barbaric, or at least, destructive activities.

These were the corners where spotters could cop an ancient rarity, before it vanished for ever, or was consigned to an open wagon in large pieces. On my first visit to Swindon, I even saw one or two engines which did not appear in my ABC, which was itself over a year old, so they must have been long since condemned

Not so far away stood a very elderly relic, in the form of a pair of 8 foot 10 inch (2.69m) diameter driving wheels, which had belonged to a former Bristol and Exeter broad gauge locomotive. At the time, I wondered if they would meet the cutter's torch one day, given the vandalism bestowed upon the two broad gauge engines put aside for preservation, well before the demise of the broad gauge, in 1892. These engines had survived until 1906, when it was apparently claimed they were occupying valuable space. It is inconceivable that a corner could not have been found in which to store them, had the will been there. At least today we can look upon replica locomotives of the same types.

It should not go unnoticed that City of Truro, the first engine thought to have exceeded 100 mph, was given to the LNER for display at their York museum in 1931. The Great Western did not want to preserve it. Clearly the GWR's lack of

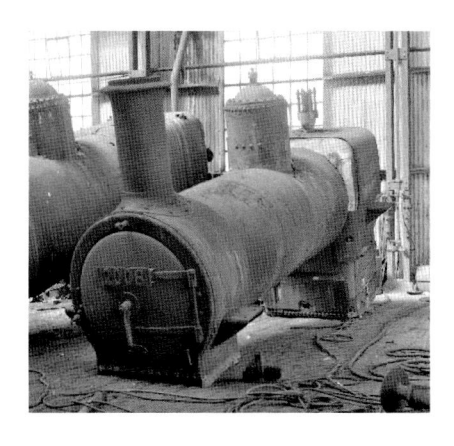

*This does not look much to be excited about but it would have been a very satisfying cop. Just in time, No.2008, with its frames near-by, were spotted in the early stages of scrapping at Swindon on 13 April 1958. Starting life as a saddle tank and later converted to a pannier tank, it was withdrawn from Birkenhead shed as the penultimate survivor of the 850 class, introduced in 1910 and extinct by 1959.*

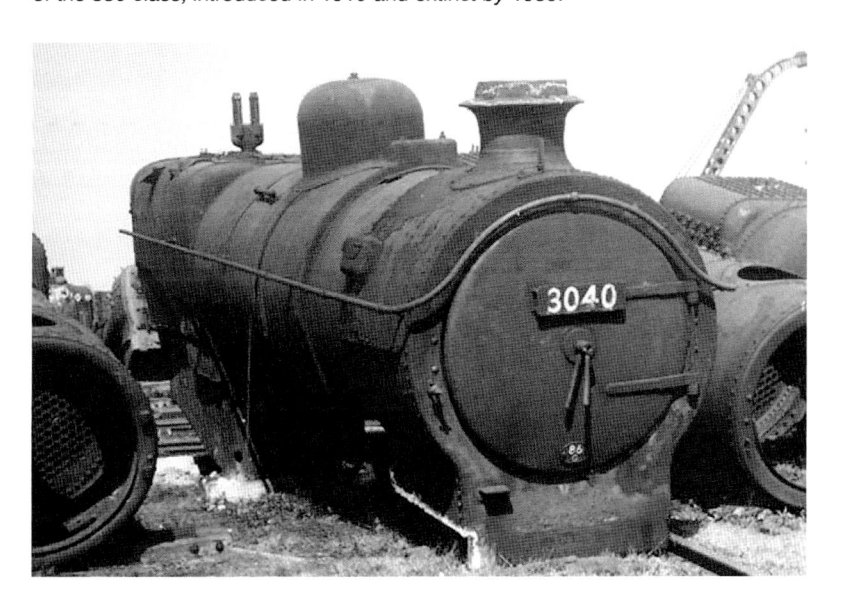

*The boiler of 3040, bearing an 86G (Pontypool Road) shed code, was spotted at Swindon on 13 April 1958. 3040 had been purchased by the GWR as Government surplus after the First World War and given Swindon brass top feed and safety valve casings. An exemple of this 1911 Great Central design survives in the National Collection.*

77

sentimentality or sense of history had not evolved very far by that date. It is good to see those enormous Bristol to Exeter Railway wheels survived the closure of Swindon works in 1985. Swindon perhaps, more than any other works, clearly displayed its nature as locomotive 'hospital, beauty parlour and graveyard'.

Having been free to explore Swindon works, we went, as if by inertia, in search of the loco sheds. Our real goal was the fabled 'stock shed', home to some more modern preserved engines. The sun was streaming in and sure enough, there, in the silence, were 4003 Lode Star and Dean Goods 2516, both bearing that now familiar dead quality of engines out of steam. Nevertheless, the fact they were both very grimy and dust covered, left them looking as if they had been there for decades. We must have felt a little like archaeologists unearthing treasures, as we stood there in the silence, marvelling for several moments. It was, then, left to the Western Region, partially to atone for its predecessor's dismissal of past achievements.

In our eagerness to enter the stock shed we had paid scant attention to what stood a short way off. Unlike the other regions of British Railways, the Western Region had inherited few 4-4-0s and they were never likely to be seen at the eastern end of the region. Nevertheless, there stood an example of the so-called Dukedogs, a rather ungainly amalgam of Duke class boilers and Bulldog class frames, undertaken in the late 1930s. They represented a curious perpetuation of a Great Western design approach from the 1890s, with their enormous steam domes and outside frames. Again, a survivor can still be seen, this time on the Bluebell Railway.

That first visit to Swindon finished with a visit to the running shed, which yielded more unfamiliar engines, but this time we didn't linger very long. The place was full of dense sulphurous smoke which slowed down our number taking and made it impossible to savour the loco discoveries we made. Of all the sheds I was ever to visit, that one remains in my memory

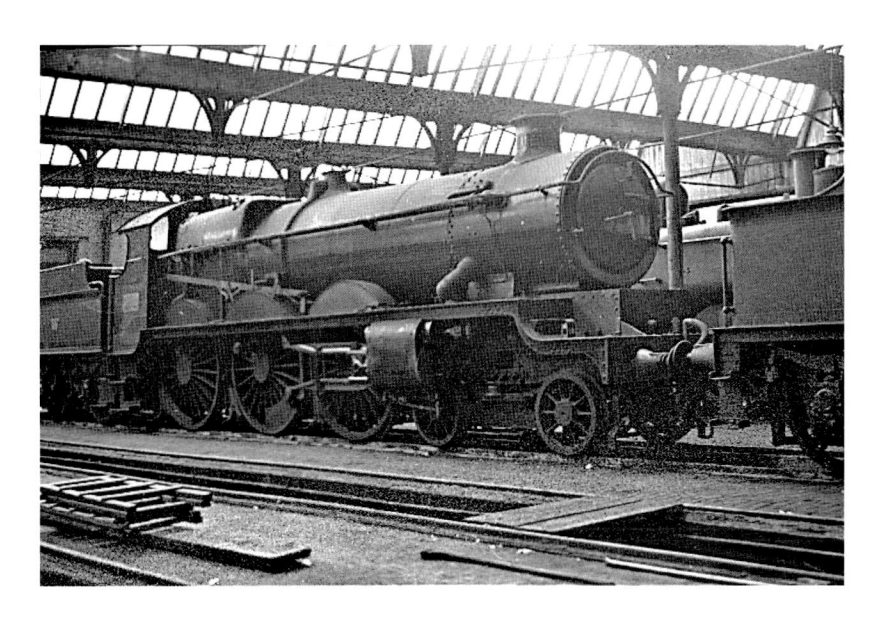

*Star class 4003, Lode Star, covered in dust with nameplates removed for safe keeping, it had not turned a wheel for some years. No longer included in the ABC and encountered rather unexpectedly in the Swindon stock shed, it conveyed a rather ghostly presence.*

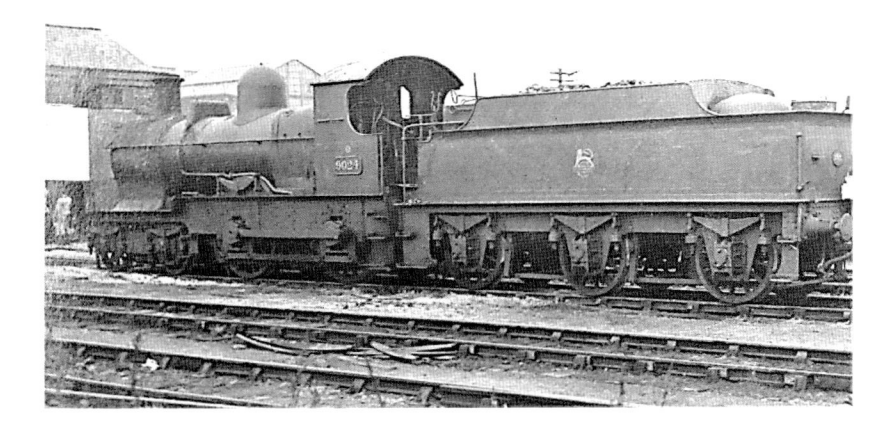

*One of the so called "Dukedogs", No. 9024, seen outside the stock shed at Swindon on 29 September 1957. Introduced in 1936 as an amalgam of Duke class boilers and Bulldog class frames, their huge domes and outside frames belonged more to the 1890s. They were mostly to be found on the former Cambrian Railway lines. Wales was a long way from home, so sightings like this were a treat for a spotter from the South East.*

79

as the most disagreeable railway environment I was ever to encounter.

If Paddington and Swindon epitomized the Western Region locomotive scene, then it followed that other important centres would capture the spirit of their respective regional locomotive stock.

We may not have had the internet but we became avid magazine readers, we poured over maps and we chatted with fellow spotters. It took little time for us to expand our explorations, both in depth and geographically. Having said that, Liverpool Street, Euston and Kings Cross also became our regular haunts.

There were good reasons for this. London based spotters may have had thirteen terminal stations at their disposal but only these four, along with Waterloo, could offer more or less non-stop steam activity. The others were dominated by electric traction or, in the cases of Marylebone and St Pancras, did not offer a lot of action. In fact trains seemed to slip in and out rather discreetly as if apologising for disturbing the prevailing silence. St Pancras provided an imposing setting and could at least rise to hosting 'Jubilees' and rebuilt 'Royal Scots'.

Consequently, a visit was almost invariably tacked on to a visit to Kings Cross, prompted by the possible spectacle of a 2P 4-4-0 double heading a Black Five, which was worth seeing. Other than that one had to persevere to find further interest. On just one occasion I did manage to watch some capstan shunting of a couple of wagons which were being manoeuvred onto the wagon hoist which then stood between the platform ends and the signal box, a short way off. The cellar below platform level was originally designed on a modular basis, the module being a barrel of Burton beer. On this occasion the two open wagons concerned appeared to have no connection with that trade.

The departure of a Manchester express, or even the Thames-Clyde Express, never seemed to generate the fluster of activity associated with the busier stations. Word had it that

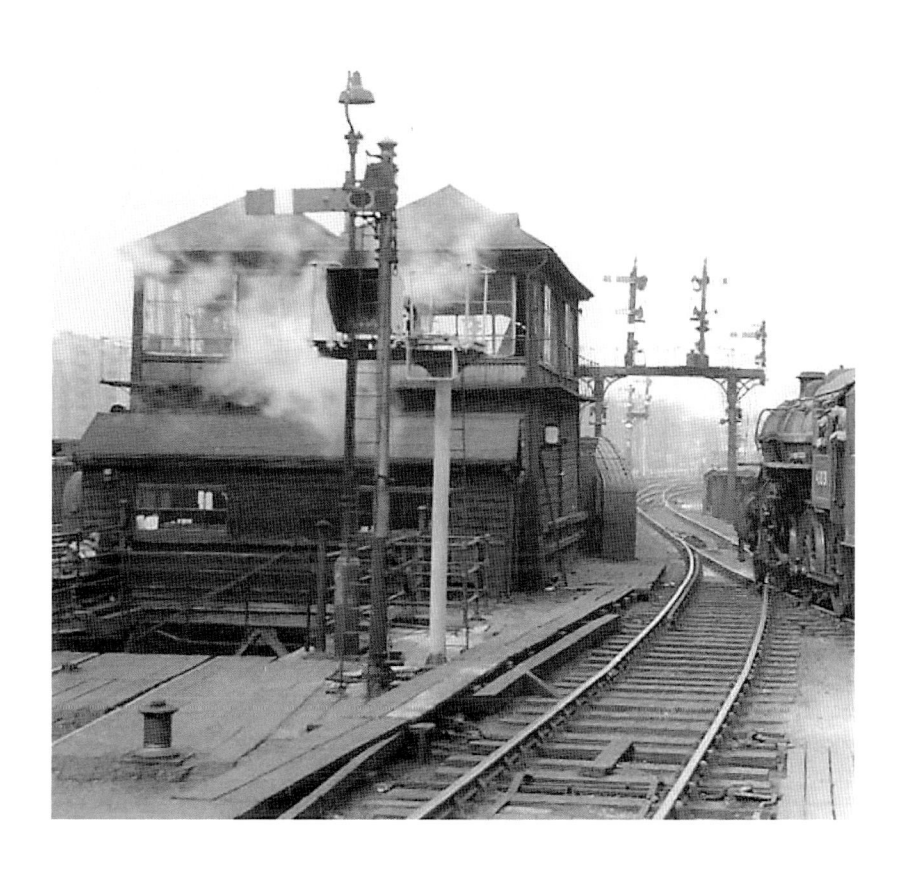

*The 11:40 am P&O Tilbury boat train stands ready to leave St Pancras on 16th March, 1957, behind 43031, a London Midland 4MT 2-6-0. The signal box, just beyond the platform ends controlled the numerous semaphore signals in evidence. In front of it is the wagon hoist which was to remain in occasional use for a further 10 years or so. It served the cellars below, which were famously laid out for the storage of Burton beer barrels. Only on one occasion was I surprised to see capstan shunting in action. The wagons were manoeuvred using ropes and powered capstans, like the one seen in the foreground.*

some of the rare 50,000 numbers might be seen if one took a local train to Hendon, and so it proved. One or two examples of venerable former Midland Railway 0-6-0 freight engines, not venturing far from their Kentish Town home depot, could be spied up on over-bridges or behind wagons being shunted.

Overall, it seemed odd to a Southern boy that there was so little of the bustling suburban busyness associated with all the routes south of the Thames. Anything seen on these St Pancras sorties was indeed hard won.

What was lacking was the background interest of loco movements and the bustle of a frequent steam suburban service. Marylebone could be positively somnolent between trains. Consequently, when diesel multiple units were introduced, both there and at St Pancras, to displace the 2-6-4 tanks which had hitherto held a virtual monopoly of the suburban traffic, then they all but lost any appeal as spotting venues. Fenchurch Street, on the other hand, had no space for anything *but* 2-6-4 tanks, which minimised its spotting appeal exactly for that reason.

As I became familiar with the locos of each region, the different sections of the combined ABC started to take on a character of their own. The first 9,999 numbers covered the Western Region, a decision determined by the fact that the Great Western was the sole railway to have continued the early railway practice of applying brass number plates to its engines. That was still the practice when the last Great Western designed steam engine left Swindon works in 1956. These were followed by a block of some 20,000 relatively unused numbers, presumably reserved for all the diesel and electric locomotives anticipated for the future. Only then did we turn to the 30,000 block for the Southern Region. The Midland Region used both 40,000 and 50,000 whilst the 60,000s went to the Eastern and North-Eastern Regions. The Scottish Region, embraced numbers in the 40, 50 and 60,000s. At first sight, it had seemed reasonable enough

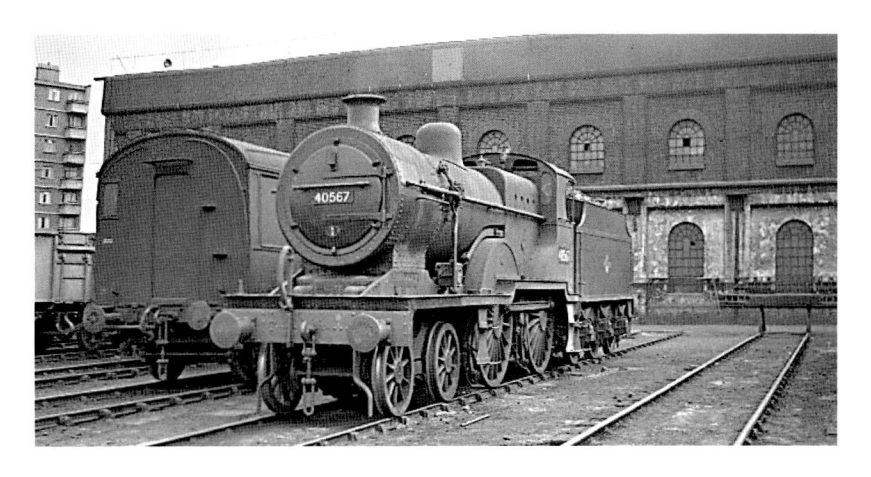

By 1957, most engines at Devons Road shed were 'jinties' – 0-6-0 tank engines, employed largely on dockland freight work. The following year Devons Road became the first shed to be all diesel. The adjacent Bow works lingered on into 1960. It had long undertaken work on a sprinkling of engines from further afield in addition to regular freight loco types and former London Tilbury & Southend locos. Nevertheless, it was a bit of a surprise to stumble upon recently outshopped 2P class 4-4-0 no. 40567. As a London and North Western section engine, based at Crewe North (confirmed by its 5A shed code), one might have expected it to be maintained at Crewe works. In the London area it was a type more associated with the Midland section, double heading Black Fives out of St Pancras.

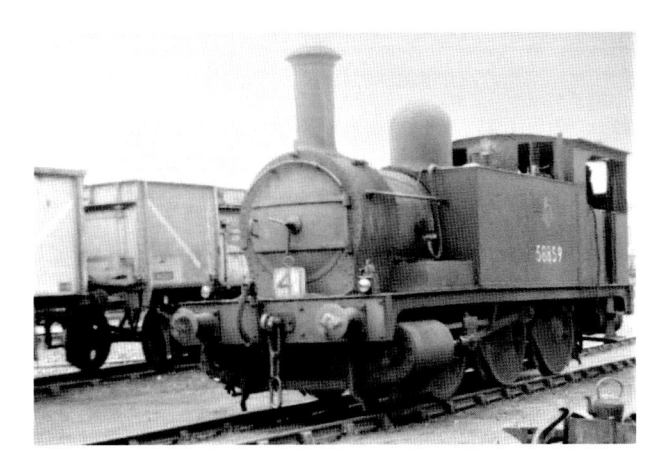

The last survivors of former North London Railway locos were 0-6-0 tanks. This example, being in the 50,000 series was unusual enough for that reason alone. Seen here shunting on 2 September 1957 at Devons Road, Bow, it was to be withdrawn the following month. Devons Road became the first all diesel depot the following year.

but upon reflection, it represented a fuzzy sort of logic. Whilst it made sense for the number blocks to relate to the steam loco stock of the 'Big Four' pre-nationalisation companies, it was strange to introduce the discontinuity of numbers 10,000 to 29,999, allocated to a relatively small number of existing diesel and electric locos and as yet unidentified future ones.

That of course did not take account of the 70, 80 and 90,000 series, reserved for all the British Railways standard steam types, for use on all regions and again representing an over generous reserve of numbers. To add to all that, the Southern Region maintained a separate series of 36 numbers for engines allocated to the Isle of Wight, a practice inherited from the Southern Railway.

If all that sounds complicated, then in practical terms, it meant that the Scottish pre-grouping companies furnished a good source of cops in the 50,000 series, and remaining engines in that number block were mostly still at work in the areas of their respective pre-grouping company origins, Lancashire and Yorkshire and Midland Railways.

I wonder if I was alone in feeling each block of 10,000 numbers had a certain magic of its own. I think it must have been to do with associations with history and regional geography and perhaps the overall design style of its locomotives. For example, the Western Region series seemed the most defined and consistent, as if going about its business in its own distinctive way, independent, self-assured and self-reliant, rather like the Great Western Railway of its origin. The 30,000 block of the Southern had a soft approachable character, their roots much associated with green countryside, seaside holidays and summer days. Even the first digit '3' was rounded, chubby and friendly.

The 40,000s seemed a bit proud and a bit impersonal and detached, as if by a business-like 'take us or leave us' quality. Was that an echo of the former London and North Western's sobriquet, 'The Premier Line'? The 50,000s were dainty and elusive, perhaps feminine, whilst the 60,000s were purposeful, hard-working and with a sense of traditional solidity.

Most of this was, of course, fanciful, subjective nonsense and if others saw loco numbers in such terms, their responses would probably have been quite different. The point is however, spotters did seem to have favourite regions. If, in the case of big cities, where there was easy access to more than one region's locomotives, a conscious choice of spotting location would be made according to the mood of the moment. Elsewhere it may have been a little different.

There had been performance comparisons made between pre-nationalisation main line locomotive types by way of the 1948 Locomotive Exchanges. Some of the knowledge gained no doubt had a measure of influence on the development of British Railways' Standard designs which followed. However, in spite of nationalisation, the regional system worked against much homogenisation of the historic loco stock, as opposed to the later Standards which did move more readily between regions, as required. Even so, there were certain isolated famous long standing exceptions like the original ex-Great Eastern B12s which worked on the former Great North of Scotland lines from 1931 until 1954.

One can understand the inertia of familiarity – "If they are suitable, why switch engines around?" and, in terms of maintenance it was probably sensible to have them in the hands of the works and local fitters who knew them best. There were tentative moves away from traditional territories, typically to replace older engines lost to scrapping. One thinks of ex-LMS 2-6-2 tanks on the Southern, standing in for elderly defunct Southern tanks, especially in the late 1950s. There were too the ex-GWR pannier tanks used as Lickey Incline bankers. Those examples reflected an administrative regional boundary change in 1958 when the Western Region took over from the London Midland, rather than any technical reason to displace the ex-Midland 0-6-0 tanks which had been working alongside the resident 9F Standard, itself unaffected by the change. Generally, regional transfers were made on a pragmatic basis, to meet a need, rather than any overall effort to optimise the distribution of motive power across the United Kingdom.

Temporary transfers to meet emergencies were in another such category. A dramatic example of this was in the aftermath of the 1953 Crewkerne mishap, involving a broken driving axle. With Bullied pacifics temporarily withdrawn for checks, V2s, B1s and Black Fives were memorable replacements on the South Western mainline. Not in the same category, but noteworthy in terms of territorial change, were the 13 Western Region pannier tanks disposed of to London Transport, the last of which continued to work until 1971, three years after the conclusion of main line British Rail steam.

This gave rise to an amusing incident when a former spotting friend, who had then recently moved to Metroland, telephoned me in a state of mild panic to say how much he was still upset by the demise of steam and he confided that he was having worrying withdrawal symptoms. He explained how he often awoke at night with his head full of steam engine sounds. He was overjoyed when I suggested he must have missed out on the news that London Transport had purchased engines from British Rail and so perhaps he was not having nightmares after all. Because of the tendency for engines to remain in their historical territory, loco spotters generally knew what to expect in each region. To a large extent that even went back to pre-1923 Grouping days, where older engines were still likely to be identified with their originating company territory.

If spotters wanted to see very specific engines, then long journeys might have been involved. Typical examples were those last three remaining Adams 0415 class 4-4-2 tanks, which had survived because they had proved particularly well adapted to the tight curves of the Lyme Regis branch and were therefore closely associated with their particular location, something which could have a special appeal. There was a feeling such examples would be permanently there and, sooner or later, one would get round to seeing them. Alas, that was of course, not to be, so we are lucky to have some of those examples preserved.

More famous engines, closely identified with one location, included the unique LNER Beyer-Garratt articulated 2-8-8-2, with its memorable number 69999. Another was the 0-10-0 Lickey Incline banker, nicknamed Big Bertha, again bearing a memorable number, 58100, at least until 1956, when both were withdrawn. The former was employed on banking coal trains on the Worsborough Incline whilst the Lickey banker assisted trains northwards from Bromsgrove. Both locomotives had almost mythical status and I was aching with disappointment when I most narrowly missed seeing Big Bertha.

That occasion had been during an Ian Allan works visit to Derby back in 1956. Following the group I was in, we were led alongside some wagons, beyond which I glimpsed the top of a loco smoke box, crowned by an unusually large triangular lamp iron. At that time I thought no more of it but later, waiting on the platform for the train home, a fellow spotter asked me if I had seen Big Bertha. Then, the penny dropped. The engine had not long been withdrawn and in its working day had, almost uniquely in Britain, carried a search light to assist with buffering up to the rear of passenger trains. Why else had I noticed that outsize lamp iron? Oh! The unimaginable frustration. I could hardly even say I had glimpsed the engine. I had certainly seen neither frames, cab nor wheels and the engine had at least one spare boiler anyway. Nor even had I seen its number, so I had to settle for a very near miss. What chagrin! At least I had the small comfort of having seen another unique number, 60700, the rebuilt version of Greasley's experimental high pressure 4-6-4 streamliner of 1929. Unlike the other two, it was not usually confined to one locality but it seemed to spend lengthy stretches out of use, so it remained a rarity from that standpoint.

Another example of searching for particular engines came in a more positive sense in June 1954, when the excited word went round of a new batch of Britannias appearing on the 'Royal Mail', 8:30pm departure from Euston.  For several weeks, new engines, allocated to Holyhead, and numbered 70045 onwards, but not yet sporting their nameplates, were appearing on this turn.  The Royal Mail from Kings Cross departed at 8:20pm so I would wait to see its engine back on and then make for Euston.  Trouble came when the loco emerged from Gasworks Tunnel as little as 4 or 5 minutes before departure time.  Then there would be nothing for it but a brisk jog to Euston, just in time to see the latest Britannia departing.  By this time, I suspect my grandparents had given up all hope of ever understanding what railway interest could keep me out so late.

By the time I arrived at Euston, mail sorting on the train would already be under way, whilst postmen on the platform manhandled the last mail sacks from trolleys into the Travelling Post Office vans.  This might be to within very few minutes of departure time, so there could be a last minute flurry, were a post-office lorry to arrive late with its load.  All this occurred on platform Number 2 next to the main taxi road which, in the daytime, looked very different as a mainline arrival platform.

Instead of busy postmen there were then numerous porters in evidence.  They could be seen at most bigger stations, often chatting in twos and threes, mostly near the arrival platforms.  Certainly at Euston they would almost swarm from all directions towards an arriving mainline train, especially on platforms 1, 2 or 3, some pushing barrows, and all in anticipation of picking up tips from grateful passengers struggling with heavy baggage.  Porters were to disappear everywhere during the 1960s, sometimes to be replaced by do-it-yourself trolleys, on the lines of airport baggage trolleys.  Even the demand for these decreased with the development of such a small thing as wheeled suitcases.  It was this progressive erosion or evolution of the traditional railway scene which was to transform the context of loco spotting activities.

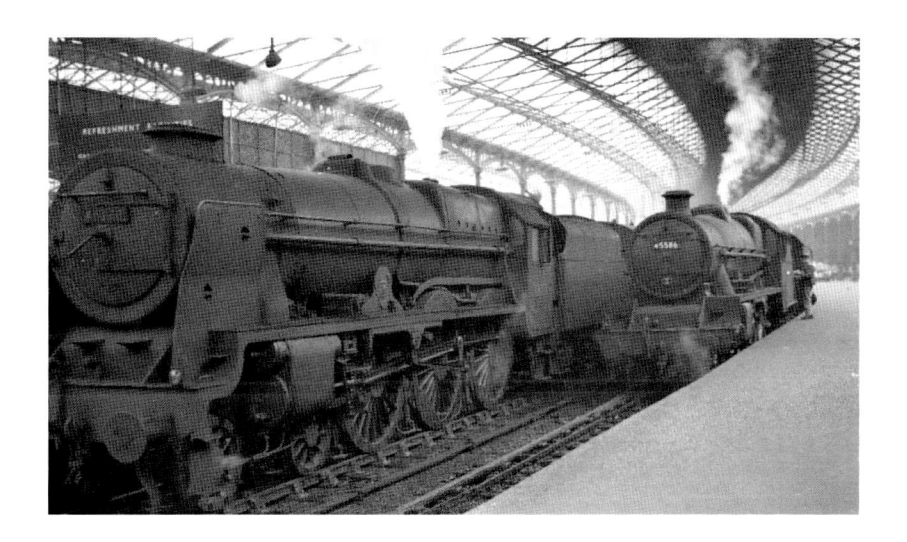

*The old Euston Main Line arrivals platforms 1 (on the right) and 2, with rebuilt Royal Scot 46170 British Legion and Jubilee 45586 Mysore. 46170 was a rebuild of the 1929 experimental high pressure loco, 6399 Fury. It broadly conformed to the taper boiler rebuilt Royal Scot format, and was included in that class.*

*Note the sign behind 46170, indicating the whereabouts of refreshment facilities,. They were scattered around the station and one wonders how many travel-weary arriving passengers were desperate enough to seek them out.*

*Later in the evenings, platform 2, which bordered the taxi road, became a hive of activity in preparation for the departure of the Royal Mail travelling post office train.*

I recall in the early 1970s seeing newly felled telegraph poles, like so many dead trees lying at intervals along embankment sides, along the Great Northern main line. It was an aspect of decluttering which came with modernisation and contributed to growing blandness across the entire railway environment. The relative silence of continuous welded rails was fast replacing the clickety-clack of rail joints and the rise and fall of telegraph wires was giving over to radio and electronic communication. Semaphore signals were becoming rarer and wayside stations had been fast disappearing since the late-1950s. The die-hards, who went on to find satisfaction in spotting diesel and electric locomotives, would have experienced even more dramatic changes as modernization progressed, including the demise of the Travelling Post Office trains themselves, in 2004.

Following nationalisation in 1948, there had been attempts at formulating a house style, but it did not go much beyond the allocation of regional colours and the universal application of the double sausage shape station name signs. It was not until new standard locomotive types were introduced from 1951, that loco spotters could think more in terms of British Railways, rather than the old company names.

Just occasionally one could still enjoy a little treat as a reminder. For example, as late as 1954, I was delighted to see a conspicuously well turned out Gresley varnished teak corridor carriage, amongst the standard carmine and cream carriages of a departing train at Liverpool Street. Then again, Euston one day provided the unexpected sight of a single LMS maroon painted carriage, conspicuous within an otherwise standard suburban green electric train. How these had survived so long in that condition remained a mystery. Perhaps they had more recently been prepared for filming or exhibition purposes? Less obvious throw-backs could sometimes be detected amongst locomotives too. There was a tank engine appearing sometimes at Paddington, on which one could still make out GREAT

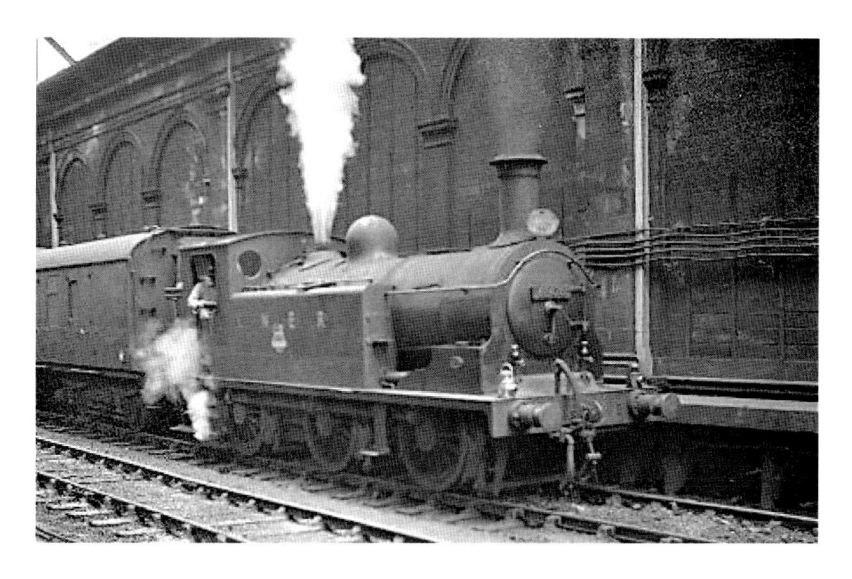

*Still proclaiming its pre-nationalisation LNER identity, along with its British Railways markings, this J83 No.68478, presented a rather startling sight when it was spotted at Edinburgh Waverley in 1958. It was one of a handful which had once been painted light green in 1947 for pilot duties.*

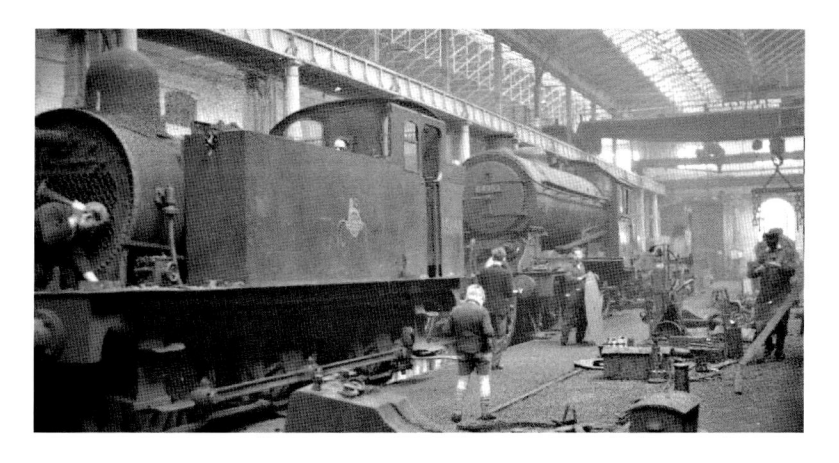

*The spotters in this April 1957 view, taken on a Stratford works visit, would have noticed nothing in particular about the J68 class tank 68660, seen in the foreground. Only on examining this photograph did the trace of the number '7034' become apparent on the side tank. This had been the number carried prior to the LNER re-numbering of 1946 and its subsequent British Railways. re-numbering in 1948 – a rare survival indeed. The engine in the background is J39 class 64953.*

WESTERN below its British Railways paint, but such examples were rare and hard to spot.

These tenuous links with the past intrigued me no end. It was like a forbidden glimpse into a time warp which corroborated the authenticity of all the historic equipment which so fascinated me. Meanwhile, British Railways were doing their best, by which we were supposed to recognise only the corporate nationalised image.

Gradually one became familiar with the details of many stations but never more so than with those of the capital's terminus stations. Initially it was the simple question of locating the best vantage points. One could build up a real attachment to some of those stations, especially if one made a point of getting to know their history and evolution. All manner of nooks and crannies and constructional details were there to be enjoyed, if one knew what to look for. Liverpool Street was one of my particular favourites. I would usually arrive on a Circle Line underground train from the Kings Cross direction. Just before the train stopped, I would always catch a glimpse of the bricked up tunnel mouth which, until 1904, had marked a rail connection between the Metropolitan/Circle lines and the main line station. It gave me a certain secret satisfaction to know I was possibly the only person on the train to recognise it. Then there was a bay platform which, in off-peak times, provided storage for some elderly brown painted Metroland coaching stock. As this was used mostly at rush hours, it sat there ignored most of the day, the compartment lights off, like some abandoned train from the past. It seemed to echo the pre-Second World War Metropolitan Railway, which had even included Pullman cars in its City service and reached the outer limit of that company's lines in rural Buckinghamshire, at Verney Junction.

From the Underground platforms I knew exactly which passage to choose to access the main line station. My favourite exit brought me out at the head of the original main line arrival platform, which extended a short distance under the station

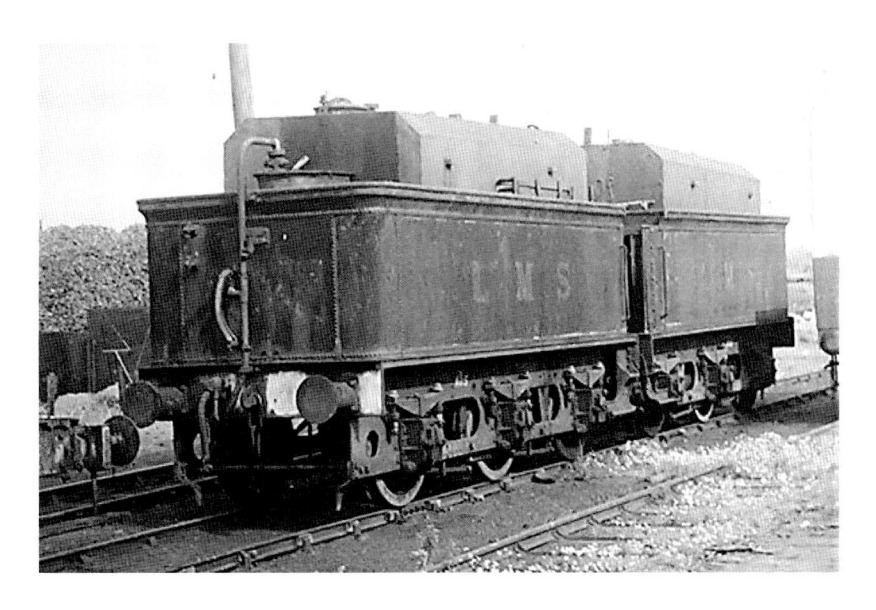

These pre-nationalisation relics made exciting finds in Eastleigh works yard on 6 August 1958; two tenders, each still bearing LMS initials, and converted for oil carrying. The left hand example, in its weathered black livery, was numbered LNWR 1484. The other, in faded LMS red, bore LNWR 1566. Oil burning was last tried in 1947 but soon curtailed after nationalisation. Three questions remained to be answered: What engines did they come from? What had they been used for in the last ten years or so? and, why did they finish up at Eastleigh?

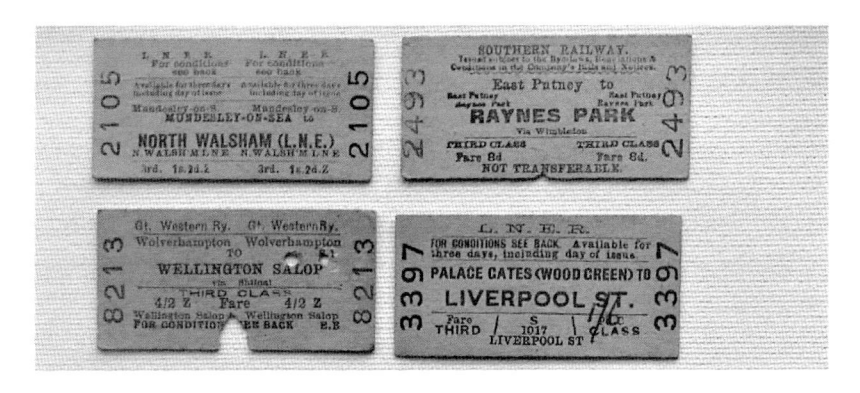

Big Four tickets could turn up long after Nationalisation. Serious collectors could come up with a more interesting range, yet these examples were collected without any effort. They date from 1953 to 1958 and remind us of just how much the loco spotting environment was transformed by the closure of certain routes and significant stations. It is a pity to think modern ticketing will not leave such an interesting record.

hotel. There was always a sense of anticipation as to what would be standing there. It could be anything from an elderly B12 class 4-6-0 to a recently delivered new 'Britannia'. These handsome machines were the most powerful main line engines to have worked the Great Eastern section, and we were keen to cop the newest arrivals as they entered service – Boadicea, Hereward the Wake, Robin Hood, and so on.

Some of the attraction of Liverpool Street lay in its strange layout and the way passenger movement was at two levels. When the Great Eastern outgrew its Bishopsgate terminus, it had involved a descent from Bethnal Green for the new line to Liverpool Street, in order to pass below the former route to Bishopsgate. This in turn led to trains terminating one floor below street level. Whilst not the most convenient for travellers, it was a delight for explorers like me. The initial station of 1874 had been extended on the east side in 1894 and although invaded by electric trains to Shenfield after 1949, this was one spot where we expected to find rather more modest engines than the 'Brits'. Typical were the B1 and Sandringham classes of 4-6-0s, regularly used on the semi-fast and Southend services. The Britannias may have largely displaced these from the top jobs but the Sandringhams had a particular attraction for spotters. This could be put down to their usually smart green turn out and the fact they were 'namers'. Many carried the names of famous football clubs, which no doubt widened their appeal. The majority of them, however, carried names of stately homes and other historic locations – much less eye-catching to the average lad.

At the country end of the platforms was a turntable and servicing area for main line engines. A detailed view of this was not readily available. Even so, the top of the taxi ramp leading down from the Skinner Street over-bridge was a popular, if somewhat hazardous viewing location. We had to squeeze up against the railings, as a constant stream of cabs drove past, if we were to see most of the trains coming and going on the

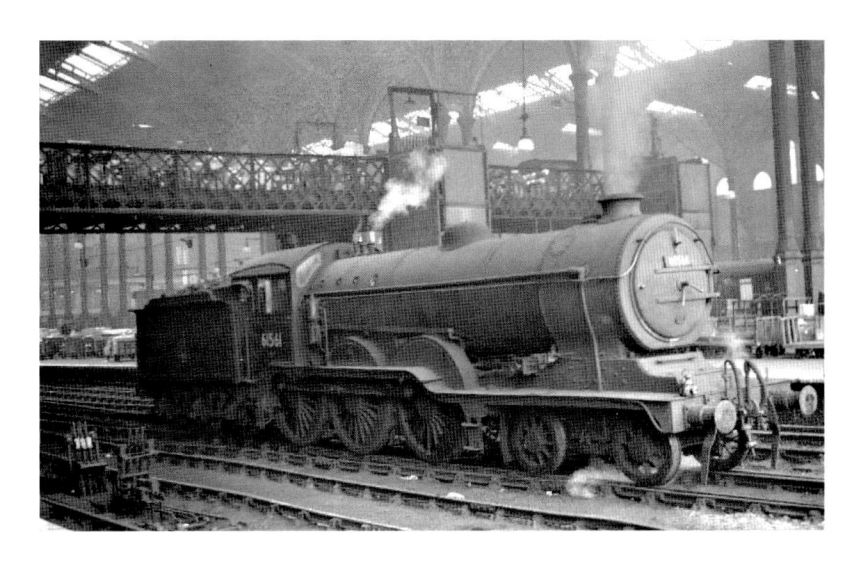

*Class B12/3 No.61561 stands on the Western side of Liverpool Street. One of the class, No.61572, has survived in preservation. Any reference to Liverpool Street immediately conjured up images of 'Sandringhams' and B12s, both classes having been designed for the Great Eastern section. In due course some two dozen Britannias, shedded at Stratford and Norwich, progressively displaced both classes from the premier duties, until they had all gone by 1960.*

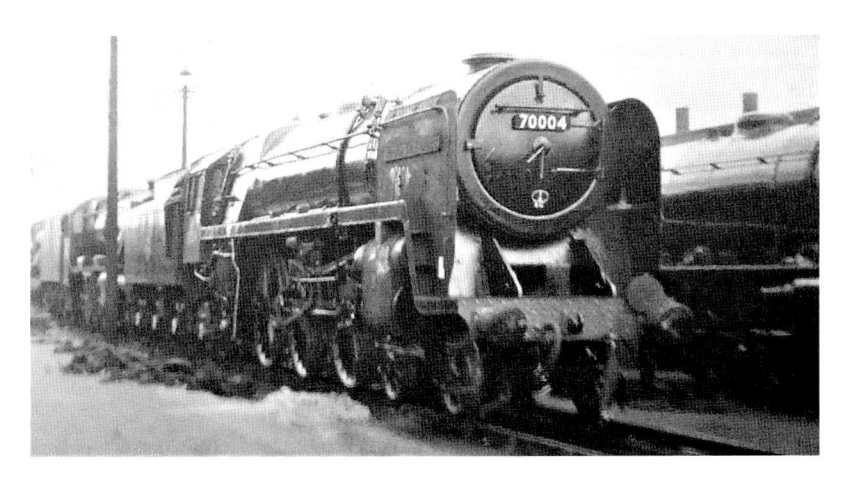

*British Railways standard class 7P6F, or Britannia, 70004 William Shakespeare at Crewe works in April 1959. First thoughts were how shabby it looked compared to when it was displayed in new condition at the Festival of Britain in 1951. Subsequently, Stewarts Lane shed had regularly turned it out in sparkling condition for working the Golden Arrow.*

western side. That included the frequent local and outer suburban trains. These consisted almost exclusively of 0-6-2 tank engines hauling dull cherry-red painted compartment carriages. These would have made up the train which we had raced up Bethnal Green bank on that early holiday trip to Mundesley. These carriages had the peculiarity of operating in groups of five, whereby the carriage ends shared a common four-wheeled bogie. Forming an articulated quintet, they were known as 'Quint-Arts'. I never knew if this was an official designation but there were numerous bits of railway terminology like that which gave one a feeling of being in the know. The world at large, of course, had not the slightest interest but, as in any special interest group, an inside knowledge reinforced a sense of participation and gave a real or imagined sense of validity to the activity, in this case of being a knowledgeable spotter.

Meanwhile, high above the west side retaining wall, one had an occasional glimpse of a North London Line electric unit coming or going from Broad Street station next door. Since most Liverpool Street suburban trains left from the far west side of the station, anyone approaching as a pedestrian from Bishopsgate Street, on the opposite side, was faced with numerous options. The first might be to enter the street level booking office, descend to the east side concourse, cross the taxi rank road and turn left under the station hotel, to gain access around the ends of the two platforms that terminated there; then continue on the opposite platform past the large newspaper stand and under the impressive arrivals and departures board, to enter the main station concourse, turning left in front of the various ticket barriers, before reaching the suburban side.

Alternatively, one might follow the overhead pedestrian way, which linked the 1894 east side of the station to the far western side, threading its way around to shortcut the deviation under the hotel, but missing out on the newspaper stand, down at platform level. Either choice was convoluted but at least the

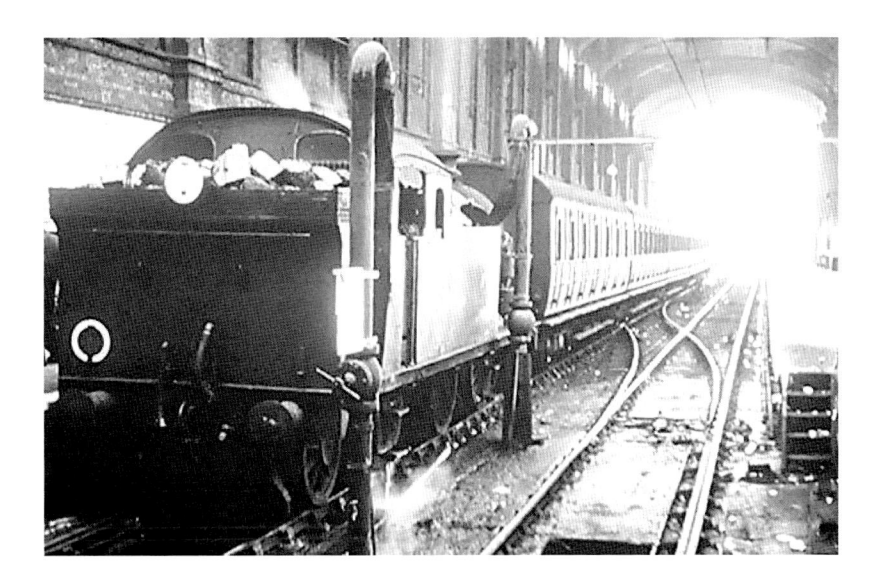

*The closing days of steam suburban services from Liverpool Street see a class N7 0-6-2 tank engine taking water at platform 1, having uncoupled from its Quint-Art set. The second water crane would have been used at busy times by an adjacent engine. The overhead wires are already in place in this 1960 view. By 1920, demand had necessitated the introduction of an intensive service. Then, at the busiest times, trains arrived at a platform every 10 minutes, stopping for as little as 4 minutes, whilst their arrival engine had just a little longer to take on water.*

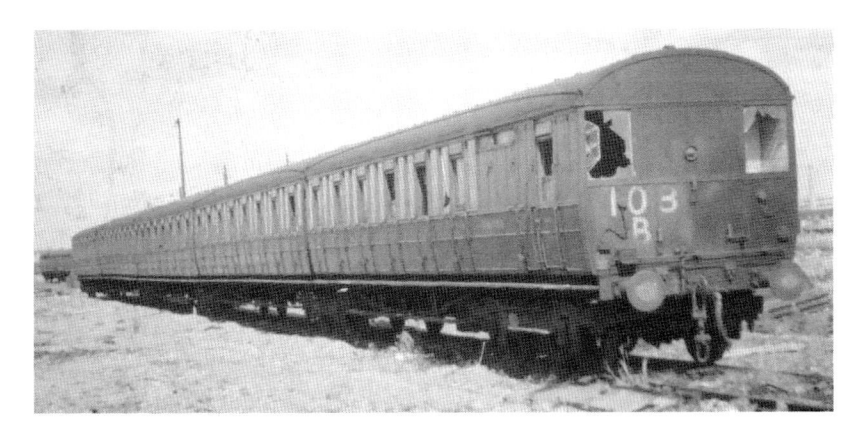

*A forlorn Quint-Art set, dating from 1925 onwards, displaced from Liverpool Street suburban services, when these were electrified in 1960. These were never very comfortable but must have been a significant improvement on the four-wheel gas lit carriages they had replaced.*

second choice gave an elevated view and led past the high level tea pavilion, along with its own views onto the activities below and which was beloved of the late poet laureate, John Betjeman. There were flights of steps down to platform level but one could continue right through the station, still at street level, to arrive in Sun Passage, the narrow pedestrian alleyway which flanked the west side of the building, separating it from Broad Street station.

  It is hardly surprising that all this was considerably simplified during the extensive rebuilding which occurred in the early 1980s. Whichever path one selected, Liverpool Street could be full of subtle impressions of changing light and shadow, changing smells and changing sounds. It was here at the suburban side where arriving tank engines would sit simmering patiently, awaiting their next turn of duty. Well before reaching them, their presence would be announced by sudden eruptions of their Westinghouse brake pumps. These would sporadically burst into life with perhaps half a dozen "pert*oo*mpah"s followed by a languid "pal*oooo*phtar" or two, before finally subsiding into a wheeze, all of this in an aura of hot oil, steam and the sulphurous whiff of burning coal. Incidentally it was beyond the buffer stops here that the line once emerged at the tunnel mouth giving onto the Metropolitan line.

  Above all this was the attractive iron roof of the 1874 station, which essentially survives within the now much modified station layout. As a successor to Brunel's Paddington, Cubitt's Kings Cross and Scott's St Pancras, Liverpool Street was something of a disappointment in terms of its vistas and clarity of layout, but there was no escaping the peculiar charms of its eccentricities, never quite throwing off its Great Eastern identity. Even officialdom reinforced this by re-painting one of the two station pilot locomotives in dark blue Great Eastern livery. These were maintained in immaculate condition and spotters were quick to point them out.

  In complete contrast, at the end of one day's spotting, we were standing on the east side concourse while a postman busied

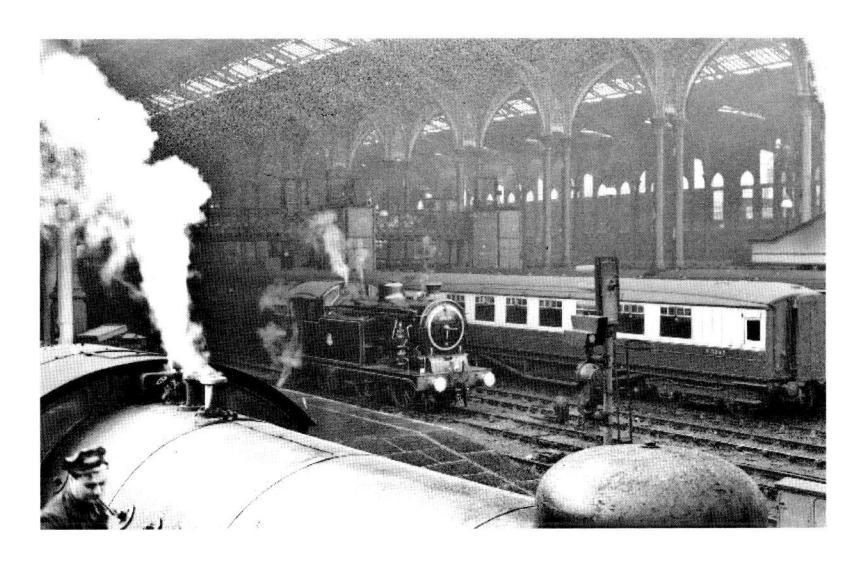

*The West side pilot at Liverpool Street from 1956 until its withdrawal in 1960 was N7 class No.69614, seen here from the Skinner Street taxi ramp. It carried a fully lined out BR black livery with the addition of red-painted coupling rods and burnished smoke box door ring and buffers. The crews of the station pilots are said to have received a supplementary payment for keeping their engines in immaculate condition.*

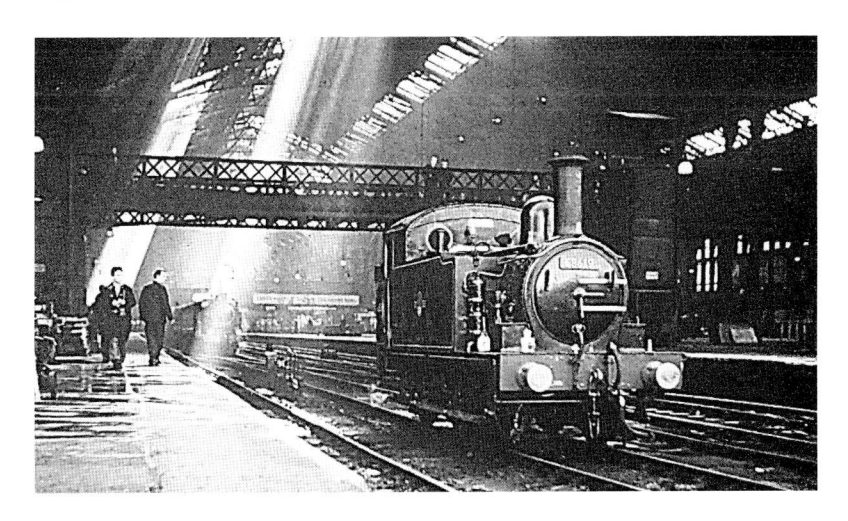

*Liverpool Street station pilot, class J69 No. 68619, painted Great Eastern dark blue in September 1959, seen sheltering from the rain between duties. Although another J69 survives, 68619 itself was withdrawn in October 1961 and scrapped at Stratford.*

himself emptying a nearby letterbox. To our surprise, he turned to ask, "Do you want to see my railway?" He led us through an inconspicuous iron door, no more than a narrow gap in a row of advertising posters, then down steel stairs to the Post Office railway platform below. This was a different world where we watched for several minutes as mail bags were manhandled and the driverless trains arrived and departed, sent on their way by the press of a button.

As often as not, a visit to Liverpool Street would be followed up by a brief stop at the adjacent Broad Street station. Only during rush hours was there the likelihood of seeing a steam locomotive or two. It was a place which exerted a certain modest attraction in its own right. Maybe it was the ghosts and echoes of the past. In its peak year, 1896, it had handled more than 46 million passengers, but then declined inexorably under the challenge of buses and trams until its eventual closure in 1986, when it was handling something nearer 300,000 passengers a year.

We would usually enter by the steps at the front of the building. Arriving at the concourse level we would pass what looked like a closed refreshment room, or perhaps an enquiry office, its heavy dust laden polished wooden counter still in place and visible through grimy windows. Beyond that the empty silence was barely punctuated by an occasional arriving or departing electric train. On one occasion a member of staff was randomly sprinkling white disinfectant over the concourse from a large watering can, an apparently futile gesture which seemed to reinforce the hopelessness of the whole situation. Indeed, out of the rush hours, we could complete visits without observing any movement at all. We might lavish a penny on the operating model of a North London Railway locomotive, which was housed in a glass case, but unless we were planning to take a train to Willesden Junction, that would be the end of our visit. We always returned to street level by way of the open arcaded staircase on the outside of the building which overlooked

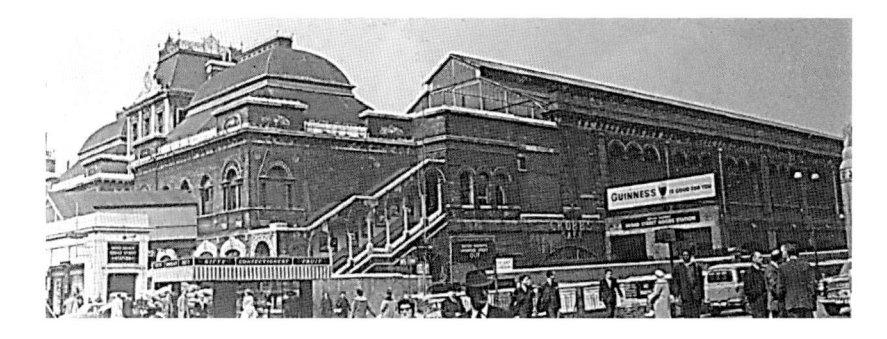

*Broad Street station as it appeared in 1964. The cluttered frontage hid the main entrance stairs but the open arcaded staircase, overlooking Liverpool Street's entrance, on the right, is clearly visible. The extensive train shed was progressively cut back and platforms de-commissioned before the station's demise in 1985.*

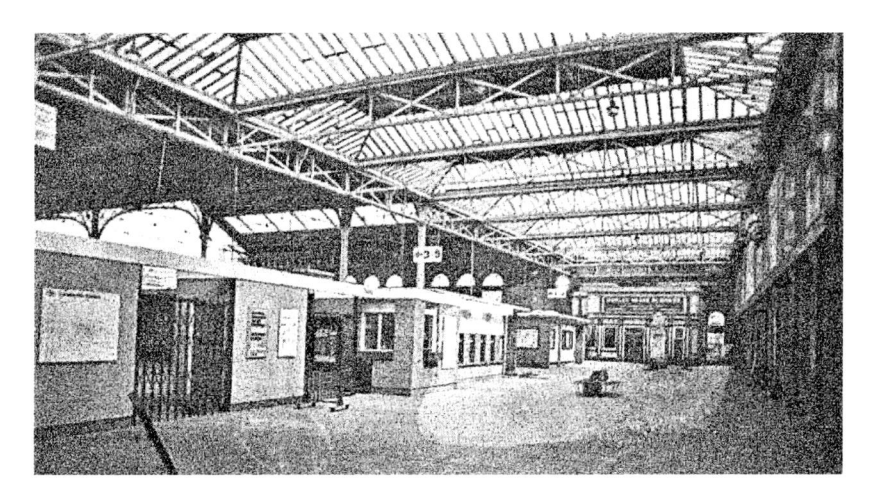

*It is hard to imagine in this 1958 view of the Broad Street station concourse that about 27 million passengers had passed through in 1902 alone. By 1906 there were about 80,000 passengers using over 700 trains a day, representing about 24 million passengers a year. The subsequent decline was inexorable so the new brick ticket and enquiry office and gents toilets, seen here, were too little and too late when they were built in 1957. At the time of closure in 1985, passenger numbers had dropped to about 312,000 a year.*

*Access to the arcaded staircase, leading down to street level, was by the modest arched opening at the far end of this view of the concourse.*

Liverpool Street station next door. There was a certain novelty in this and the worn steps attested to the millions of footsteps which must have passed that way over the previous ninety years or so. The steam railway oozed history and we loved it.

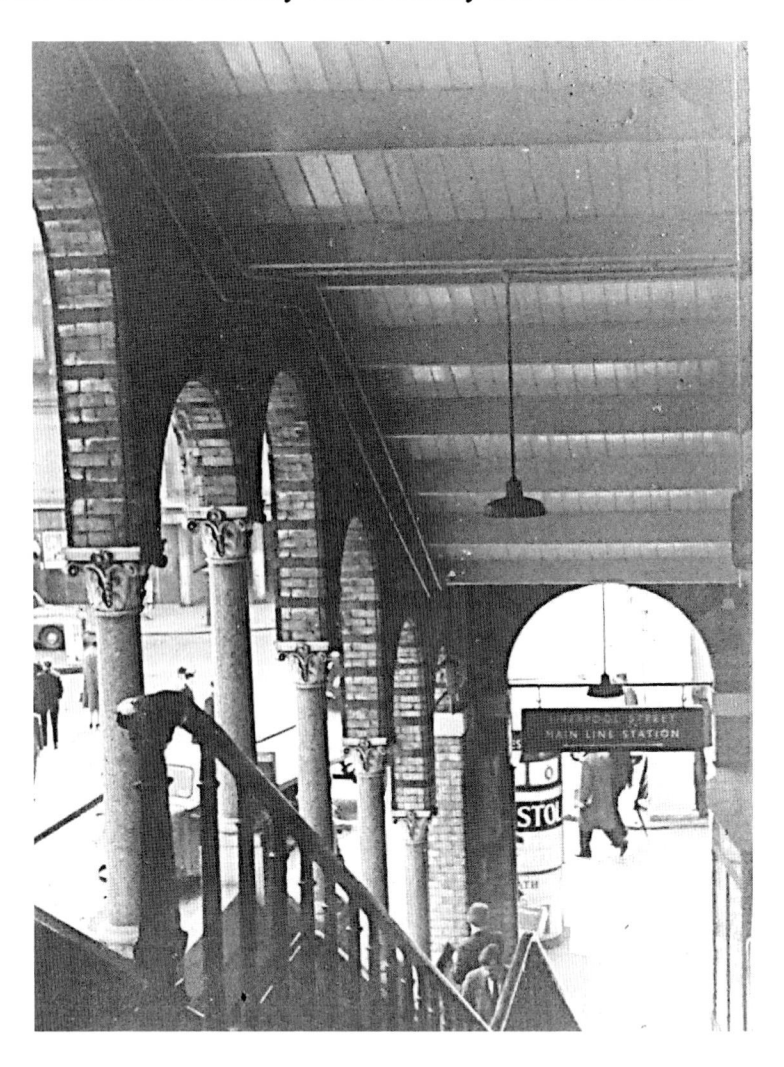

*The open arcaded staircase flanking Broad Street station was a simple attraction. Its deeply worn steps attested to the days when the station had handled up to 46 million passengers a year, achieved in 1896.*

# CHAPTER SIX                              Rambling Around

Not all spotters recorded their sightings indiscriminately. True, some of them did no more than collect numbers, which always struck me as a hollow exercise. Others were very discerning and collected only 'namers'. Some stayed in one region or even at one particular location, but many moved around. To me the attraction of stringing together two or three locations in a day's spotting made it all the more rewarding. One could sample the different characters of locomotives of diverse origins and dates, one could physically observe some of the historical geography of the railways and one could see trains in action. We may not have thought about it in terms of aesthetics at the time, but there was undoubtedly a visceral excitement to be enjoyed from all this. Another point in favour of travelling around a little was the simple avoidance of monotony. After all, not all locations, even in Greater London, offered non-stop entertainment.

Many of us would fill the gaps by noting the electric sets we had seen. There was some interest to be derived from this on the Southern Region, where there was a long history and quite a lot of variety, both between and within train types, but elsewhere this was less so.

Variety or not, there had to be something special about an electric train if a steam enthusiast was to take much notice. A case in point was Bullied's so called double deck carriage seating, introduced in 1949, to increase passenger capacity. The carriages, which retained the traditional slam door compartments, were formed into two 4-car trains which had an almost fabled reputation in that nobody seemed ever to have noticed them. One day, at a time when I had seen very few Schools class 4-4-0s, I opted to wait at London Bridge where I knew I could see them on the services to Hastings. There, at least, I would see more electric trains whilst I was waiting.

Unexpectedly, in came the double deck train, which was too much to resist. Significantly, it was during the afternoon and not during the rush hour, because the design had not been perpetuated due to the time it took to load and unload passengers. Unhesitatingly I climbed aboard, immediately to realise how claustrophobic an environment it would be when full of passengers. The space normally found above the traditional luggage racks over the seats, was impinged upon by the upper deck seating. It was a narrow squeeze up a few steps to the upper level and once there the low roof profile and fixed windows maintained the claustrophobia. I doubt the design would pass muster to-day as far as health and safety concerns were involved for, in truth, there was no double deck but just double level compartments. There was no alternative way out from the upper level. As it was, these units remained in service until 1971.

At the first stop I took a train back to London Bridge and resumed my wait for the arrival of a Hastings bound train. When it came, it contained a couple of ex-South Eastern and Chatham Railway match-boarded carriages.

It was enough to be noticeable but it never struck me as anything remarkable since one could still occasionally encounter pre-grouping vehicles throughout the national system, at least until the mid-1950s. I wonder if those particular examples laboured on until the arrival of the 'Thumpers', the diesel electric multiple units which replaced steam on the Hastings line in 1957.

Strictly speaking, it was this observation of entire trains which represented train spotting, as opposed to engine spotting. There was, in addition, a small band of spotters whose interests revolved entirely around London Underground trains. That system, its history and rolling stock, together made a worthy enough package in its own right. Nevertheless, the corporate conformity was strong, and when all was said and done, it took steam to bring the hobby to life.

One of my earliest recollections of underground travel was at a very young age when I was being taken by my mother and grand-mother to the famous Kensington department stores, by way of a Circle Line train from Moorgate. Our carriage was still in wartime grey livery and had hand operated sliding doors. A man who was a little worse for wear, was lolling around dangerously near the doors, which had been left open, as we rattled along. He got out after a stop or two, to everyone's relief. I still wonder why nobody shut the doors.

That recollection returned to me some eight years or so later, when friend Roger introduced me to those vintage electric trains from Broad Street. They too had wide hand operated sliding doors and spacious saloon interiors. They had been introduced in 1914 with Siemens electrical equipment, but the outbreak of hostilities with Germany had necessitated a rapid switch to the Swiss Oerlikon company. The last of them survived to the very end of the 1950s.

From Broad Street, there would be very few, if any, steam engines to see before reaching our destination at Willesden Junction and the interest lay in identifying defunct stations en route, lost to war damage and subsequently closed for good. The triangular layout of Dalston Junction station was still intact enough at that time to hint at its former importance. It was once the dividing point for North London Railway operations, heading east towards docklands, and west towards genteel Richmond. In our day only freight trains operated on the east side.

Willesden Junction main line station was another place which hinted at past glories, and in fact it was not to last beyond 1962, when it was totally demolished. Until then, it was just possible to spot in the time-table, the odd main line train which still called there. This was where we would eschew further travel in the Oerlikon stock, bound for Richmond or Watford, in favour of one of these main line trains which arrived a few minutes after 1 pm on a Saturday. It had probably come from

Rugby or Northampton and it gave us the thrill of travelling the last five and a half miles to Euston, non-stop behind a 'Jubilee' or a 'Black Five' locomotive. There was a minor bonus too, because the main line passed a little closer to Camden loco shed than did the suburban tracks. This afforded a better view of the more glamorous express engines stabled there, before we cruised down the 1 in 77 bank into Euston.

One of the delights of frequenting the railway system was the discovery of unexpected corners, and sometimes almost secret places, not usually accessible to the regular traveller. Euston was a classic case in point. It was perhaps the most chaotic of all London's termini. As the first main line terminus in London, dating from 1837, it had grown piecemeal over the decades. Plans for its replacement were already afoot until the Second World War interrupted further progress.

The station included some architectural gems but they were of more interest to the aficionado and the railway enthusiast than to the long-suffering travelling public, who had to navigate around and through them, to locate their trains. In the centre of the whole complex was Philip C. Hardwick's Great Hall. Originally it performed as a huge waiting room, capable of handling the crowds and the paraphernalia of Victorian travel, and it was essentially designed to feed passengers onto a single flanking departure platform. That feature remained disguised, but visible to the enquiring eye to the very end, when the entire station was eventually rebuilt in the early 1960s.

By that time the Great Hall was surrounded on three sides by numerous platforms and sidings. Parcels traffic was mixed up with passenger traffic and the separate arrivals and departures sides limited operational flexibility. For passengers, the sign posting, the location of arriving and departing road vehicles, the connections with the Underground network, the fragmented buffet facilities and everything else that one needed for a smooth journey, appeared to be completely random. As an aside, there were by 1958, seven catering establishments at

Euston, none very memorable, even if you had managed to find them. For many years a sign above the main arrival platforms was provided to give clues to their whereabouts. Local knowledge was definitely an advantage and it was that which appealed to railway enthusiasts, if to nobody else.

In the 1950s there had been a number of desperate attempts to improve the passengers' lot. One of these was the construction of a small cinema-like waiting room beyond the buffers of the main arrivals platforms. Not much appreciated by either travellers or loco spotters, it was in fact a useful source of information on both departures and expected arrival times. Armed with this information, which could be noted down in comfort, a spotter could identify the origins of arriving trains and their locomotives, the anticipation of which enhanced the interest of merely recording numbers.

On rare occasions, access was available to the Shareholders' Room. This magnificent room was reached by way of dramatic double flights of steps, which rose from the north end of the Great Hall. The room had been restored and re-decorated in its original colours in 1953 and it was a special treat to visit this holy of holies of the former London and North Western Railway Company.

The occasion I recall was an exhibition of 'The Steam Locomotive'. I never knew what prompted the event and I was puzzled as to why so many of the superb models on display were devoted to the works of the former Great Western Railway. Nevertheless, I was delighted to see in three-dimensions, models of machines I had only read about or seen in photographs. Their running numbers too were interesting because they explained some of the number series missing from the ABC.

On a separate occasion at Euston, some minor works had necessitated the closure of the toilets. The alternative facilities were very well sign posted, and just as well. A devious route involved the length of the Great Hall, slipping through an insignificant door below the Shareholders' Room, two or three twists and turns in gloomy passageways and finally arriving at one's very unprepossessing destination. All this was punctuated at every stage of the way by handwritten messages and encouraging arrows, all chalked on random pieces of cardboard.

A little further exploration was to reveal an almost forgotten area, which still retained a section of roof of the type which covered the tracks in the earliest years of the station. It has to be explained that the original arrival-side roofs were raised six feet by the simple expedient of sitting their supporting columns on tall iron bases. This happened in the early 1870s.

The introduction of increased areas of glazing further enhanced the sense of spaciousness. In contrast, the boarded roof of this rather obscure area, tucked away behind the Great Hall, was an unexpected reminder of the small, and by modern standards, claustrophobic scale of the original station sheds. After the monumental scale of the original waiting room, in the form of the Great Hall, the train sheds must have seemed a pronounced anti-climax. What pioneer third class passengers made of the open trucks they then boarded, can only be imagined. It was such chance discoveries which added unexpected interest to loco spotting excursions.

Paddington too had its own exclusive room, normally inaccessible, and that was Queen Victoria's waiting room. On one occasion I stumbled upon an open day and have to acknowledge I found the interior of the room most disappointing. I had certainly anticipated something grander and more decorative and I wondered if, a century or more before, it might have contained heavy furniture and drapes, for example. Nevertheless, the high level view across the station shed was impressive. The room was eventually to become an executive travel suite.

Like all the larger London termini, except perhaps Waterloo, Euston was dominated by main line locomotives. This applied to parcels traffic as much as to passenger trains. There were of course tank engines, on empty carriage workings,

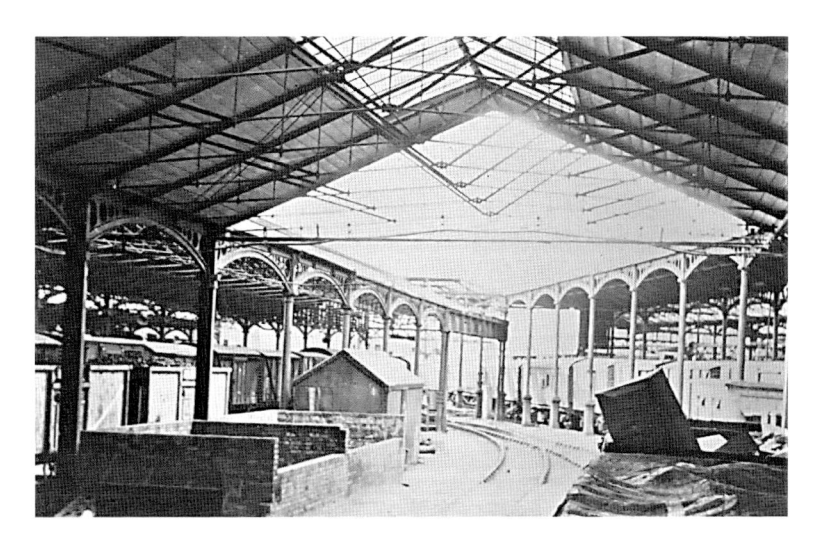

*At Euston, beyond the north end of the Great Hall, lay a small area of the original boarded roof design. In 1871, all the other roofs were raised by six feet by the simple expedient of inserting a tall column base under each column, as seen on the right. Exploring obscure corners could uncover fascinating details for those who went beyond simple number collecting.*

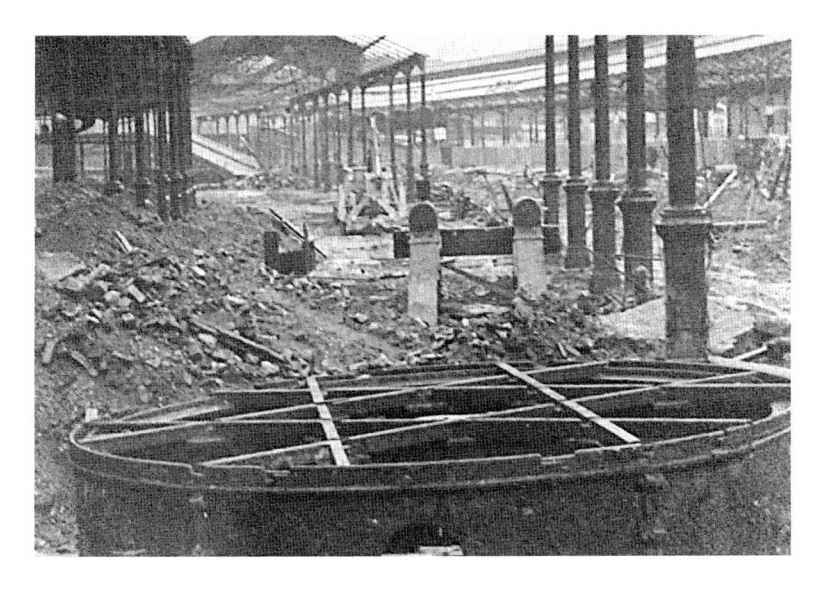

*The demolition of Euston in the early 1960s revealed this turnplate, used to marshal the earliest carriages from 1837. Its discovery was every bit as exciting as a rare cop.*

and they regularly performed the extra job of banking the heavier trains; that is, giving them a hearty push to get a departing train underway.

Much as the large stations provided regular spotting venues, we were automatically drawn to sheds and works if we wanted to cover a balanced range of loco types. Beyond that, we made specific trips to more obscure corners, to track down locomotives which were known to operate in particular areas.

I was sharp enough to know my immature hand-writing might not elicit a positive response from shed masters, so my Dad, as helpful as ever, got permits to visit Brighton Works, Brighton shed, including the electric train depot, along with Three Bridges and Redhill sheds, all in one day. For the Southern Region that sort of intensity was necessary, if we were to get a good range of cops. Pre-planning a busy day like that was essential. Otherwise, we seemed to see mostly the same old engines. This was the only occasion I undertook a 'shed bash', spotters' jargon for a day of concentrated visits to several sheds in succession. As time went on, it became apparent just how generous most shed masters were in granting entry to their depots; I do not recall ever being refused. There were indignant rumours of sheds which were difficult to bunk, but after all, we had no automatic right to be there anyway.

With several subsequent trips over the years, Brighton was to become quite a favoured locale, until the shed closed in 1961. It gave us a good boost of Southern steam to counteract the pervasive electrics back home. As if to prolong the experience, we would usually return home via Horsham, by way of the Shoreham to Christs Hospital line. It would be a largely eventless journey, with few passengers joining or leaving the train of elderly compartment carriages. If we tired of watching the countryside slip by, we would spend a minute or two examining the framed pictures displayed beneath the luggage racks. They were predictable and rarely captured the imagination. There would usually be a map of the Southern

Region network, still showing the Bisley branch, closed back in 1952, along with idealised views of seaside locations. I remember very few details except that views of the Cinque Ports seemed regularly to crop up, which at least were better than the dreary brown photographs we encountered in some Western Region carriages.

On the other hand, we were never to be treated to colourful pictures of locomotives of the kind we encountered on the London Midland Region, for example.

All in all they created a feeling of irrelevance to the few passengers using that slow cross-country route. One was hardly likely to be inspired to journey to the places illustrated. Consequently the pictures seemed to be there because they had always been there, if for no other reason than to decorate the compartment.

In contrast, friend Roger planned one of his circular trips, this time from Kings Cross to Cambridge on the ex-Great Northern route, returning to Liverpool Street on the ex-Great Eastern route. That immediately paid off when we saw several of the quaint E4 class 2-4-0s, which did not seem to travel much further from Cambridge than Mildenhall, for example. It was a far cry from the days when they once handled the bulk of the Great Eastern semi-fast or long distance trains. After spending an hour or so on the foot bridge over the shed yard, it occurred to us to venture down to the shed master's office for permission to explore further. After all, he could only say, 'No'.

Hesitating at the open door of his office we caught his eye and were welcomed in. He obviously knew what we wanted and asked us to hang on a moment. As we glanced around, we took in the parquet floor, probably impregnated with a century's worth of oil and coal dust and buffed up by the boots of hundreds of footplate men. It was swept to a dull sheen; one could not say polished. The walls were decorated with framed photographs of former Great Eastern engines. One or two of the photographs

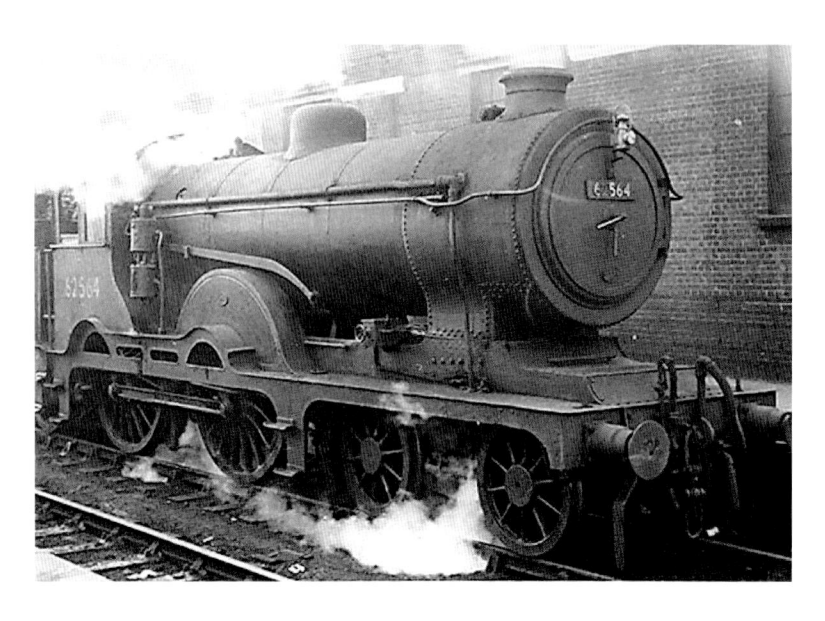

*Claude Hamilton class D16/3 62564, seen at Cambridge on 26th February 1957. This example displays the original perforated valencing over the driving wheels, a peculiarity we looked out for.*

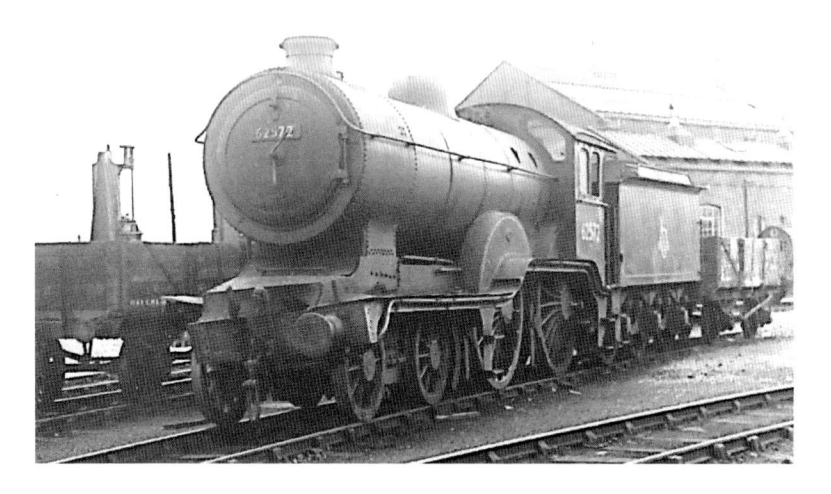

*Recently withdrawn from 31B, March shed, class D16/3, 62572 is seen on 3 August 1958 at Stratford works. By that date a buckled front end was enough to condemn an engine, with little hesitation. The tender was empty and the coupling rods already removed. This was one of Gresley's rebuilds from 1933 onwards, of the D15s of Great Eastern origin. They carried his round topped boiler and raised footplating.*

112

had turned sepia and only the odd one represented a familiar type of engine.

The shed master was a very gentlemanly fellow who led us to the nearby mess-room, where half a dozen loco men sat around a table, this time decorated with tea mugs and an ash tray. Asked if anyone would like to see us safely to the end of the yard and back, there was a volunteer, probably happy to leave the cigarette smoke behind for a few minutes. We were delighted at the outcome. Amongst the cops was one of the 'Claude Hamiltons' with the original perforated footplating, which was something new to me, but what was even better was to discover, deep within the shed, another F6, just like the one I had ridden on at Mundesley.

Following the Cambridge shed visit, Roger suggested we track down further examples of the F6 or very similar F5 2-4-2 tanks. If the rarities were not going to come to us, we had to seek them out. Alongside the ABCs, Ian Allan also published a Locoshed Book. This gave the shed allocation of every engine, which in turn was marked on an oval plate, near the bottom of the smoke box door. The problem was the need for laborious updating every month, from information published in the Trains Illustrated magazine. Both publications were still beyond my resources, though Roger had discovered there was a fair sprinkling of F5s and F6s allocated to Stratford, something I had not noticed on my first visit there. He had seen pictures of them at work on the Epping to Ongar steam shuttle, which was a Central Line Underground outpost.

Having spent some time at Stratford, watching the main line expresses passing through, along with the occasional freight from the direction of Temple Mills marshalling yards, we decided we had had enough of the all-pervading stink which filled the air and we took to the Central Line, which reached the surface at that point. The sickly sweet smell, which could vary in intensity but was rarely absent, engulfed the whole district and

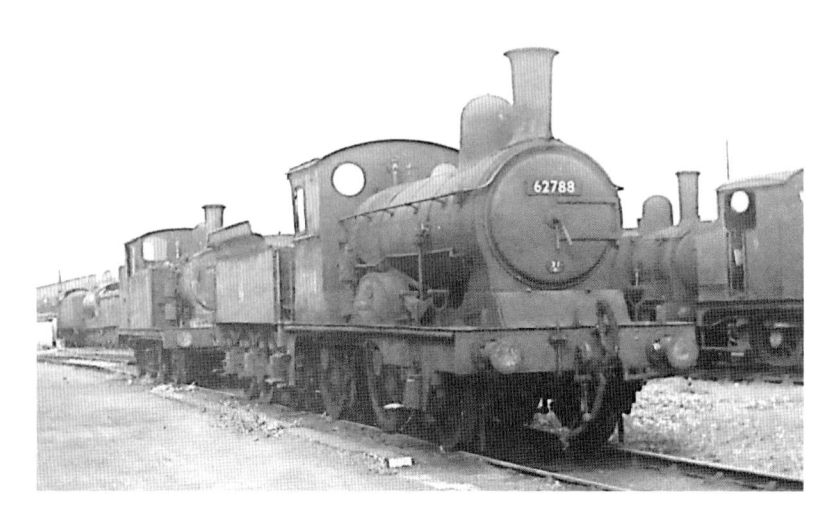

*E4 class 2-4-0, 62788 in the company of other condemned engines in the Stratford shed yard in September 1958. It had been withdrawn from Cambridge shed the previous March. Cambridge was their last stronghold. 62788 was one of six fitted with side window cabs in 1936 for working in the bleak winter conditions over Stainmore summit, between Darlington and Kirkby Stephen.*

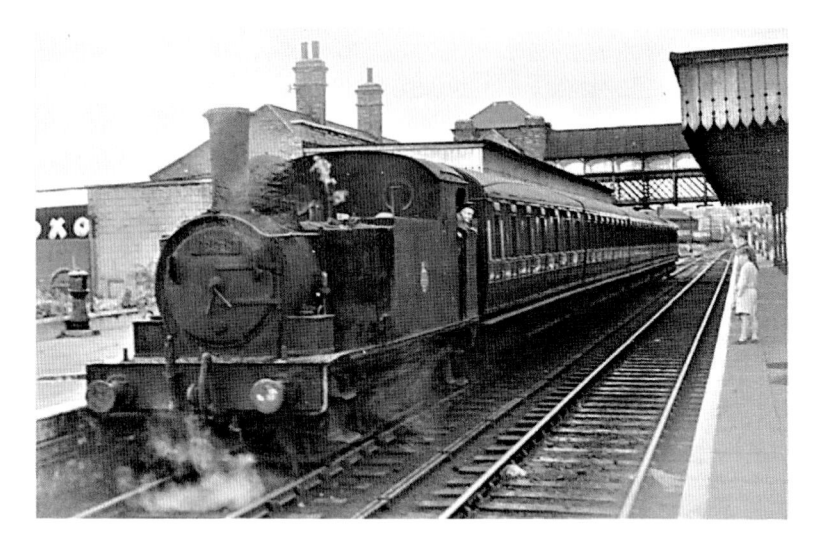

*The driver of class J69, No. 68636, chats with two interested lads whilst awaiting departure time from Palace Gates, bound for North Woolwich. Classes F5 and F6 2-4-2 and N7 0-6-2 tanks, and even L1 2-6-4s also regularly worked this service, though the mostly empty carriages were well within the ability of the J69s.*

was rumoured to emanate from a soap factory or tallow works in the neighbourhood.

Reaching Epping we were rewarded with the sight of two F5s and, having come that far, we took a ride behind one of them to Ongar and back. Nobody boarded nor left the train at either North Weald or Blake Hall station and only two people got out at Ongar.

However, the hunt was not over. Briefly facing the olfactory horrors of Stratford once again, we set out on another one of Roger's circular tours, this time joining the train from North Woolwich, bound for Palace Gates. Sure enough, it arrived behind an F5, before embarking on its somewhat tortuous journey across North East London. Leaving from the low level platforms, the train swung left and then right in a great arc around the whole loco shed and works complex of Stratford. It flanked coal heaps and groups of stored and condemned engines which, to our delight, included numerous elderly specimens, E4s, Claude Hamiltons, J15s and even yet another F5.

Onwards through Temple Mills, with the day's mission accomplished, we settled down to enjoy the rest of the ride, which included the protesting squeals of grinding wheel flanges as we negotiated the twists and turns in the South Tottenham area, before reaching Seven Sisters. Once at Palace Gates, it was not far to walk to the main line station at Wood Green, and thence back to Kings Cross by a suburban train. Rather like our Basingstoke and Reading circuit, this was to become a familiar if less ambitious jaunt.

When school finished for the summer that year, we decided on another circular trip, but with a difference. This time we were to take an electric train to the end of its route at Alton, and then retrace on foot the route of the Alton to Basingstoke line, which had long since been lifted.

The last leg was to be from Basingstoke to Waterloo, a steam hauled trip along that familiar stretch, but in the reverse direction from usual. I do not remember now what prompted this new activity but I do recall studying an old ordnance survey map which clearly showed the dotted path of the route. We started by scrambling up the embankment to the former trackbed, just a short way from the point where the line had once left the Winchester line at Butts Junction. Initially the route was obvious and before long we climbed a little way up the side of a cutting and settled down to our sandwiches. Already, we were musing on the fact that at this point, London and South Western tank engines would once have been passing in front of us.

The only real challenge was to fight our way through a stretch of bracken. There was a moment too, when the route turned across a wide open stretch of farmland in a sweeping curve, with no further clues as to where to head for. Whether it was pure luck or skilful judgement I do not know, but we did quickly pick up the trail again, and plodded on. If anything, we held hopes of finding the remains of one or two of the intermediate stations. In the event we found nothing more than the odd concrete post and bits of platform edge. That was slightly disappointing and we were getting tired when the grassy track we had been following abruptly changed into a black cinder path. Even better, we quickly reached a buffer stop, from which a single railway line was still in place. I was sorry when, after a hundred yards or so, it curved round to bring us near to the end of the goods yard, close to the main line, west of Basingstoke station.

None of that adventure brought us any cops but it had been fun following the old route which had apparently crossed little more than empty fields and should have been predictably unviable, even in its day. One observation remains. It was experiences like that which unleashed the imagination and added to the charm of the railway hobby – the bit that went beyond number collecting. Perhaps it could be seen as the rural equivalent of exploring the forgotten corners of the big London stations.

# CHAPTER SEVEN                    Digging Deeper

When school resumed in the autumn of 1954, our headmaster decided that friend Roger's academic prowess merited his accelerated passage through school, so it was decided he should skip the forthcoming year. Inevitably there were few opportunities to plan spotting trips since he needed to concentrate his time a bit more on school work.

All was not lost however. For one thing, I had been a confident lone traveller from the age of twelve, but then that was over sixty years ago. That is not to say it was not more fun to go spotting with like-minded friends and indeed, I soon found two or three others at school. Better still I discovered my next door neighbour, Blair, was more than interested. Like me, he too must have been absorbing train sights and sounds since the cradle.

However, my first new travelling companion from school was Paddy. He was the lad who was fascinated by tennis statistics. His version of engine spotting was biased towards the simple number collecting style. He was quick to locate concentrations of locomotives and pointed out how close to each other were Willesden and Old Oak Common sheds. There were differing reports on the grapevine regarding both official and unofficial ease of access to Willesden. What was constant however, was the message that the obvious way into Old Oak Common was via a hole in the fence, next to the Grand Union Canal. Just about everyone I spoke to seemed to know about this, so it invited exploration. Only a ten minute walk or so from Willesden Junction, and there it was. Sure enough, the infamous hole in the fence had been patched up, but a brand new one had been cut next to it.

Clearly the authorities knew about it and were not over concerned, for it remained unchanged for a long time, if not to the end of steam and beyond. As sheds went, or, to give them their proper designation, Motive Power Depots, Old Oak was very special, possibly unique. Consisting as it did of an interconnected group of four turntables, each radiating twenty or so tracks, it represented a serious concentration of locos, particularly on a Saturday afternoon or Sunday, when fewer were out on the road.

The first thing any spotter did when choosing to bunk a shed was to locate the foreman's and related office area. At Old Oak it was fairly easy to avoid being noticed and by standing within each of the boarded turntables in turn, it was a rapid process to note all the engines present. That was not all though, because there were always quite a few more to be found outside in the yard. Given Willesden's uncertain reputation, we chose week-ends, visiting both sheds on a few occasions without ever being challenged.

My first experience of Willesden had been during the International Railway Congress in late May, 1954. The roundhouse shed had been transformed for the occasion with a boarded-over turntable and whitewashed walls. These walls remained unnaturally clean for two or three years afterwards, evoking recollections of the event.

In spite of its poor physical state, from its inception in 1948 until 1952, British Railways had been paying its way. From that point it sustained increasingly heavy losses, which prompted the announcement of the British Railways Modernisation Plan in 1955. Even at my tender age I was aware there were overseas countries fast developing diesel and electrical haulage, modern stations being built, and faster services with new types of rolling stock. In Britain, the years of austerity might have been over but the years of abundance had not arrived. Coal was still plentiful and the costs of widespread electrification were daunting. Nevertheless a programme of new steam engines, to continue for another few years, did seem to be missing the obvious, much as we might enjoy them for their own sake.

For spotters, it had been exciting enough to see examples of new British Railways standard classes of locomotives, and especially a glamourous 71000, Duke of Gloucester, and an impressive 2-10-0 freight loco, 92014. There was also novelty value in some of the new diesel locomotives displayed, but other examples had been around for some time, and were really just experimental or developmental engines.

Meanwhile, the contrast between Old Oak Common and Willesden was striking. Old Oak was, for the most part, always full of clean express engines, whilst Willesden was devoted to mostly dirty freight engines. Even so, it was not unusual to find a few express passenger engines present, which always looked a bit out of place. Sometimes a visit would be enhanced by, for example, the presence of an elderly London and North Western 0-8-0 freight loco, of the type jokingly called 'Wheezers', on account of the sound they made when on the move. On one occasion I counted myself lucky with a sighting of 45500, the first of the Patriot class, which was conspicuous by the unusually large central bosses of its driving wheels, inherited from a long defunct 'Claughton'. Such little highlights provided some compensation when we might otherwise return home to find our note books had revealed only a few cops.

There was quite a difference too between Willesden and its express passenger counterpart at Camden. Willesden kept many of its engines outdoors and seemed a spacious place. Camden, in comparison, always looked crowded. This was confirmed when a small group of us turned up, permit in hand and eyes agog at all the glamorous machinery around us. I immediately anticipated we would be escorted around for safety's sake, given the amount of loco activity within such close quarters. Instead, there was little more than a casual, 'OK, be careful, it's busy', and that was it.

If you are aware of potential danger you do not take risks. In a quieter shed we sometimes jumped across an ash or inspection pit between the rails, but never when the gap between

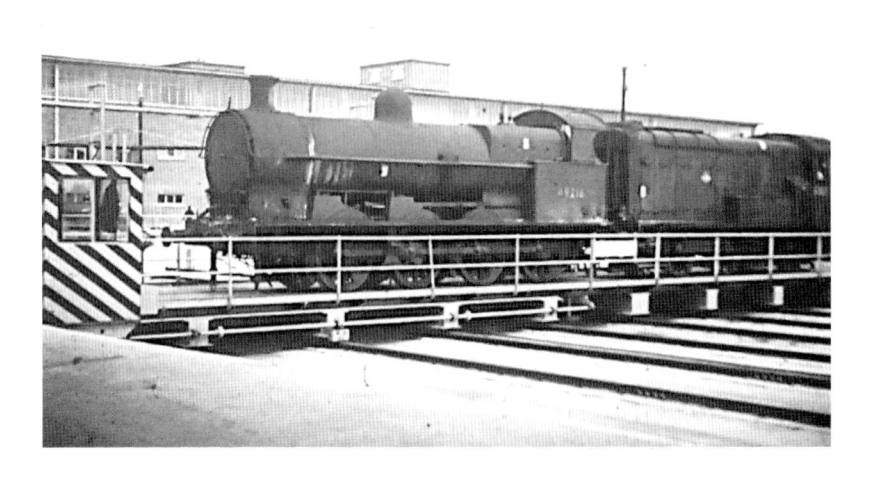

*A 'Wheezer', 49216, without its tender, on the traverser in Crewe works yard, 12 April, 1959. These seemed rather brutish, lumbering engines, with their long front overhangs, but they did have a very distinctive personality which held our attention.*

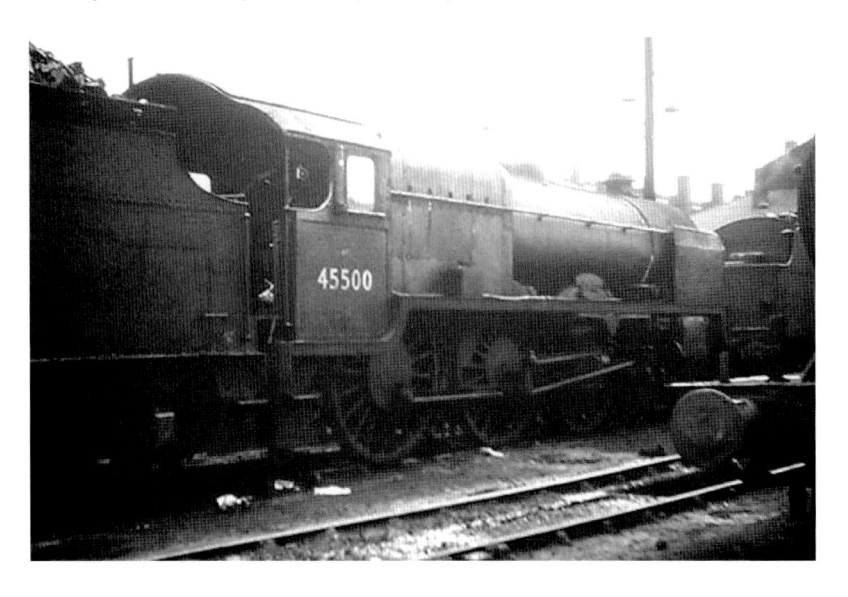

*The first two Patriots were nominally rebuilds of LNW Claughtons, which explained the large wheel bosses. Such distinctions made them interesting to the keen spotter. 'Patriot' is seen here on 29 March, 1959, hidden amongst the predominantly freight and mixed traffic allocation of Willesden m.p.d.*

engines was only a few feet apart. The menace of those buffers at head height was always enough to make us check there were no loco movements affecting the immediate area. Here at Camden though, that was out of the question. It felt anything could move at any moment, and so it did. At the north end of the shed, just where the spaces between the tracks narrowed towards the turntable, an engine, a short way off, started purposefully towards us. It was certainly not the moment to try crossing the track and the other side was blocked by stationary engines. A second's thought and it was obvious there was adequate safe space. All it needed was not to be intimidated by those heaving coupling rods passing just a couple of feet away. It was a useful reminder never to get into a position of risk and always to be extra vigilant in tight surroundings.

There were sheds where fitters might thoughtlessly leave pieces of valve gear or tools, obstructing the walkways between tracks. It was easy enough to trip over such obstructions but I am not aware of any spotters coming to harm, which is perhaps surprising, given the distraction of one eye recording numbers with the other eye looking out for the running foreman! Come to think of it, I do not recall ever encountering other spotters when visiting a shed, other than on open days or as fellow members of an organised group. That is strange, considering I understand there were something like 230,000 members of the Ian Allan Spotters' Club by 1955 and no doubt abundant non-members. Few of those, I suspect, took the club rule about not trespassing too seriously.

If the non-enthusiast showed even a passing interest in railway locomotives, it was most likely to have been the smartly turned out express passenger engines which caught his attention. Indeed, those were the ones which held the gaze of the typical spotter too. Spotters though, were on the search for numbers and could not afford to dismiss freight locomotives. Indeed, for spotters with less access to main line express routes, they naturally became the more knowledgeable observers of freight engines at work.

If St Pancras played second fiddle to Euston, which was served by Camden and Willesden sheds, it too was served by a largely passenger loco shed and a predominantly freight loco shed, in the forms of Kentish Town and Cricklewood respectively. Both sheds were easy to access and offered a possible sighting of an elderly ex-Midland Railway freight loco in the 50,000 number series, something otherwise unusual in the London area.

By and large, freight engines offered a lot of interest but not much glamour. They did however, tend to score in terms of the rolling stock and loads they handled. As a visual spectacle there were those freights which stood out and some were impressive enough to become widely known by nicknames. This was the case, for example on the former Great Central mainline, where fast freights south from Annesley, usually hauled by Standard class 9Fs, came to be known to enthusiasts as 'Windcutters' and to their crews as 'Runners'. If, as a spotter, one was content with frequenting terminus stations or certain other large stations, then all that freight interest could be missed. For that reason it was worth the journey to a shed like Cricklewood.

When we made trips to St Albans, we would be impressed by the large articulated Beyer-Garratt 2-6-6-2s which could be seen plodding steadily south with their lengthy coal trains from Toton marshalling yards, near Long Eaton, on the Midland main line west of Nottingham, to Brent sidings, right opposite Cricklewood sheds. Once there, however, they seemed to dematerialise, much to our disappointment. Because there was no turntable to accommodate their length, they had to be turned for their return trip north, on a reversing loop, which connected the east side of Brent sidings with the loco shed yard on the west side.

Somehow, these manoeuvres must have been taking place regularly out of sight, with never a word being mentioned about them between spotters. I rather kicked myself later when I discovered the loop line in question when studying a road map. As it was, I never managed to photograph the Garratts satisfactorily, having to contend with a difficult shot of one of them, seen outside of its natural territory at York motive power depot, in 1956. Had it stayed put long enough it would have made a worthy exhibit at the National Railway Museum, now on the same site.

Generally speaking, one could never be too sure where a freight train was heading. Next to Cricklewood shed was Brent Curve Junction where the inter-regional freight-only line, via Dudding Hill and Acton Wells Junction, led towards the Southern's Feltham yard. This would regularly produce a few cops and because engines operating on the Southern carried route head code discs, one could in these cases, determine their destinations. Strange to say, I never saw any traffic in the opposite direction, which remained one of life's little mysteries.

If freight engines tended towards the dirty and unglamorous, they nevertheless had their endearing characteristics. Just the act of pottering around in goods yards or carriage sidings, provided pleasurable distraction between watching through trains, either expresses or local 'stoppers'. What is more, some of them made very distinctive sounds. Some of the ex-Great Western classes were notable for their farting, popping and sniffing noises, shared with some of their passenger types, incidentally. Meanwhile the ex-LNWR 0-8-0 Super Ds or 'Wheezers' have already been mentioned, along with the WDs or 'Dub-Dees', with their distinctive "clinky-clank" motion. Spotters knew them as 'Clankers' just as, at the other end of the scale, the A4 streamlined pacifics were known as 'Streaks'. Some nicknames were usually fairly universal but I did notice the ex-LMS 'Princess Coronations' or 'Duchesses' were often called 'Semis' in the Midlands and North. The only explanation I ever heard was that it was short for 'semi-streamlined'. Some of the class had indeed once been streamlined, so that when this was finally removed by 1949, the curve of their smokebox tops was slightly flattened where it had once followed the streamlined profile of their casing. Nevertheless, try as I might, I could never see anything slightly streamlined about them.

The formal naming of freight engines was quite rare, though the last WD 2-8-0, number 90732, carried the name plate 'Vulcan' on its cabside. Sharing the same grimy state of most WDs, its name unsurprisingly, had to be pointed out to me when I found myself standing next to it during a visit to Stratford, in 1956. Some of the ex-North British class J36 0-6-0s were given painted-on names, related to the First World War, when they returned in 1919 from service on the continent. 'Somme' and 'Mons' had the odd distinction of sharing names with examples of the ex-Great Central class D11 4-4-0s, but as passenger locos, those latter at least had the distinction of brass number plates.

The more lowly J36s tended to have their names obliterated when they received repaints on passing through the workshops. Happily No. 65243 'Maude' has been preserved by the Scottish Railway Preservation Society. Perhaps it should be noted that Maude was a First World War military commander and not a French lady, as many a spotter seems to have assumed. Another group of freight engines, fourteen of the Southern's B4 0-4-0s, also carried painted names, this time of French towns, when they served in Southampton docks, but they lost this distinction when they were displaced by the USA tanks.

Even the background to names of grubby freight engines could therefore hold a fascination for the spotter who bothered to read up a little on their history.

As time went on, it became obvious that the number of cops available at any given location, would progressively decline. This would apply to freight engines as much as it did to passenger types, which remained the bigger attraction. This was the case when I had been staying with my grandparents and I made three consecutive Saturday morning visits to Paddington. Each time I returned, my grandmother asked if it had been a good visit, and I had to acknowledge it had yielded only four or five new sightings. Continuing like that could consume too much time and too much pocket money for little reward.

Nevertheless, activity at Paddington was generally enough to provide steady compensating interest and things seemed to flow like clockwork throughout the day. As trains got underway, it was rare to see a locomotive slipping, as was more likely at Waterloo, for example. However, what did catch the eye, was the parade of destination place names strung out along carriage roof lines and repeated, carriage after carriage, as the train moved out. Some of these stuck in the memory and the imagination;

Paddington Birmingham Shrewsbury Chester & Birkenhead
Paddington Oxford Evesham and Worcester
Paddington Cardiff and Fishguard Harbour
Paddington Exeter Plymouth and Penzance…

and so on, fanning out from north-west to south-west across the country.

Destination boards of this kind always struck me as a rather clumsy way of guiding passengers, to say nothing of physically moving the boards themselves, between trains. The other regions too, used destination boards of this kind, though I wonder if platform announcements were not more useful and more reassuring. The continental method, which I had seen in films, looked altogether more practical, where painted metal lists of destinations were attached next to carriage doorways. Today, of course, we do see printed variations of that approach in use in Britain.

Obviously not all spotting was done at terminus stations, so that at through stations with less background activity between passing trains, one was inclined to notice surrounding details which might otherwise have gone unobserved. Typical was the presence of weighing machines at many a station. What a wonderfully evocative Victorian term that was – a *machine* for checking your weight. These heavy cast iron scales required one old penny (that was worth about 20p by 1920) in a slot before they displayed one's weight on a large clock-like face. Before that stage could be reached it was necessary to step up almost *into* the machine which might have a wobbly platform to stand upon, enclosed both sides by projecting hand-rails. The ironwork of some of these machines was quite decorative. I used to imagine rather prosperous and portly Victorian gents steadying themselves into position, before parting with the required fee. Who else would have paid so handsomely, at that time, to know their weight? Contrarily, I cannot imagine many ladies of that era gathering up their skirts and squeezing between the handrails, only to risk displaying their weight to the world.

On the subject of spending a penny, the brass coin-operated locks on many a station toilet door were also rather splendid pieces of old mechanical ironmongery, albeit on a smaller scale, which did not escape notice. They used to operate with a reassuring mechanical precision not matched by today's flimsy aluminium door bolts.

Another piece of vanished station furniture was the cast-iron platform ticket machine, usually placed near platform entrances. One old penny again was charged, this time for a card ticket resembling a train ticket. They had been introduced on the GWR in 1912 to keep platforms clear. They were marked with figures 1-12 along their edges so they might be clipped at the appropriate point to record what time one entered the platform. After all, one penny purchased you only one hour's worth of access to the platform. Needless to say, ticket collectors clipped them at random, if at all. By all accounts,

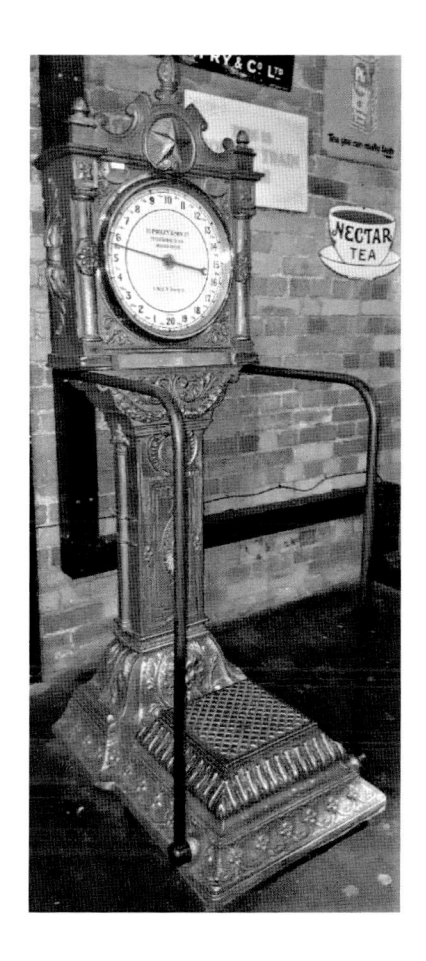

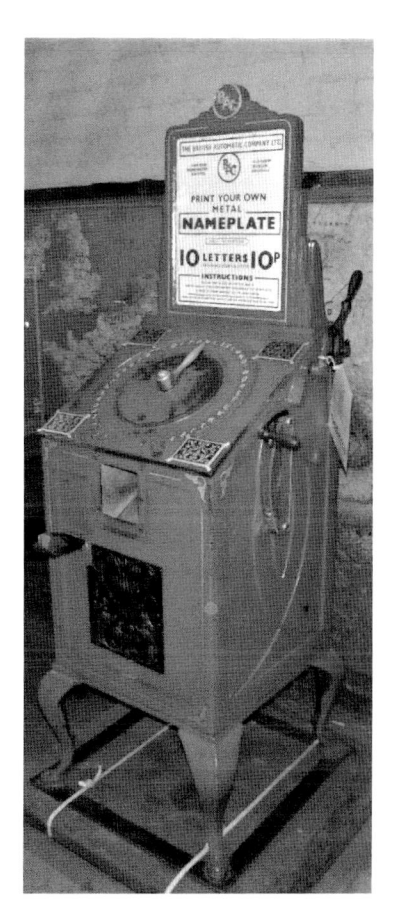

*Weighing machines came in many variations and were more associated with busier stations. Some had very decorative cast iron casings. They were frequently painted green or red but this example is in golden paint. A less frequently encountered machine was for embossing lettering onto an aluminium strip. Letters and numbers were selected by rotating a hand on the large dial and were then impressed by pulling the lever on the side of the machine. It was a laborious process. Having tested the novelty of it all, it is questionable if many users found a use for the embossed strip they had produced.*

platform tickets did not pay for themselves even when the price was doubled to 2d from 1958 onwards. At the London termini most favoured by spotters, the best observation points were reached along the open access taxi roads. Kings Cross was an exception, but the celebrated platform 10 was open access anyway.

In places where platform access was required, uncontrolled entrances often meant the purchase of a platform ticket was unnecessary. When a ticket machine had to be used, there was a certain modest satisfaction to be had from tugging on the heavy handle which slid smoothly with a click to deliver its ticket. This had not been the case when it came to the chocolate vending machines of my early spotting years. During the Second World War when chocolate was unavailable, the coin slots had all been sealed with strips of metal firmly wedged into them.

I used to be disappointed that the promise of chocolate, suggested by the cast-iron lettering crowning these machines, was not to be trusted. When I spotted a machine without the telltale wedges in place, I drew my mother's attention to it each time we had occasion to pass it. Those old cast iron machines lacked a window or indicator to show if they were full or not. Nevertheless, my mother eventually popped in the required coin and was, I think, as amazed as I was to receive a modest chocolate bar. I suspect that might have been in 1949 when post-war sugar rationing was suspended for a few months, before being re-imposed.

The experience of getting one of these machines to operate again, after so many years, seemed to unleash in my mother a minor spending frenzy. Chocolate in hand, she spotted a similar vending machine dispensing books of matches, from which she immediately made a purchase and rarely failed to do so whenever we later passed that way. There must have been a ready market for matches when smoking on trains and stations was so widespread, but what my mother, a non-smoker, did with them was a puzzle.

Whilst not served by vending machines, there were plenty of good non-platform viewing points to be found. The footbridge above the shed yard at Cambridge shed has already been mentioned. Another classic example was along the footpath crowning the retaining wall above Leicester, London Road engine shed and yard. This gave a grandstand view of the station as well as the loco activity in the foreground. A famous location near Tamworth was in a field, but it did offer good views of the LNW main line and the Midland Derby to Birmingham route, which crossed over it. Obviously the diversity of choices was endless and spotters were not slow to discover the best vantage points.

Nevertheless, the effect of diminishing returns applied to most locations, to the point where it was necessary to travel further afield if appreciable numbers of cops were to be achieved and if interest were to be sustained. Maps, books and old magazines were studied to locate the best destinations and in doing so, all manner of further background information was encountered. This was perhaps the point where many spotters became railway enthusiasts, as these wider interests gradually overtook mere number collecting.

Without necessarily being aware of it, railway photographs contributed hugely to our knowledge and appreciation of places, trains and above all, locomotives. As we saw greater numbers of photographs of engines at work, we might have associated specific types with certain classic landscapes. For example, 'Castles' on the seafront at Dawlish, 'Duchesses' tackling Beattock bank, LMS 2P 4-4-0s double heading Southern 'West Country's on the Somerset and Dorset, LNER A4s crossing the Forth bridge or a more homely LNER E4 2-4-0 at Mildenhall. Those classic images could be imprinted on one's awareness long before ever seeing them in reality. Conversely, whatever one's mental image of a particular loco type, those images could be reawakened from deep in one's memory, whenever a particular loco type was encountered.

One built up impressions and mental images of locomotive classes or, in some cases, of individual engines. One of the by-products of this was an aesthetic engagement, a development of personal responses to particular engine types, which went hand in hand with observations on the track. It was a matter of time before one had a short list of favourites, hard to justify, but nevertheless firmly held preferences.

Perhaps then, as it became harder to harvest many cops, it was little wonder that photography became another aspect of railway enthusiasm which attracted many a loco spotter. For the most part, it was not a widely exploited subject area for amateur photographers generally. One observed that when it grew out of loco spotting, the emphasis was on taking shots of locomotives in isolation, portraits as it were. It seemed to be less to do with capturing the moment but more a case of trying to capture the personality or essence of a particular locomotive type, just as one might do with a person. Observing spotters at work with a camera, and even trying oneself, this type of photography was clearly more difficult than it first seemed. One saw some enthusiasts struggling to get a good angle and the light in the right position, but for the most part it seemed like casual snapping away, just for the sake of having one's own picture record. What made us do this, I am still not sure, since good illustrations of all types were not generally hard to come by. In any case, as a last resort, there was always Lens of Sutton!

Others stood back and went for shots of engines in their working context and this would typically show the train behind, sometimes with much less emphasis on the engine itself. These were the shots better suited to capturing the day to day atmosphere of the location and the locomotive's place within it. Seen the other way round, the astute photographer chose the location to bring out the character of the engines. What was interesting was the fact that seen from the loco crew's perspective, there was no particular glamour to be seen. They may well have had professional pride and satisfaction in the job but the immediate reality was that it could be plain hard work. The view from the cab, by definition, was very different from that of the loco spotter.

Few teenage loco spotter photographers, who, incidentally, were much in the minority, were likely to have had such thoughts as they snapped away with their cameras. In retrospect one can guess it was the somewhat more mature enthusiast who may have thought about these things and he was probably no longer a spotter in the sense of number recording. To take satisfying pictures involved a different eye, a different mind-set from loco spotting. In any case, for moving subjects it could be difficult to concentrate on a viewfinder, as well as catching a number or enjoying the sight of the passing train. Spotting and serious photography tended to be different activities.

Perhaps the pictures with the most interest for fellow spotters were those which captured departures from usual practice. For example, unusual double heading loco combinations, ex-works or newly turned out modifications, or haulage by very unexpected engines or loco types seen at unusual locations; all these had a wider interest than simple portrait or context shots. If we ourselves were unable to record such views we had to resort to magazines where the best of them tended to be published.

Less specific still, were the 'arty' shots, which fell much more into the realm of the creative amateur photographer. They would embrace dramatic views with smoke, steam, extremes of light and shadow, difficult weather and so on, but they had less appeal to the focussed number takers.

As usual, the question of costs entered into the process. Younger spotters might depend on borrowing a family holiday snapshot camera, not technically advanced and therefore limiting them to static subjects in good light conditions. Black and white roll film was costly by the time prints had been made, so naturally care was taken in selecting subjects. In due course one acquired a better camera with much the same running costs and then progressed to a 35mm film camera. That could bring colour photography within reach but again, costs pushed one towards transparencies for projection, rather than coloured prints. It was all a question of what format and what budget matched one's needs. Only much later, in today's digital world, does one click away, unconstrained by the technical and cost limits of steam days. It is quite extraordinary now to contemplate the quality of some of those amateur shots taken even before the days of roll film cameras. Those tripods, heavy cameras and glass plates would surely have sent some of today's station managers into apoplectic fits.

    Thankfully, all that effort yielded the rich pictorial records we subsequently enjoy. I was reminded of that twenty years after the demise of main line steam when I had to attend a conference centre. Arriving in good time I parked the car some distance away in the landscaped grounds and strolled towards the building where the meeting was to be held. Then, with no warning, a cloudburst sent me scampering for cover – any cover. Dodging cars and deep puddles and diving through the first available open doorway, I stood disorientated, breathless and dripping in my own little puddle. I reached for my handkerchief to wipe my steamed up glasses and looked up. 'Coo, you're wet', said a voice from behind. I had already noticed that, but more interesting was the display of photographs coming into focus in the corner of an otherwise pretty dreary room. For a brief moment it reminded me of the sort of display I had seen once or twice in loco shedmasters' offices, tucked away in gloomy recesses of Victorian motive power depots. They were like private portrait galleries of steam locomotives. 'Umm, er, where is this?' I mumbled, still a bit confused. At that second I would not have been surprised had he said Top Shed or Nine Elms. 'It's the post room,' came the reply. There were no clip boards on the wall, no chalked up rosters, no oil lamps and no coal dusty floors. He was right, it was a post room. 'You interested in locos?' I ventured crassly. The response was a cautious, 'Yer'.

A minute or two later I knew I had struck a vein of gold. I did not learn his name but I did hear how he had joined the London and North Eastern Railway as a lad, how he had worked at Stratford shed during the Second World War and how, on one occasion during that period, he had, at the age of sixteen, stood in illegally for an absent driver. I smiled at the thought of those passengers, toe to toe, shoulder to shoulder, squeezed into an overcrowded suburban train in the blackout, blissfully unaware who was taking them home to Enfield or Chingford or was it Ponders End, their carriages pressed to their creaking limits?

He told me about bomb damage and hard times and eventually, leaping ahead twenty odd years, how there had been enginemen who had retired in tears at the end of British Rail steam, and others who had died within a year or two of heart break from the total dislocation of their lives. I could feel the truth of that because there was me, a former steam railway addict, now deprived of my regular fix and only coming to terms with it yet another twenty years on.

Still damp and dishevelled I remembered I had a meeting to attend, somewhere upstairs. Looking back now the significance of that meeting totally escapes me but I do know that meeting downstairs unlocked a great tide of memories, nostalgia and quizzical reflection.

# CHAPTER EIGHT          Collecting the Memories

As time went on one might look a little more closely at the details of familiar engines. Some people became quite intense and recorded variations like the type of tender in use or even the type of chimney fitted. If engines bore names, they too might be scrutinised more carefully. For the most part, those names did not seem to mean much. An engine had to 'earn' its name through history or association, if one was to recall it, or feel at all interested in seeing it again. For example, Flying Scotsman would be noticed as would Mallard, which, as the world record holder for fastest steam locomotive, would always be special, but what was one to make of names like 'Call Boy' or 'Sandwich'? 'Spearmint' did not seem too impressive either. An indiscriminate application of names to locomotives (racehorses in these cases) could invite ridicule.

Western Region naming had known better days and by the 1950s their names, for the most part, read like a check-list of National Trust properties. The Southern names seemed more varied, if a bit deferential, celebrating respected shipping companies, public schools, Battle of Britain squadrons and Arthurian legend. Quote a few names from that last group and you could be well in with your English teacher at school.

The London Midland loco names consistently reflected the military, Empire and national pride and generally felt as if they had been drawn up by a Home Office functionary. Only when they appeared to run out of ideas and resorted to mythology, did things come alive. Bellerophon, Cyclops and Thunderer were always more appealing to me than names like 'The Boy Scout' – sorry, lads. There was something appropriate about those names from classical antiquity. They seemed to suggest the elemental qualities we might perceive in steam engines – beauty, strength, speed, agility, doggedness and so on. That surely would have explained the

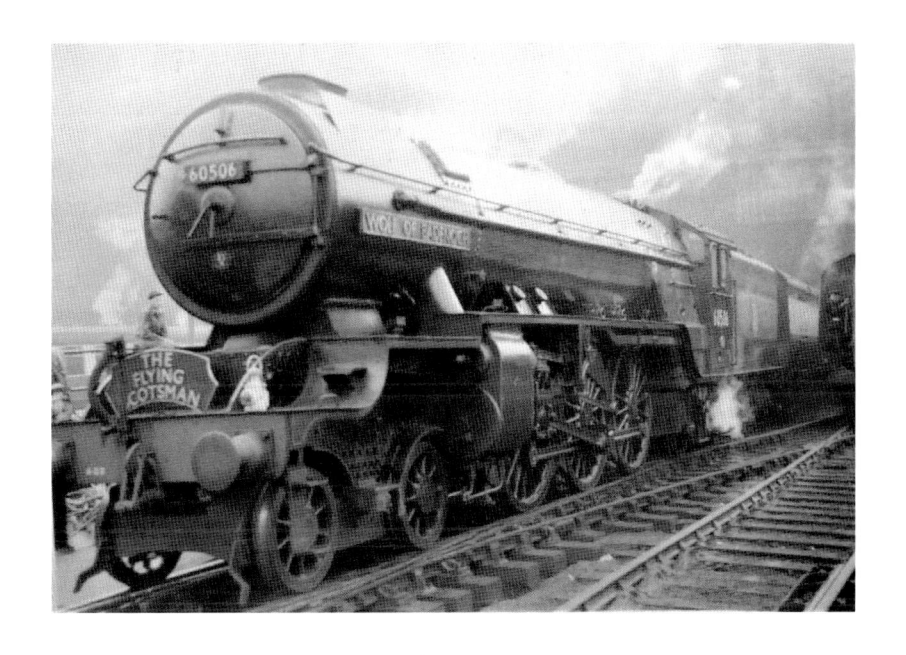

*Class A2/2, No. 60506, Wolf of Badenoch, heads The Flying Scotsman at Kings Cross, early in 1954. Introduced in 1943, this was one of the six 4-6-2 rebuilds of Gresley's P2 class of 2-8-2s of 1934. One wonders just how effective were the minute smoke deflector blades, visible just below the chimney. 60506 and sister engine, 60504, both briefly worked this turn out of New England shed at that time. Note the Doncaster practice of indicating the loco class on the buffer beam, (to the left of the coupling).*

widespread use of names suggesting these qualities during the early decades of steam locomotion. It was said that a 'Comet', 'Phoenix', 'Samson', 'Goliath', 'Vulcan' and an 'Atlas' were to be found on nearly all lines at that time. On a lighter note, none of this stopped us enjoying names from the Scottish Region like 'Jingling Geordie' and 'Wandering Willie'.

On the question of place names, there were stories that early rail travellers were prone to reading a locomotive name and confusing it with the train's destination. How true could that have been? Surely, passengers were not routinely inclined to walk to the engine to see where the train was heading. That said, photographs do show us some engines carried place names which were painted on, large and clear. Examples from the former London, Brighton and South Coast Railway come to mind. Perhaps then, names like 'Leatherhead' or 'Epsom', arriving from Victoria, might have created some confusion, but elsewhere, I doubt that many passengers would have been fooled in that way by names like 'Bombay' or 'Pretoria'.

Favourite locations were all important to spotters. Paddington, Euston and Kings Cross, along with Liverpool Street, usually had a posse of spotters present on Saturdays and at holiday times. At Kings Cross we congregated at the end of Platform 10 (today's No.8) which was one of the few locations I recall where a notice forbade spotters from continuing towards the platform end. It was of course universally ignored. Adult enthusiasts were inconspicuous but youthfulness and our sartorial style – or rather lack of it – gave away us youngsters. Only once did I see a station official insist on applying the ruling. There was a bewildered shuffling of feet in which the whole crowd of us, some fifteen or so, described a large circle and arrived back in much the same position from which it had started. The man in the suit disappeared to disturb us no further.

There could be far bigger obstructions to deal with, back along the platform. That was apparent when, for example, the Yorkshire Pullman was preparing for departure. Trolleys and

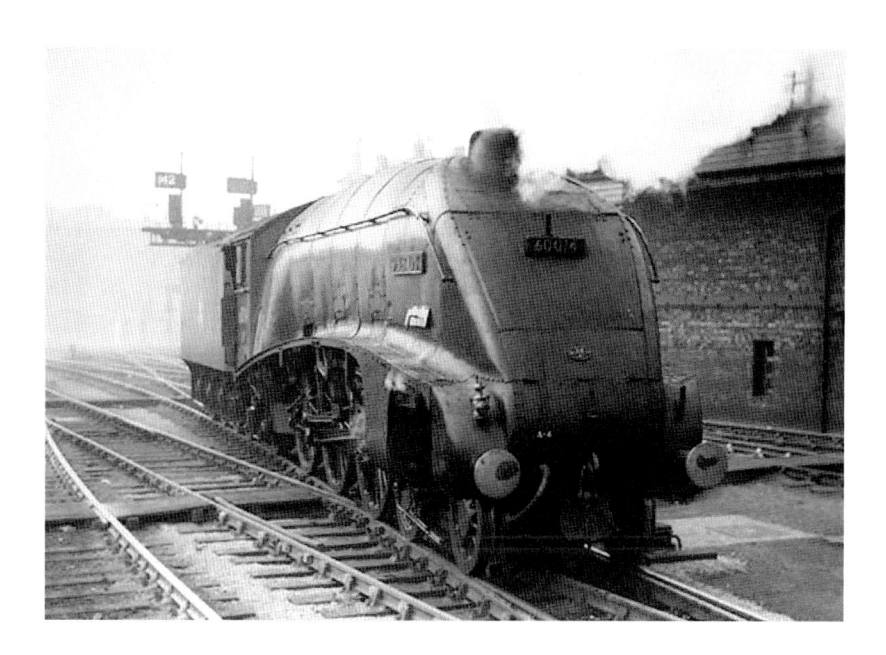

'Streak', or more correctly, class A4 60014 Silver Link, backing out of Kings Cross towards the smoky portals of Gasworks Tunnel. This was the engine chosen to head the inaugural run of the new streamlined Silver Jubilee service from London to Newcastle in 1935. It was a sister engine of Silver Fox, also built for the Siver Jubilee service. The latter was graced with the decorative stainless steel fox plaque shown below, here displayed at the NRM.

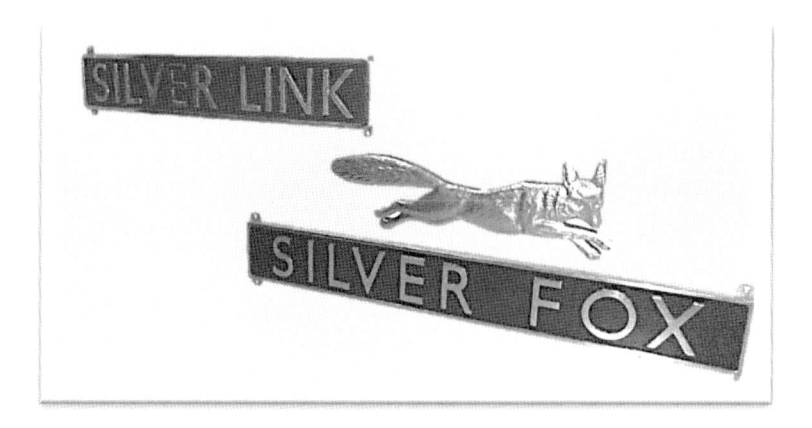

The Silver theme was continued with similar locomotives named 'Quicksilver' and 'Silver King'.

137

wicker hampers would be strewn across the platform, laden with supplies of table linen and all the accoutrements of Pullman travel. Smartly uniformed Pullman attendants would be hovering around and one could get glimpses of cutlery and menu cards being arranged inside the cars.

Meanwhile, back at the platform end, there was ongoing entertainment to be had. Gasworks Tunnel, which trains to-day still enter immediately on departure, was well named, for in those days there was a continuous sulphurous haze emanating from its portals. As engines backed out of the tunnel tender first, to join their trains, all eyes were turned in anticipation. If the chime whistle of a streamlined A4 Pacific was sounded just within the tunnel, the melodious note would send up cries of, 'Streak!' and necks would be craned to identify it by name and number. Most engines from Kings Cross shed were well turned out but that changed in the closing years of steam, which was the same for all the main line sheds. Meanwhile though, we came to notice grimy express engines were not often from 'Top Shed', as Kings Cross was known. I was particularly disappointed when V2 2-6-0 Green Arrow, 60800, came bustling in from Hull in an appalling and apparently irretrievable state, as dirt encrusted as any freight engine imaginable. The V2s were well proportioned machines with their own characteristic three cylinder exhaust beat and to see that very locomotive to-day in the National Collection, spotlessly preserved, still gives me a sense of relief.

Between the arrivals and departures of the more important trains, suburban trains were coming and going from their own platforms on the west side. Occasionally one of these emerged up the steep gradient from the Metropolitan Widened Lines from Moorgate. They would pause for a while, seemingly exhausted, the enveloping smoke and steam gradually dispersing, as if the whole train was gathering its wits before plunging again, this time into Gasworks Tunnel. Various big engines entered and reappeared from the tunnel as they

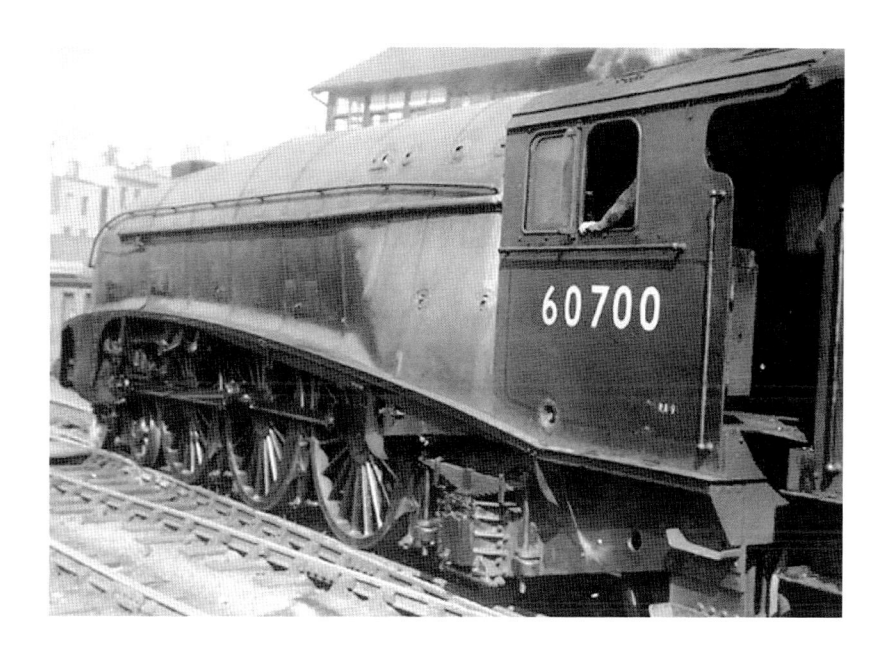

*Class W1, 4-6-4 60700, awaiting departure from Kings Cross. It was a long stretch for the fireman between tender and firebox. This was the 1936 rebuilt version of the unique 'Hush-hush' of 1929, generally following the lines of the A4s. It was a bit special for spotters and not frequently seen. There had been suggestions to call it 'British Enterprise' or 'Pegasus', but it remained 'the un-named streak' until withdrawal in 1959. The 'RA9' displayed in the bottom corner of the cabside, was a reference to route availability. '9' was the most restricted category. The Western Region used their own cabside codes, using letters and coloured discs, refering to loco power and weight.*

manoeuvred towards the turntable and servicing area on the suburban side, adjacent to the tunnel mouth. Sometimes the view of all this secondary activity was obscured by the presence of a departing Cambridge buffet express, typically waiting for its B1 or Sandringham/Footballer to back down – types of engines which perhaps looked more at home at Liverpool Street.

Another obstruction to the overall view was the substantial bulk of Kings Cross signal box, eventually demolished in 1976. Although it very rarely hid engines for long, it could distract from the passing of a suburban train bound for Moorgate. These had their own 'York Road' platform just outside the main body of Kings Cross itself, and were served by tank engines equipped with condensing apparatus to reduce the effects of smoke and steam in the tunnels. Eventually curiosity won us over and we made the smoky Metropolitan Widened Lines trip to Moorgate and back. It did not yield any cops but it did give us a hint of what the original steam hauled Metropolitan might have been like.

Apart from the obvious railway centres favoured by spotters, there were lesser places which could compete as personal favourites. One of mine was Brighton. On my very first visit to the motive power depot, I had been struck by the sheer variety of locomotive classes represented. The Brighton Works shunter, an 1878 veteran A1X 0-6-0, could usually be spotted during a visit, and sometimes it could be seen close at hand, in the shed yard. It might have gone unnoticed, except for its odd number, DS377. More immediately obvious was its distinctive livery, a golden ochre colour, described as Improved Engine Green.

Introduced by William Stroudley, the Chief Mechanical Engineer of the London Brighton and South Coast Railway, there has been speculation as to whether he had a colour vision defect or whether this colour description was Stroudley's way of getting the Board's approval for the adoption of the ochre colour he had previously used on the Highland Railway.

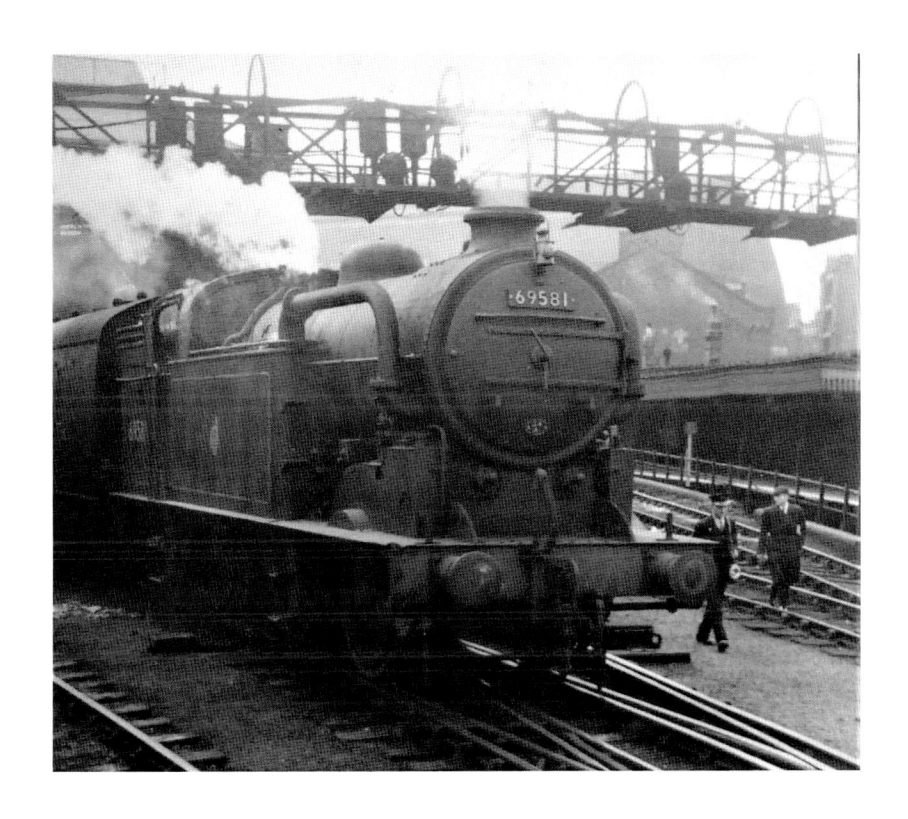

*Class N2, 0-6-2 tanks were the mainstay of Kings Cross suburban services: No. 69581, with condensing gear for working the Metropolitan widened lines, is seen at the head of a departing suburban train from Kings Cross, in 1957. The connection from the Metropolitan line from Moorgate emerges on a steep gradient at the platform behind the two figures on the right.*

Railways, per se, rarely featured on television at that time. However, in February 1956, King Arthur class 30740, Merlin, appeared in a BBC programme, in the Saturday Night Out series. The Longmoor Military Railway arranged a demonstration sabotage derailment. Outside broadcasting, in fuzzy 405 line black and white, in night time conditions, was barely up to the job. An animated commentator did his best to sound excited but it was a complete anti-climax. The locomotive just hopped off the track and slumped to a halt. Inside Brighton works a month later, I was surprised to see Merlin. Although its buckled front buffer beam was the only sign of damage, it was clearly a candidate for imminent scrapping. Two years later, on 13th April 1958, the last 4-4-2 express passenger locomotive in Britain, returned to Brighton shed for the last time, having hauled a farewell special from Victoria to Newhaven harbour. This was the ex-LBSC Railway H2 32424, Beachy Head which, forty two years later, the Bluebell Railway undertook to rebuild in replica form. I was pleased to have seen the original for the last time, a few days after its arrival at Brighton, for it was not long before it left for Eastleigh works, under its own steam, on its very last journey.

Both these examples became lasting cameo memories. Inevitably the rate of making cops gradually declined. Thoughts drifted back to those first visits to Rugby and Swindon, when seemingly prodigious numbers of cops had been achieved, to say nothing of loco types we rarely saw in the London area. Paddy was already starting to think on the same lines, so our thoughts turned towards ranging further afield. Expense and time were major constraints, even assuming we could get the necessary shed permits. Particular attraction obviously lay in the railway works which, by their nature, drew together a concentration of engines from a wide geographical area. They offered us both abundance and novelty. Unfortunately, from time to time, Paddy was unavailable for spotting trips. If he annoyed his father he risked having his ABC confiscated for a week. Since

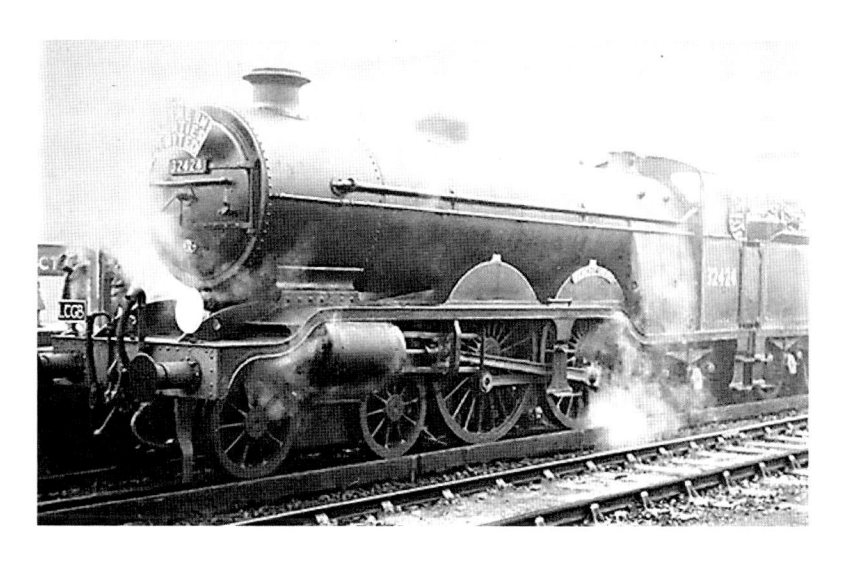

*Class H2 32424 on the Locomotive Club of Great Britain 'Southern Counties Limited', at Clapham Junction on 24 February 1957.*

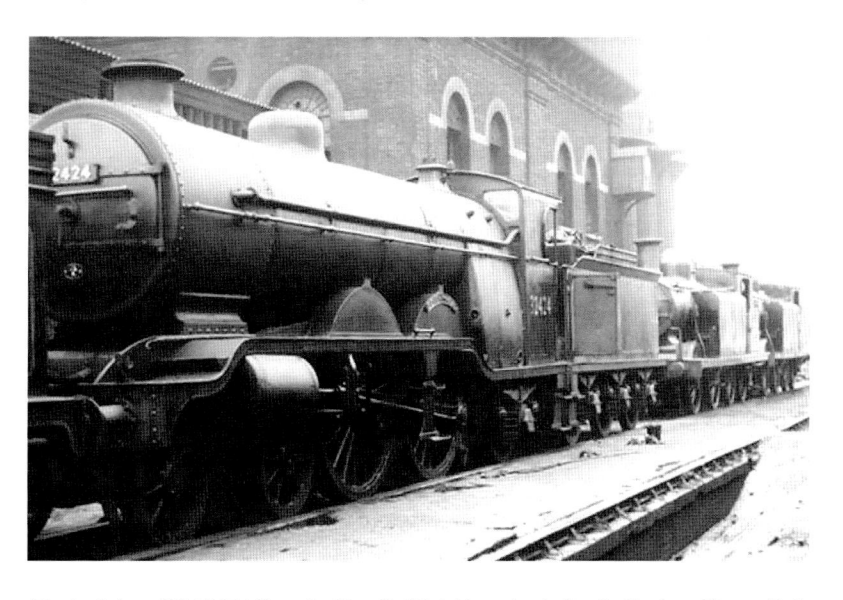

*The last class H2 32424 'Beachy Head' at Brighton shed after its final working, a Railway Correspondence and Travel Society tour on 13 April 1958. It is a happy thought that some minor components have been incorporated into the Bluebell Railway's recreation of 32424. With its tender gate flapping in the breeze and not a whiff of steam in sight, it is every bit 'dead', compared to the the last illustration*

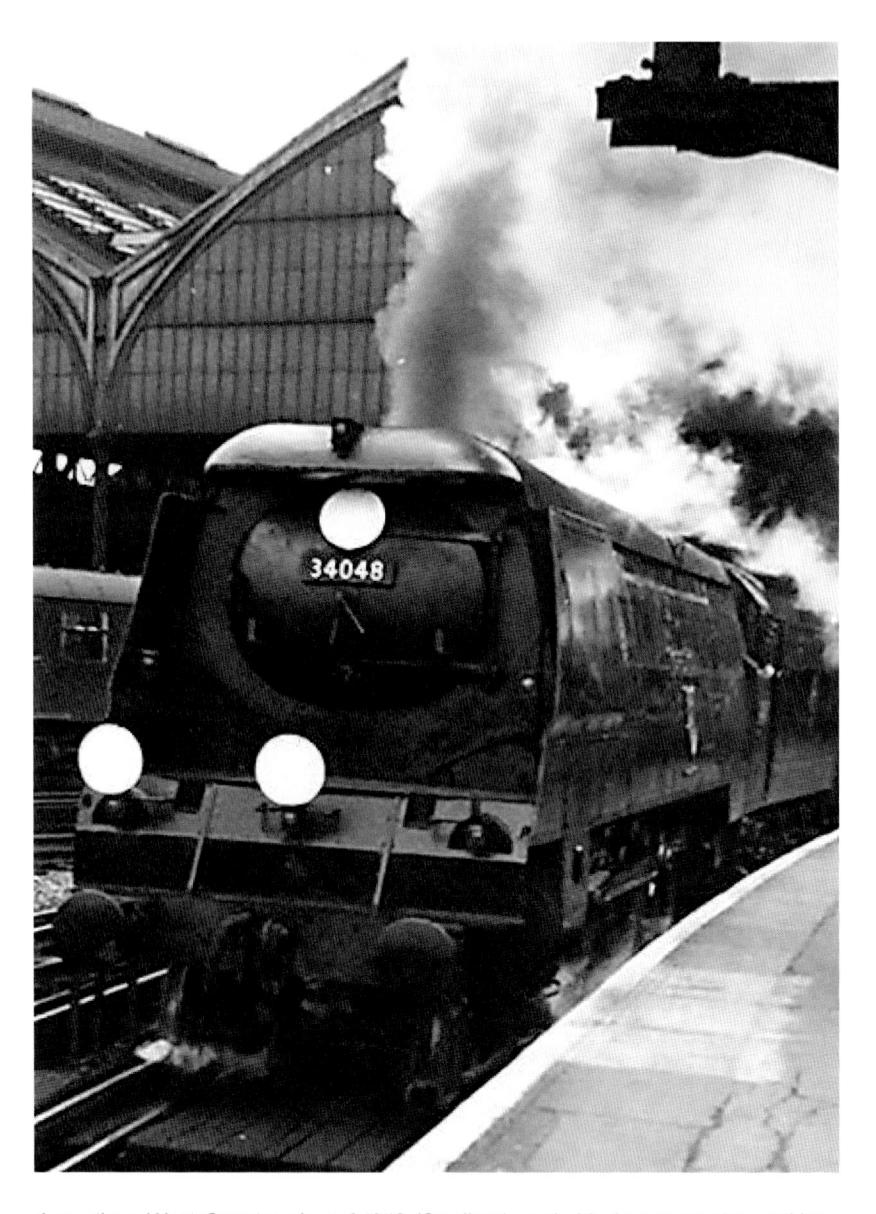

*A spotless West Country class 34048 'Crediton', probably just ex-works, making a spirited departure from Brighton on a train bound for Salisbury via Southampton Central, according to the headcode discs. They were certainly not historically conventional in shape and one can see why some wits nicknamed them 'Spam cans'. Note the fixed electric route indicator lamps for night use.*

a loco spotter without his ABC was as comfortable as a shirt with no buttons, he seemed gradually to lose interest and plunge himself deeper into his tennis statistics, and I found myself exploring alone more frequently.

It was on one of those occasions at Kings Cross, when a fellow spotter asked me if I wanted to join a small party to visit Doncaster shed and works, a few days later. I must have emptied my money box that week because I remember the trip vividly. The shed yielded 0-8-4 and 4-8-0 tank engines, both unusual configurations, and the works introduced me to numerous unfamiliar classes of engines. The abiding memory was that of immaculate ex-works express locos in the paint shop. As our train made its way back in the dark to Kings Cross, I reflected on what an enjoyable outcome had derived from that chance encounter at the end of Platform 10.

Shortly afterwards, when Ian Allan announced a circular day trip to Eastleigh and Swindon, I jumped at it. This was to be my first foray with my neighbour, Blair, from next door. It turned out to be a circular excursion par excellence. We were to be hauled by an elderly T9 4-4-0, following an unusual route which included stretches not usually taken by passenger trains. From the early start from Victoria it was clear the engine was struggling so, by the time we reached the Virginia Water area, it was forced to stop for a good half hour to raise steam. From then on the schedule was never recovered. Having said that, it was a wonderful day. Eastleigh did the trick by hosting all manner of Southern engines we never saw at the London end of the region and Swindon was as exciting as it had been on my first visit. We eventually staggered into Liverpool Street's Platform 11 around 10 o'clock in the evening. The engine crew had certainly earned their overtime and I wondered if everyone would manage to get home that night.

Opportunism did play its part for loco spotters and I made the most of it when Dad proposed a week's cycling tour around Cornwall. His intention was to cycle up to London, take

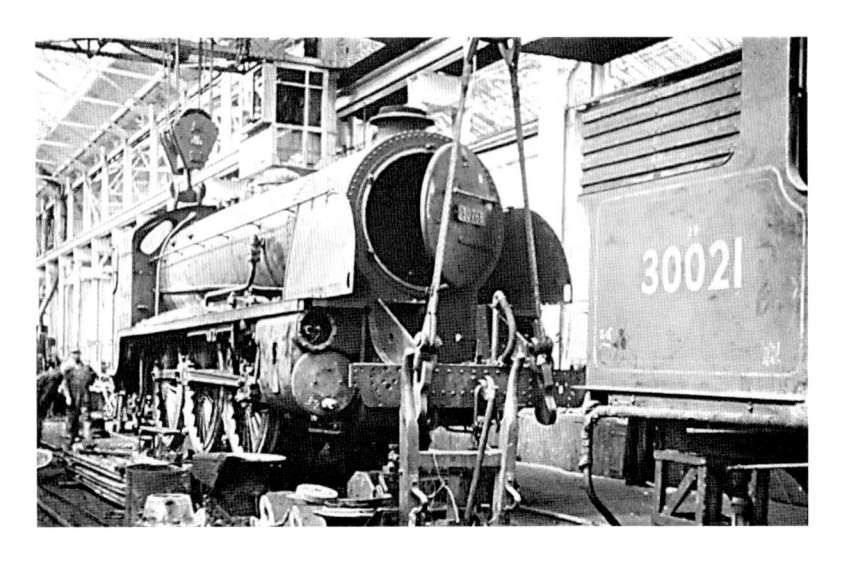

King Arthur class, 30768 Sir Balin, on the overhead crane at Eastleigh works on 3 August 1960. It was during works visits that one was reminded of the number of heavy and awkward to handle components which went to make up a steam locomotive. Sometimes the number of fitters engaged on a single engine was a further reminder of just how expensive it was to maintain a fleet of several thousand steam locomotives. That was before considering the need for both drivers and firemen and the labour required for routine maintenance.

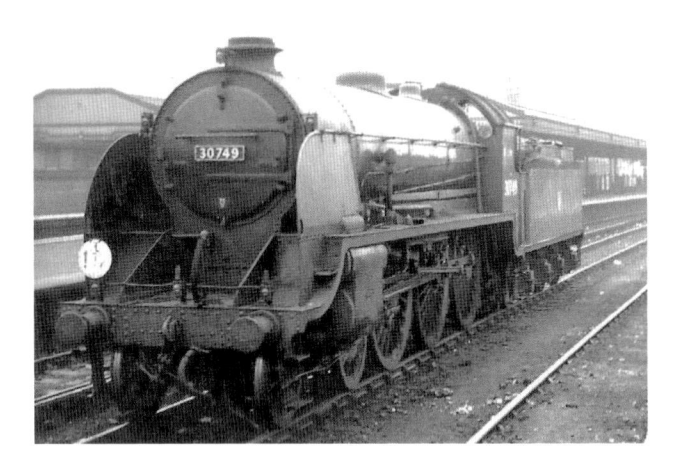

King Arthur class 30749 Eseult, at Clapham Junction in the mid 1950s. The 70D shed code, on the bottom of the smoke box door, indicates it was allocated to Basingstoke shed and the white headcode disc suggests it had worked a Southampton docks train of perishable foodstuffs on the mainline to Nine Elms goods yard.

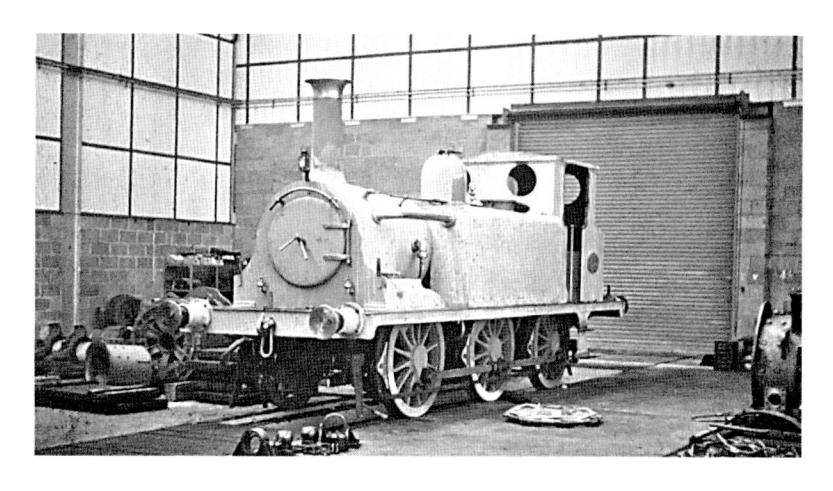

*Former LBSCR class A1, No.82 Boxhill, was withdrawn in 1946 and put aside for preservation. It is seen here in primer in Eastleigh works diesel shop, on 3 August 1960, undergoing a repaint in its original livery prior to.display at the , Clapham Transport Museum and then at the NRM, York, from 1975.*

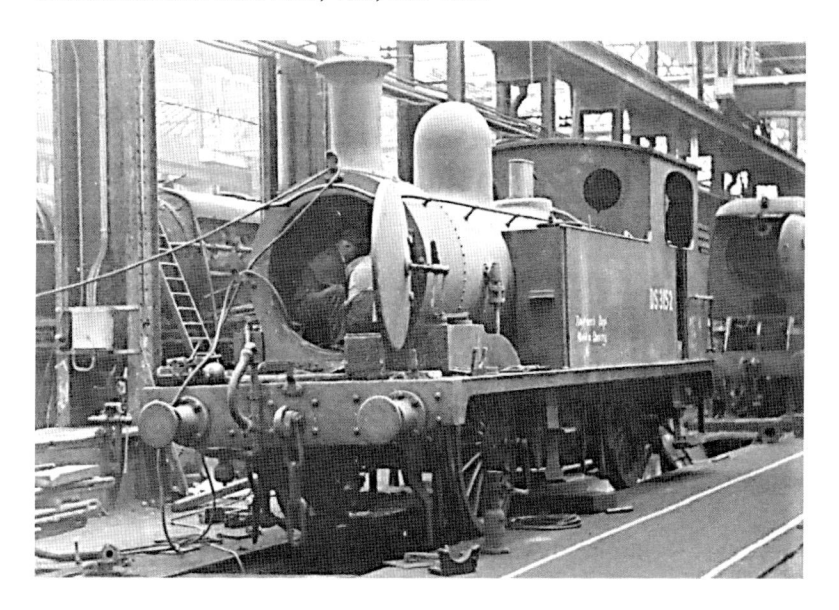

*Class G6, DS 3152, was a service loco from the Engineer's Department, Meldon Quarry. This example, again seen in Eastleigh works on 6 August 1958, dated from 1897 and was withdrawn in 1960. Two men are working in the cramped conditions of the smoke box. Even that was better than for those who had to squeeze through a firebox door to work in the claustrophobic confines of the firebox.*

our bikes on the 'Cornish Riviera Limited', non-stop to Plymouth, and then spend the week in Cornwall. I think his choice of train was probably to please me, and he certainly did not hesitate to write to the shed masters at Plymouth Laira and Plymouth Friary, on my behalf. Both replied positively within a few days and I could not wait to get started.

There was a minor disappointment when we discovered the 'Cornish Riviera' was fully booked. However, I was pleased to learn there was a relief train following only ten minutes later. That too was heavily booked but we managed window seats and all was well. I was of course familiar with the route as far as Reading, but beyond that the number of locos to spot seemed to decline abruptly, with flurries of interest around Westbury, Taunton and Exeter. Having said that, I was finding the Great Western railway architecture, and overall railway environment, of particular interest. Adding in the highlights like the overall roof of Exeter St Thomas, the coastal line at Dawlish, and a passing glimpse of the preserved broad gauge engine 'Tiny', at Newton Abbot station, then I was more than satisfied by the time Plymouth was reached. What was more, I was pleased to have made the non-stop journey behind a 'King', a former Great Western Railway class of loco and still the most powerful and prestigious on the Western Region.

In complete contrast, at the humble end of the scale, Plymouth Friary yielded 30757, Earl of Mount Edgcumbe and 30758, Lord St. Levan, a unique pair which had spent most of their lives associated with the little Plymouth, Devonport and South West Junction Railway. In terms of mystique and long term association with a particular shed, they were perhaps the West Country equivalent of Guildford's 'Ironside'.

It is easy to recall such sunny summer days discovering something new, watching trains go by, the anticipation of an imminent cop, and failing that, the sure knowledge that something novel would turn up in good time. Did we share comparable sentiments not just with bird watchers but with

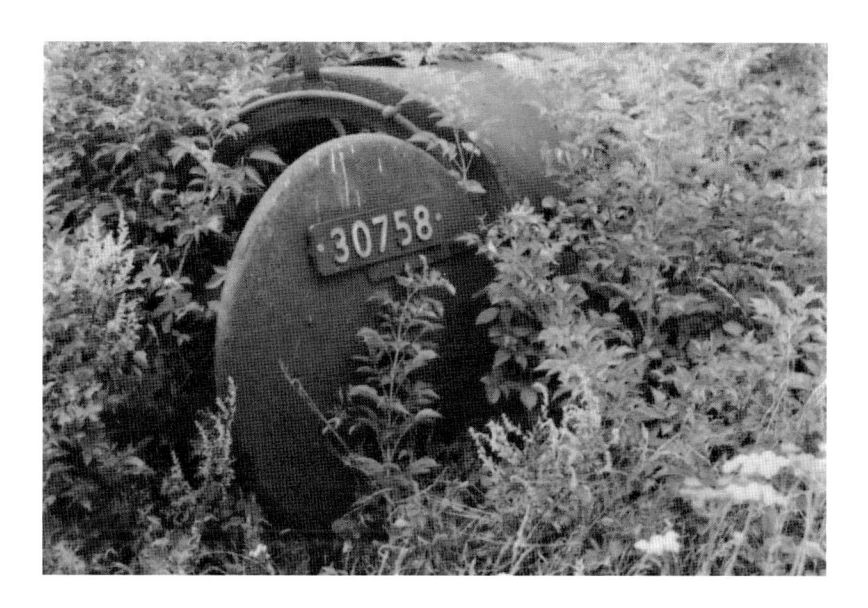

*The boiler of 'Lord St. Levan' in Eastleigh works yard in 1958, the engine having been withdrawn some 18 months before. It was not unusual in a works yard for the occasional boiler to linger on for several years, as if there was a reluctance to finish the job of disposal. Such discoveries could evoke poignant memories of happier days.*

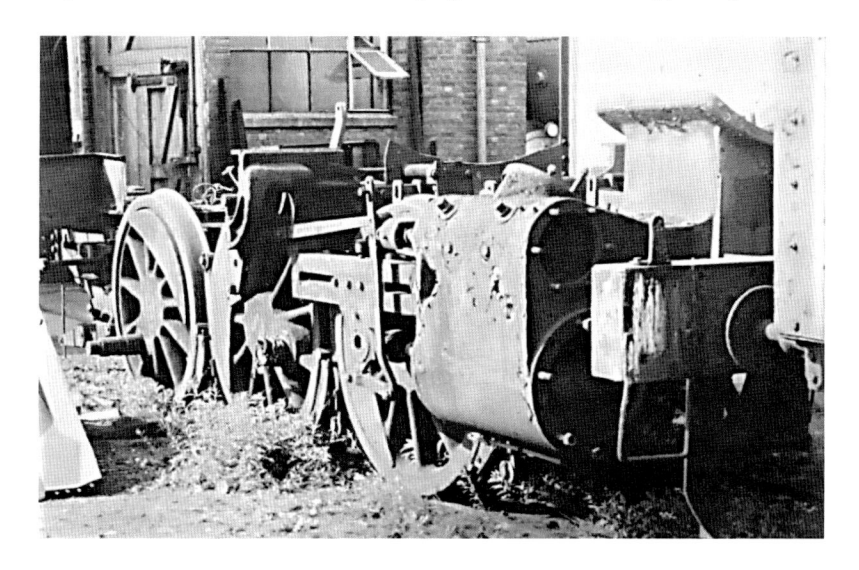

*When the Southern Railway bought 15 USA class locos from government war surplus in 1946, one example was retained for spares, seen here at Eastleigh works in 1958.*

anglers too, watching the movement of water, anticipating a worthy bite but unfailingly optimistic if it were slow to materialise?

It was nothing like that when I found myself on a snow covered platform at Romford station during one Christmas holiday. I saw a single down express behind a grubby B1 4-6-0 and, much to my delight, an ex-Midland railway 0-4-4 tank, arriving on a train from Upminster. That at least was one of those unusual specimens in the 50,000 series. Other than that, nothing, before my duffle coat gave up the struggle to keep me warm and without further perseverance I took the next electric train back to Liverpool Street. What had possessed me to choose Romford in winter as a spotting locale I shall never know.

There was also a trip to Salisbury on the 'Atlantic Coast Express'. The destination had been chosen because that was as far east as some west of England engines ventured, so there was a fair likelihood of some cops. I made my way to the loco shed where I could see rows of engines from the entrance doorway and then, again for some inexplicable reason, I lost all courage to bunk round. No matter how hard I tried, I stood there for about ten minutes, rooted to the spot. I did not see a single railway man and still just could not make myself go in.

Disappointments could equally result from impetuosity. I was enjoying the scene at Oxford on one occasion when I thought it would be a good idea to take a train past the loco shed to obtain a better view. Subsequently I alighted at Handborough (described on the platform time-table as Long Handborough and re-spelled Hanborough since 1992), only to find there were no return trains for several hours, and no other means of transport back to Oxford. I ended up sitting in the sunshine for three hours, until a bus turned up. During all that time, only three or four cars went by and the entire afternoon was a spotting disaster. Why I did not just take the five minute walk to the loco shed in the first place, escapes me. I can only assume I was mistakenly locked into a 'Southern Electric' mentality, where there was almost bound to have been a return service within a few minutes.

As school holidays came and went, the loco works at Crewe, Derby, Bow, Longhedge (Battersea), Ashford and Stratford were added to the list, to say nothing of repeat visits elsewhere, but Darlington and the Scottish works always eluded me. It was a close run thing. I started detailed timetable planning for a trip around Scotland and even had the necessary shed and works permits to hand. Then a school friend invited me on a trip to Germany to stay with his aunt and uncle during the summer holidays. So it was, with a mixture of regret and curiosity that I ended up on a boat train which plodded from Liverpool Street to Harwich. It seemed to promise a good deal less excitement than my abandoned trip to Scotland had done.

During the following two weeks we went to Cologne and I made a point of visiting the main station. It was impressively large but gloomy and tired looking, with not a single train spotter in sight. Several trains came and went behind large engines but they were black and grubby and did not leave much of an impression. Their small number plates set me wondering. Was it the striking legibility of the painted numbers we had back home, along with Ian Allan's ABCs, which sustained loco enthusiasm as it existed in Britain?

In contrast we had occasion to travel on a Dutch electric train and we both remarked on the smoothness and quietness of the ride. Suddenly, trains back home seemed very old-fashioned. It was another reminder that steam was not going to go on for ever. Nevertheless, that still remained hard to accept.

# CHAPTER NINE                    A Scottish Diversion

In spite of Nationalisation in 1948, the vast bulk of older locomotives still tended to be seen on the lines of their originating companies. So it was that complete classes and blocks of numbers remained all but empty in my ABC, their geographic distribution closely echoing the limits of my railway travels. Thumbing through railway books and magazines, I was awestruck by the peregrinations of the likes of HC Casserley, whose celebrated locomotive photographs were sourced from every imaginable corner of the railway system.

In my own case, as usual, I had to be opportunistic if new ground was to be covered. So it was, when the chance to see at least a few purely Scottish engines came, in 1958. A school friend, Ken, a keen geographer with whom I would go youth hostelling, but who had no particular interest in railways, suggested we undertake a hostelling trip, taking in the Glencoe area. He planned the hostels and I set-to on the travel arrangements. We could have gone directly from Euston to Glasgow, but I had my reasons for choosing the East Coast route. An early start saw us on 'The Talisman' departure from Kings Cross to Edinburgh Waverley.

Along the way I had fleeting glimpses of numerous unfamiliar engines and managed to record quite a few of them. York, Darlington and Newcastle were particularly fruitful, but it needed vigilance if nothing was to be missed. It paid off near Alnmouth, where we passed a long line of ex-North Eastern and North British 4-4-0s, looking suspiciously like imminent victims of the cutter's torch. The combined effects of an ageing locomotive stock and the growing impact of the modernisation programme, were creating a perceptible increase in the rate of locomotive withdrawals, although there still remained much to be enjoyed.

The afternoon journey from Edinburgh to Glasgow was made in a crowded and stuffy diesel multiple unit train, an indicator of changing times. On arriving in Glasgow we were pleased to have some time in hand which would enable us to stroll around and get some fresh air. We were enjoying the sights and sounds and rather appreciating the orange, green and cream painted trams, when we thought it might be fun to take one of these back to Queen Street station for our onward journey. On asking a passer-by which tram we needed, I was taken aback by a booming reply, 'AARCH! Yah dinna wanna tacka TRUM'. It turned out we had gone around in one big circle to arrive only a couple of minutes' walk from Queen Street.

It was with eager anticipation that I descended onto a gloomy and smoky Queen Street Low Level platform, from where we took our evening rush hour train to Craigendoran. The plan was to take the push and pull train from there to Arrochar and Tarbet, and then to set out for the youth hostel.

The engine was in pushing mode and to my delight the fireman was only too happy to let us ride on the footplate, which immediately revived memories of my last ride eight years previously, at Mundesley. Again, the engine number was to stick in my mind, 67474.

A few days later we were to join the 11.24am train at Dalmally, behind a Black Five, which had staggered up on the old Caledonian line from Dunblane on a wet and blustery morning. The ensuing journey to Oban was sufficient to dry us out and warm us through. There were few passengers on the train, and even fewer the next morning, when we took the Connell Ferry to Ballachulish branch train. I managed a couple of cops and on reaching Ballachulish we unexpectedly discovered we could buy a cup of tea at that remote station.

The next station we encountered told a very different story. A couple of days later, we had stumbled across the surprisingly intact remains of Invergarry station, on the route of the former Fort Augustus branch. The subway platform access

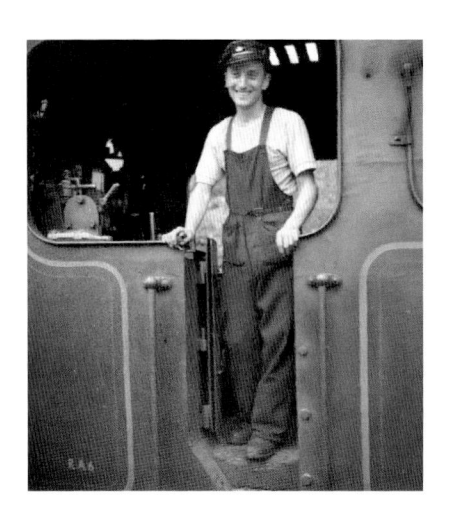

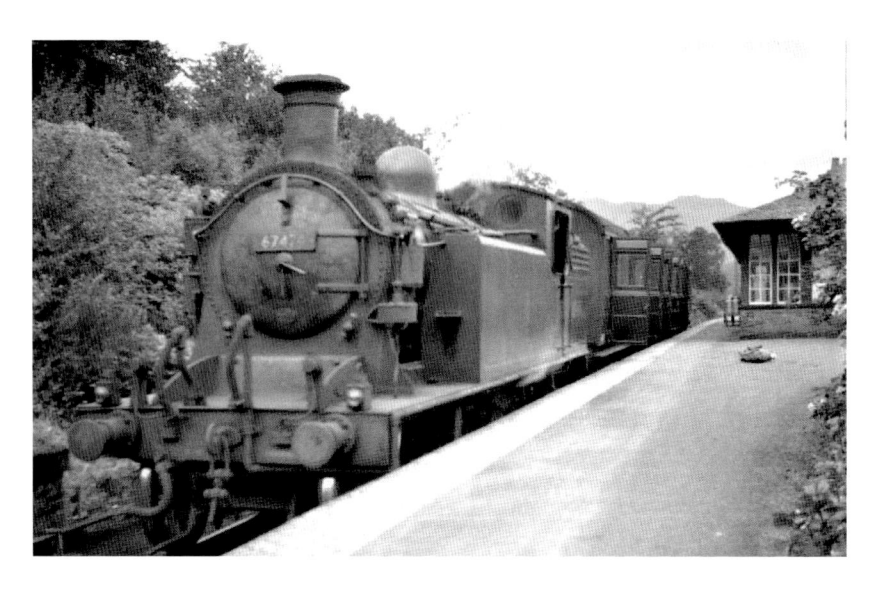

*All but two of the thirty strong C15 class of 4-4-2 tanks had gone by 1956. Nos. 67460 and 67474 lasted until 1960. They were fitted for push and pull working and were retained for working between Craigendoran to Arrochar and Tarbet. No. 67474 is seen here at Arrochar after the fireman had welcomed us in his cab for the journey. The two carriage train is seen here waiting with all doors open, giving the unlikely impression of hordes of passengers expected for the return trip. The purpose of this arrangement was unclear.*

was blocked by stones but that was no obstacle to exploring around the building and along the forestry trail which occupied the former track bed. We were both hugely intrigued and even more so on later reaching the site of Fort Augustus station.

The site of the station building there was clear enough, with the platforms themselves still intact. Looking at my note book now, I am reminded of the layout with its two-road loco shed, turntable pit, goods shed, sidings, and terminal platforms, along with the through platform serving the loch-side pier branch. It all amounted to lavish over-provision for even the most optimistic traffic projection for a line serving a small community, and even smaller communities en route. By the time we located the five viaduct supports, formerly serving the loch-side pier branch, we were questioning whether the scene amounted to historical geography or industrial archaeology. We later learned the pier branch had lasted only from 1903 to 1906, that passenger services ceased in 1933 and the line had lingered on for occasional freight until January 1947. It was all so fascinating that I put away thoughts of loco spotting for a few days.

We were to meet up with Ken's parents in Inverness. They were returning from a driving tour around Scotland and were giving us a lift home. En route, they were kind enough to offer me a short detour to the loco shed at Perth, so, with a number of elderly ex-Caledonian Railway cops in the bag, that was a good note on which to finish the loco spotting aspect of our holiday. It was fun to take the little car ferry, dwarfed as it was by the Forth Bridge. I was mightily impressed and resolved one day in the future to make the crossing by train.

On arrival in Edinburgh, Ken and I decided to celebrate the end of our adventures with a memorable supper at the North British Hotel. The high standards of the old North British Railway's principal hotel must still have been in play, as the waiters made us feel like kings. We had anticipated our travel-worn appearance might see us discretely relegated to a shadowy corner of the dining room, but not a bit of it. We mused on the role of railway catering, comparing the refreshment rooms at Dalmally and Ballachulish stations to the present silver service splendour. No doubt that particular topic too, fitted somewhere into the vista of historical geography.

It had been a trip of contrasts. For the most part one had the impression that south of the border the railway promoters had been able to choose most of their routes with the aid of relatively minor adjustments to the landscape. In Scotland, with the grandeur of much of its terrain, it was more a question of plotting routes around, rather than through or over obstacles. Either that or do not build a railway. Both the physical achievement and the speculative risks involved left their impression upon us.

If much of this was a long way from loco spotting, it did illustrate how one thing could lead to another. What I had taken as an opportunistic way to bag a few rare cops had introduced me, albeit briefly, to Edinburgh and Glasgow.

I had come to realise how railway infrastructure was not just architecture and civil engineering but that those could be just aspects of industrial archaeology. It had caused me to reflect on the social and communication implications of living in remote communities, along with the historic economics of providing them with rail links.

Finally it had facilitated a splendid hotel dining experience of a kind I would not otherwise have associated with train travel, surpassing perhaps, even that of those Pullman cars I had so admired at Kings Cross. That trip had sharpened my awareness of just how much more there was to the railway interest than simply spotting engines.

## CHAPTER TEN   Timetables, Guides and other Distractions

When we set out on circular routes, we soon became adept at finding our way through station platform timetables, tracing the stations to be passed through, noting where we would pass an engine shed and deciding if it would be more productive in spotting terms to take a 'stopper', and hence slower train, or go for the thrill of speed, hopefully offered by an express.  This was easily decided if we were planning to travel on well-served routes and if we had a long summer's day to spend.

For our purposes, printed timetables were better for armchair travel but they were expensive to buy, especially as there was both a summer and winter edition each year, to say nothing of monthly updates.  The choice lay between Bradshaws or the ABC Alphabetical Railway Guide.  Bradshaws, which was published from 1839 until 1961, was the more detailed and gave full timetable information for all but frequent interval suburban services.  It included private railways, ferry times and hotel advertising.  If it had a downside it was the sheer host of symbols and cross-references which enabled the user to ensure his selected train ran on the day of the week he chose to travel, whether it had a buffet car, where it might be necessary to change trains, how far the journey was and even whether he had to notify the guard in advance if he wished the train to stop for him to alight, at certain remote destinations.

The less celebrated ABC guides, which had appeared in 1853 and just made it into the 21$^{st}$ century, listed the departure times for specific destinations along with the fares.  They were easier to use but tended to leave nagging doubts as to whether every essential detail had been covered.

At the bigger London termini we would routinely drop in at the enquiry office to pick up leaflets which advertised cheap day excursions.  Only once or twice, when we were unsure about a journey, did we join the queue in the enquiry office.  The enquiry clerks appeared totally unflappable under constant questioning bombardment. Each of them was armed with those two guides together with all the important booklets of special notices, which dealt with cancellations, diversions, engineering delays and so on. Their fingers would flip through the pages to land all but automatically upon the exact timetable in question. The explanatory hieroglyphics would be unhesitatingly checked and sure enough they seemed to get the answer within seconds. One forgets nowadays just how necessary and important were such services in the past.

     Those excursion leaflets were sometimes the spur for our next spotting sortie. There were two issues at stake. The first was to locate a destination with plenty of loco activity and the second was the fare involved. Those criteria alone were sufficient to condemn most of those leaflets to the waste bin. One successful outing in particular was a mid-week return to Bristol, so it must have been during a school holiday. Temple Meads station came up trumps and by 4.00 pm we were fully satisfied with our haul of numbers. Deciding it was time to head home, we boarded the next London train, pleased to see it was being hauled by a 'King' and took up our usual spotting position in the corridor lobby at the end of the first coach. That gave us easy viewing access to both sides of the line.

     Not long after departing, the ticket inspector was to take a poor view of our excursion tickets, telling us they were not valid on the 'Bristolian'. Whoops! We had not noticed anything on the leaflet about return times. Fortunately for us, he did not press the point, perhaps because the train was not very full and we were not depriving anyone of a seat. On the other hand perhaps it was just a reflection of the shoulder-shrugging attitude which was fairly prevalent at that time. I rather prefer that to some of the 'jobsworths' one encounters to-day, when one reads that collecting train numbers raises security issues and is banned by some train operators, or at least requires written permission.

     How times do change! That has always been reflected

too in the kind of service offered by the railways, a glimpse of which comes from inspecting old guides. I only ever possessed one ABC guide and three Bradshaws, one of which was for 1922, the last year of the pre-grouping railway companies. It was a wonder of publishing, given the minutiae of timetable information which was constantly reliably updated throughout the year.

Initially, the sheer density of available services stood out, right down to the most minor route, with perhaps just a couple of trains per day. Immediately, one was curious to know just what locomotives were employed, whether in these backwaters or on the principal routes. One noticed just how much time many journeys took to complete. Long distance travel could have been exhausting. Timetables highlighted Luncheon Car Expresses, Dining Car Expresses and Sleeping Saloon Expresses. Not only these comforts were necessary but so was an ample supply of hotels, whether for business travellers or tourists.

Bradshaw's 1922 hotel advertisements in particular were a wonderful source of both information and unintended amusement. A number of hotels boasted Red Coated Porters meeting passengers at stations. Sometimes hotels emphasized that they met the needs of invalids with special requirements but they seemed never to acknowledge the existence of children.

Surprising numbers of hotels were advertised as re-decorated and re-furbished and the opportunity was never lost when their managers could claim them to be patronised by 'most distinguished personages'. An 'atmosphere of cultured repose' was also an asset. The commercial traveller may have seized upon promises of 'good food' or 'comfortable and clean', which were attributes so often cited. Goodness knows what the competitors were offering. Beyond that, it seems that patrons would have been very disgruntled in the absence of tennis and croquet facilities, a billiard room and golf links, along with hot and cold sea water baths. It was also nice to know a hotel had electric light and a passenger lift, even a resident orchestra. By the way, what was one to make of 'Perfect Sanitary Arrangements'? and what did the more risqué variety theatre comedian of the time make of one hotel's statement that, 'Ladies travelling alone always given most careful attention'?

The last word in Bradshaws timetable notes must go to the Snowdon Mountain Railway. 'No trains will run with less than seven passengers, or the equivalent in fares'. So, if you were a group of five, did you have a whip round to top up the company's takings?

In contrast to those ABC and Bradshaw passenger guides, I was fortunate enough to stumble across a library disposal sale which yielded a neglected 1890 Book of Rates or Carrying Charges. This had nothing directly to do with loco spotting, but it again showed how rewarding and entertaining the exploration of background information could be. In this case it helped to set the scene against which many of the older locomotives we saw had worked in their early days. After all, who could resist noting the rates for transporting black puddings or bladders? ... and what about Divi Divi, Quassia Chips or Valonia?

A little more research snapped one out of such reveries and in my case, a few trips to the local library enabled me to thumb through every page of the Railway Magazine, right back from 1897 onwards. Several visits gave me a concise overview of locomotive and railway development generally, for the previous sixty years and woke me up to closer observation, not only of the numerous older engines, still abundant enough, but to the surviving buildings and furnishings provided for the traveller.

These adventures with Bradshaw came back to mind in a very different context in 1963, when the Euston station re-building was in full swing. The poor light in the Great Hall at Euston had always prevented me from taking a satisfactory photograph. It had been a very atmospheric location, made more so by knowledge of the place's history. There it was then, being ripped apart, still recognisable in the absence of its balustrades, light fittings, direction signs and doorways. The floors were covered in splintered wood and a heavy layer of plaster dust and rubble. I had half hoped some small souvenir might have been salvageable – a baggage label, an excursion leaflet perhaps?

There was nobody around so it must have been after knocking-off time for the contractors. Nor was access blocked in any way and I drifted into what had been the main booking office. I did not know what to expect because this had obviously been previously inaccessible to the public. In fact it was too late, in the sense that here too, everything had been ripped out. There were no desks, counters, ticket racks or cupboards, just a scattering of splintered wood, smashed glass and the same dust and rubble across the floor. Surely, here, a sharp eye would find the odd ticket, but nothing of the kind. That was until a desultory kick against a broken panel revealed a glimpse of a promising piece of paper. Freeing it from the rubble I realised this was nothing less than the front page of a complete bound document of London Midland Region passenger fares. The front cover had been ripped off but it was otherwise intact. I had my souvenir, far beyond my hopes and something I can confidently claim to be the last printed item ever to leave the old Euston main booking office.

Observing the state of Euston during its demolition, I was fascinated by the way the process was a bit like peeling an onion. Layer upon layer of building accretions were exposed. There were those who wondered if it was time to demolish St Pancras too and somehow combine it with Kings Cross. If that had ever happened, Kings Cross would have been changed dramatically, which prompted me to try to get to know it in greater detail. On the face of it Kings Cross was not the warren that Euston had become. From platform 10, I took the footbridge which, at that time, linked the platforms and gave access to the regional architect's offices. Later I read that Sir Nigel Gresley himself regularly used that bridge).

My curiosity was welcomed but because the staff were busy I was given a handful of spare plans to study, covering the evolutionary stages of the station over the previous 100 years. The site of the suburban platforms had once been an engine shed, but overall, the integrity of the original layout had been preserved and most of the spaces were still identifiable.

This was too good to be true so, unannounced, I enquired at the Western Region engineer's office at Paddington, where I again received a very friendly welcome. Someone cleared a big table for me and reached into a large rack of rolled up plans, selecting several for me to study. I was given a selection of small sewn up leather pouches containing lead shot, which were to hold flat the springy rolled up drawings. With some care and initially a little bit of a struggle with the rolls, which seemed to have a mind of their own, I managed to flatten one sheet after another, to reveal the evolution of Paddington as I knew it. The story took me back to a sketch design which preceded even the previous temporary Paddington station, at Bishops Road Bridge.

Many of the drawings bore the address of Brunel's office in Victoria Street, Westminster and one or two carried his signature. It was one of those 'Wow' moments. Amongst the Paddington drawings were a few interlopers showing quite modest engineering works, small overbridges, culverts and similar unglamorous necessities. Nevertheless, every sheet was meticulously drawn and lettered and frequently would be coloured with water colour washes. No computer aided design there, no photocopies, no dyeline printing, and no tracing paper, even though that was available by the mid-1800s (but not widely used until the 1860s). Copies of Brunel's drawings had to be 'pricked through'. That is to say a pin would be used to pierce through the beginning and end points of a line onto a sheet of paper underneath. Then the draughtsman would laboriously join the dots as it were, to reproduce the image before going on to re-create the watercolour washes and annotations. Some of the drawings displayed these prick marks so that, having been immersed in some of these draughting intricacies for several minutes, one almost felt Mr Brunel was watching over one's shoulder.

So, what had started as searches for affordable loco spotting trips had taken me through Bradshaw and ABC travel guides, a backwards look at how rail services had changed and how the public had travelled 35 years or so previously, not to mention some entertaining reflections along the way. It had led me to spend time in the library, studying the history of some familiar older locomotive types, with the aid of the Railway Magazine and ultimately stumbling upon Victorian copies of the Illustrated London News, dating back almost to the beginning of the railways and hinting at another rich source of railway history to explore. As for delving into the backgrounds of Kings Cross and Paddington, well, that extra knowledge of how it all came about further enhanced my appreciation of the whole spotting scene. There was certainly plenty to maintain one's interest between loco spotting trips.

Sometimes, during his peregrinations a spotter stumbled unexpectedly upon stored locomotives of great historic significance, yet which could give the impression they had just been overlooked for many a year or else that someone on high had decreed they should be preserved, but meanwhile, they were just cluttering up the place.

Something of these impressions coloured a visit made to the Crewe works paint shop back in 1956. Not only was Midland compound No 41000 present in its early British Railways black livery, but so too was the ex-LNWR '4 ft class 0-4-0' saddle tank No. 1439, in its former ICI paintwork. Both looked disgracefully shabby, given the exalted company they were keeping. Standing next to them was 'Cornwall', along with 'Hardwicke', one of the heroes of the 1895 railway races to the north. Cornwall's claim to fame was partly its longevity, having been built originally as early as 1847, modified from a

4-2-2 into a 2-2-2 in 1858 and withdrawn from regular service in 1907. She then saw a spell of use in the engineers' department, and subsequently some rare appearances, before being permanently retired as late as 1930.

This last pair in particular wore their correct LNWR liveries, albeit rather dusty, and gave the impression they were just waiting patiently to be displayed in the manner they deserved. In due course, they were all to become part of the National collection, based at the National Railway Museum's sites at York and Shildon. The fact that none of these engines carried a British Railways running number did not matter one bit. (They did appear tucked away in the ABC however). These were celebrated engines which one was bound to learn about as soon as one's interests expanded beyond simple number collecting.

There were too, other kinds of unexpected encounters. For many years there was the notorious case of the last Highland Railway Ben class loco, Ben Alder. It had been set aside for possible preservation in 1953. Subsequently it was moved from one location to another, providing an unexpected encounter for numerous spotters, until it settled in store at Boat of Garten, finally being cut up in 1967. I am ashamed to say that was one of those engines I had taken for granted and assumed I would get round to seeing one day or another. Brief encounters too were not unknown, typified for example by a passing glimpse of No.5 Shannon, the little Wantage Tramway engine preserved in a chain link pen on Wantage Road Station, until the station closed in 1964. In due course, it was preserved at the Didcot Railway Centre.

By the late 1950s there was growing pressure for government to assign funds properly to house and present the growing collection of railway artefacts. Bearing in mind the size and physical demands of acquisitions as massive as locomotives and rolling stock, it was a while before a single fully appropriate site became available and that was apart from all the small scale items already preserved.

There were locos stored for preservation at various locations and their numbers gradually swelled, once an official list had been agreed, which earmarked future exhibits. Some survivors, along with engines newly nominated for preservation, were moved around until a permanent home could be found for them, whilst others had already been stored at different railway works for many years.

To add to all this were demands for better presentation for London Transport's collection, which itself included some standard gauge steam items. The eventual outcome was a stopgap in the form of the Clapham Transport Museum, opened in a former London bus garage, in 1963. For loco spotters it provided an opportunity to make some belated cops, even if some of those engines had gone out of use before they themselves were born. Meanwhile, by this time, the fledgling railway preservation movement was getting into its stride, learning how to undertake not only the challenges of railway and locomotive preservation but also the challenges of public operation too.

So it was, upon the opening of the National Railway Museum in York in 1975, a high percentage of the national collection was assembled in one place.

The relative contributions inherited from the Big Four's earlier collections were interesting. The former LNER led the way along with the LMS. The GWR's record did not shine for the reasons already outlined. Whilst the Southern came in last, with its Stroudley tank 'Boxhill' and its beautifully elegant Adam's T3 4-4-0. There was perhaps some excuse for the latter. Theirs was the smallest steam stock anyway of the Big Four and many an ageing class was still at work after being reprieved by the 1939-45 war.

To-day, the compilation of data covering historic main line engines is, with the aid of the internet, a relatively straight forward process. Spotting the older interesting relics in main line steam days was very much an optional extra for most spotters. The irony is, of course, that the everyday targets of those steam spotters have themselves become the surviving historic relics of to-day, whilst old spotters are only too pleased to see any steam loco they can set eyes upon.

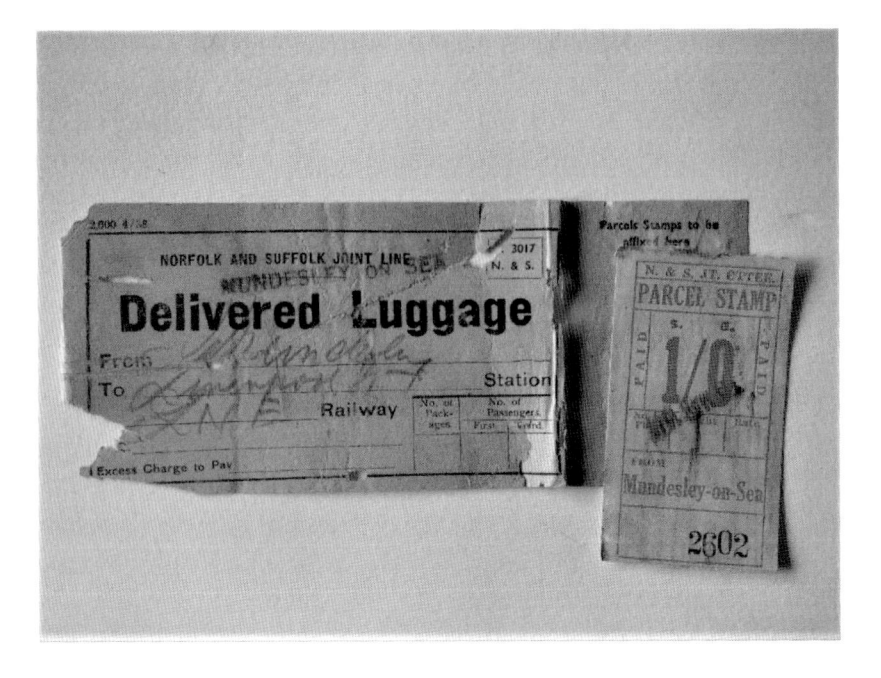

*Interesting pieces of ephemera could sometimes be recovered from old family luggage. The Norfolk and Suffolk Joint Committee remained a legal entity until Nationalisation. The code in the top left corner suggests a batch of 2000 labels was printed in April 1938 and in this case the parcel receipt for transit from Mundesley to Liverpool Street was dated March 1945. As that was during the last days of the War, one is tempted to speculate whether the passenger had been sheltering in the relative safety of the Norfolk coast up until then.*

# CHAPTER ELEVEN

## Questions of Colour and Other Reflections

In January 1959, a school friend and I were encouraged to explore Lyme Regis bay for Jurassic fossils. We managed to hitch-hike there but by the time we finished our study, we realized we had not budgeted enough for both overnight accommodation and the train ride home.

As intending passengers, we did not feel too guilty about passing the night in a second class carriage parked in the bay platform of Lyme Regis station. I do remember the next morning there was no train available to give us a bright and early start, so that by the time we eventually arrived in Axminster, our prime objective was to find something to eat. Unfortunately, our planned exploration of Axminster was spoiled by an unexpected downpour, so that instead of visiting the library to learn more about local geology (yes, that seemed quite normal before the internet) we arrived there to take it in turns to stand, dripping and steaming, in front of the one bar electric fire, as we dried out our trousers. I do not think we could have got much work done because the library closed unexpectedly quite early. In our haste for breakfast and our subsequent soaking we had not thought to enquire about train times and had rather lost track of the day.

Back at the station we were both ready to get home. As my companion, Brian, queued at the ticket office window, I watched a London bound express pull in on the opposite busy platform. By now it was dark and the rain, which had resumed, was sparkling off the station lights. The Merchant Navy Pacific stopped right opposite me, the electric cab lighting already on, as the fireman opened the firebox door to check his fire. The orange light reflecting off the inside of the cab roof created the effect of a busy room isolated in darkness. In the background, the driver stood peering back down the platform. The fireman shuffled between tender and firebox, throwing on several shovelfuls of coal, busying himself with gauge glasses and injectors, quickly cleaning around the cab floor and sweeping the debris onto the track before securing the tender gate. Finally, a perfunctory wipe to the cab window, the cab light extinguished and he was ready to go.

As I watched all that activity concentrated into a stop of perhaps 3 or 4 minutes, I was thinking just how physically demanding a steam locomotive could be on a footplate crew. The cosy cab might have seemed enviable but the prospect of heading out into the driving rain, eyeing signals and shovelling coal on a jolting footplate was less appealing. I was a bit surprised it had taken me so long to make these observations, but that was typical of the hobby; there was no end to making discoveries and gaining new insights.

As to the number of the engine, it really did not matter as I had long seen all the members of the Merchant Navy class. What is more, I had managed to have that close look at the Lyme Regis branch engine, which had eluded me those eight years previously.

If loco spotting had been strictly nothing but collecting numbers, I would have found it a banal pastime. Indeed, with some loco classes running into several hundred examples, the hope of seeing every one was a rather forlorn challenge.

The most numerous classes tended to be freight engines, with nearly 600 ex-LMS 4F 0-6-0s to see, well over 650 8F 2-8-0s and 400-plus, 'Jinty' 0-6-0 tanks. The ex-LNER gave us well over 300 01/04 2-8-0s and, on top of those, British Railways had acquired 733 WD 2-8-0s, originating from the Ministry of Supply. (935 WDs had been produced in total for the war effort. That compared with Ramsbottom's 934 DX class of 0-6-0s, built in 1858-74 for the LNWR).

Loco spotting might well have been essentially a visual pastime but the other senses certainly came into play. Growlers and Wheezers have already been mentioned and another class of engines making very distinctive sounds were these very

WD 2-8-0s. Generally known as Dub-Dees, they were all but permanently filthy, sometimes to the extent that it was hard to read the cab-side number. Their approach was frequently heralded by a distinctive metallic clink-clank to their valve gear, which did not seem to concern anybody. Apparently the moving parts of the entire locomotive were so poorly balanced that the WDs spent their entire working lives shaking themselves apart.

Given these large numbers of rather unglamorous engines, marking off a cop was not, in itself, very significant. Otherwise, what could make it worthwhile was the cameo memory which went with the occasion. It could have been an unexpected discovery hidden round the back of a shed. It may have been the last number needed to complete a class. It may have been a rare variation of a class, or perhaps the very last survivor of its type. It could be a distinctive number, or even the accidental sighting of a passing train, to punctuate an otherwise boring family outing. Any number of reasons could recall a number, just as a number could powerfully evoke memories of an occasion. Poet Ian McMillen described getting a rare number like an image that defines a moment in your life, such as where you were or the kind of day you had had. Engines which were much more likely to catch the eye, were the more glamorous main line passenger types. Their overall aesthetics, including their colour, brass nameplates and other occasional adornments and even the sound of their whistles, added to their appeal.

There were some spotters put off entirely by 'ordinary' engines, boasting of collecting only 'namers'. I must say I always suspected them, probably unfairly, of not being up to the challenge of tackling the whole picture. I wondered if they were even aware of the rare named exceptions lurking within an otherwise commonplace and not particularly glamorous class. Classic examples were the ex-LMS Black Fives, which boasted a mere four regimental names within their 842 examples, along with a single example hidden amongst the ex-LNER D16 Claude Hamilton 4-4-0s.

The Black Fives were interesting mixed traffic engines, equally at home on passenger or freight duties. Introduced in 1934, they were followed eight years later by the LNER's B1 class, intended for similar work and with the same power rating. The B1s themselves were over 400 strong, but lacked the impact of the 5s. Both classes were painted black and could appear anywhere in between a smart polished state and an abject grimy condition. Incidentally, the Black Fives are quite often quoted as having been the most numerous class. In fact that title was held by the Western Region 5700 class of 0-6-0 tanks, of which 863 were built.

The Black Fives were apparently liked by loco men, though we spotters were not generally aware of that at the time. What I think we may well have shared, was an appreciation of the aesthetics of the Black Fives. They were somehow what a modern mixed traffic engine should have been like, whilst very much echoing the lines of more overtly passenger orientated types, like the rebuilt Patriots and the Jubilees.

They may not have set the pulses racing, but they seemed purposeful and willing, and turned up everywhere. Although black painted and commonplace, they at least compared favourably with the B1s, which looked more old-fashioned and demeaned themselves by obscure and slightly comical animal names like Bongo, Puku or Gnu, carried by the first forty-one members of the class.

A Jubilee, or 'Jube', could be seen as a somewhat beefed up and more glamourous three-cylinder version of a Black Five. The application of express passenger lined green livery and a brass name plate, never struck me as totally convincing. I remained somewhat indifferent towards them. There was a lack of conviction in their naming which started off by scraping every corner of the British Empire, which even then was heading for rebranding as a Commonwealth. We knew Canada and Quebec, even Kashmir and Basutoland, but how many spotters had heard of Gwalior or Central Provinces and how did Eire and Palestine sneak in?

When territorial names ran out, we were treated to a run of some forty names of empire builders – old sea dogs like Hawkins, Drake, Nelson and Jellicoe, along with numerous obscure and forgotten names. Next came the traditional resort of all locomotive naming committees, that of classical mythology. Names from the earliest days of steam engines re-emerged, not for the first time, giving us Ajax, Bellerophon, Minotaur and so on, for a dozen or so examples, before desperation set in. The next thirty or so engines borrowed the names of Royal Navy ships – most inappropriately, I thought.

The question of train and locomotive colours was never entirely resolved and did itself add variety to the spotting scene. During some of my earliest journeys to Waterloo I sometimes saw a Bullied Pacific in the experimental blue livery tried out during 1949 – 51. I was not impressed and nor apparently was officialdom, who duly reverted to green. About the same time, I saw a train of 'plum and spilt milk' carriages on a couple of occasions, but they looked gloomy, so that colour experiment was also abandoned.

Elsewhere, the colours described as carmine or crimson lake and cream, or, as most wits preferred to call them, blood and custard or rhubarb and custard, became the standard coach livery, whilst the Southern stuck steadfastly to green for both electric and mainline steam trains. There were, I recall, two exceptions to be seen at Waterloo. The first, best forgotten, were the Tavern Cars, appearing in 1949 and lasting only a year or two. These were a bizarre attempt to replicate a pub on wheels, where the largely windowless exteriors were painted with an unconvincing brickwork pattern, along with a painted-on inn sign. These vehicles understandably raised an eyebrow, even though I was too young at the time to know what a tavern was. The thought of someone trying to down a gin and tonic, in an eighty miles an hour olde English tavern, still raises a smile. The Eastern Region also tried the experiment but sent them back to

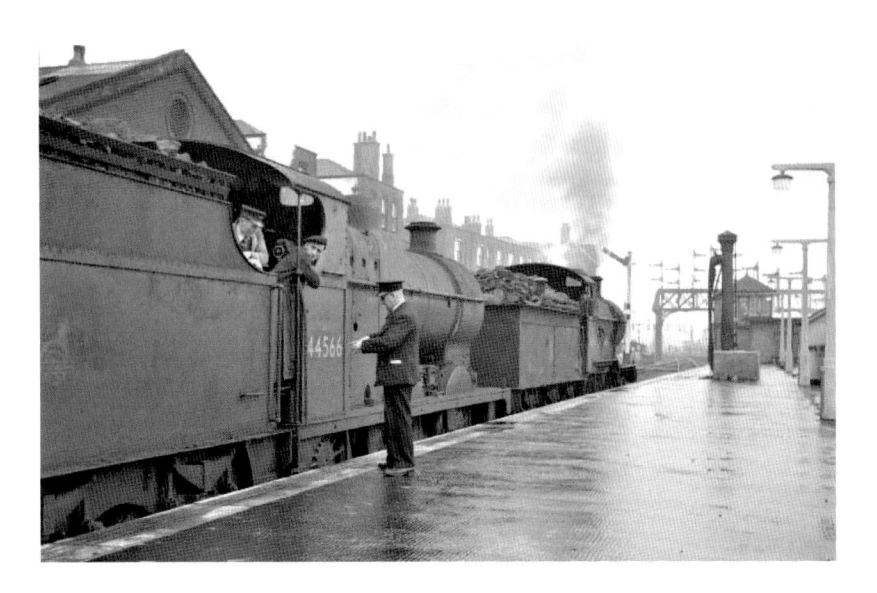

*A stopping train to Worcester awaits departure from Derby Midland in September 1956. As a double header, the lower power engine would lead the higher power one, in this case a 2P 4-4-0 passenger type heading a 4F 0-6-0 freight type. The guard is having to brave heavy rain as he gives the driver the train load details. The water column near the lead engine is of classic Midland Railway design. The long drooping leather hose, or 'bag', would have needed a big stretch to reach a loco tender and required a degree of respect if a fireman were not to get a soaking. Both engines are in the fairly uniform dark grey state into which most nominally black painted engines seemed to lapse.*

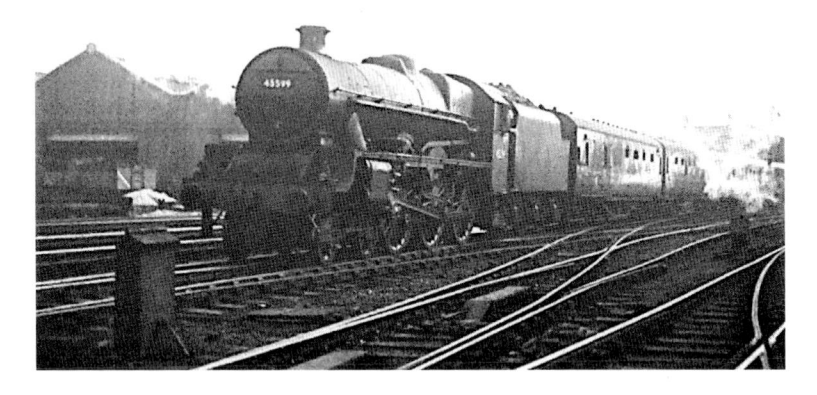

*Jubilee class 45599 Bechuanaland, tops Camden bank on 12 April 1959. The driver appears to be reviewing activity on Camden shed before tackling the serious business of building up speed. Departures from Liverpool Street and Kings Cross were equally faced with demanding gradients before trains could make more rapid progress.*

the Southern a year later and by 1951 the brickwork patterns had been painted out.

The other exception from Southern green, was provided by the umber and cream Pullman cars. These were always turned out smartly. The first class ones bore girls' names, whilst the third class cars had to contend with just a number. Incidentally, third class was re-designated as second in 1956. When an entire train consisted of Pullman stock, it was rare if its locomotive was not equally smartly groomed. Perhaps the most splendid example of this was the turnout of the Golden Arrow, between London Victoria and Dover. With national pride at stake, Stewarts Lane depot regularly produced a magnificently prepared engine. Hardly less impressive were the Bournemouth Belle and the Devon Belle, trains which were visible from my garden at home. Many a football game was interrupted by a cry of, "Pullman", as soon as it came into view. Corresponding cries of, "Diesel", went up when Southern 10201 or 10203 went by, or the former LMS 10000 or 10001. Their black and polished steel livery did not match a green 'steamer', but they did score on novelty value.

Spotters did not seem to make a special effort to see colourful or unusual liveries, though they would certainly have noticed them. There was a huge number of freight engines which lived most of their lives in a livery of grime grey. Unfortunately, this could extend to passenger types too, and it was particularly depressing when a nominally green, named express engine, appeared in a filthy state. I felt some sympathy for the lads in other parts of the country who saw a high percentage of dirty workhorse locomotives. Later, of course, during the final year or two of steam, that was to become a near universal state of affairs, made worse in numerous cases by missing loco nameplates, reserved, sold or perhaps stolen.

Meanwhile, British Railways tinkered at the edges in a half-hearted effort to modernise its image. Spotters undoubtedly noticed the crest born by engines, which changed from what was jokingly called 'the cycling lion'; that is a lion straddling a locomotive wheel, to its 'ferret and dartboard' replacement, from 1956 on. There were changes to carriage colours too, so that something near LMS red displaced 'blood and custard' and the Western Region adopted a version of the former GWR brown and cream, for selected trains. These seemed to cause little comment, as did the appearance of a deep red livery for some of the former LMS Pacifics. Eventually, the Southern Region seemed to suffer most from these changes, as examples of all these carriage liveries impinged upon its traditional green policy, not unusually producing a ragbag of colours within one train. The effect detracted from any suggestion of electrical efficiency or rolling green West-Country scenery, both aspects of the Southern's image.

If anything, this added variety only detracted from any corporate identity. Spotters would more likely have been interested in the anarchic gestures of certain sheds and works who might, just occasionally, give a smoke box number plate a red background or a white painted border. Needless to say, these did not always last long, once noted by officialdom.

Within two years of the Scottish trip, I had made what turned out to be my last three works visits. As a student in Manchester, I was well-placed to join the Railway Society's visits to Gorton and Horwich, both of which left indelible memories. There was a growing awareness that these opportunities had to be seized, since it was becoming apparent that the rate of locomotive scrapping was relentless and gradually accelerating.

At one fortuitous student lodging, the whistle of approaching trains provided just enough time to leap to the window, to catch an oblique glimpse of expresses heading for St Pancras. Many a rebuilt Royal Scott was seen in this fashion, before I decided that kind of athletic manoeuvre was perhaps becoming a bit too obsessive.

Horwich offered the unusual spectacle of a handful of

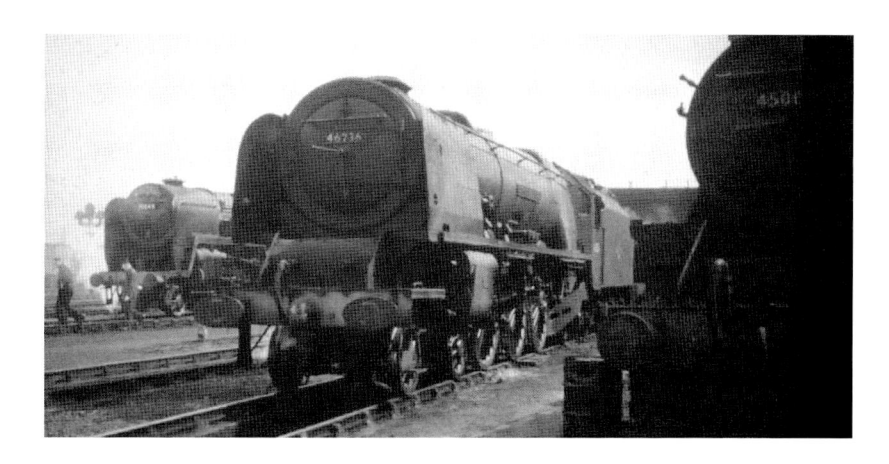

*Princess Coronation or Duchess class 46236 City of Bradford at Camden in April 1959. It was built in streamlined form in 1939. The streamlining was removed in March 1948 and the locomotive represented the London Midland Region in the locomotive exchange trials of that year. When the streamlining was removed, these locomotives initially ran with a partly flattened smoke box door profile which had accommodated the curve of the streamlining, later rectified as shown. In July 1958, 46236 was repainted in British Rail lined maroon as seen here. It was repainted in LMS lined maroon in November 1959, withdrawn in March 1964 and scrapped at Crewe the following month.*

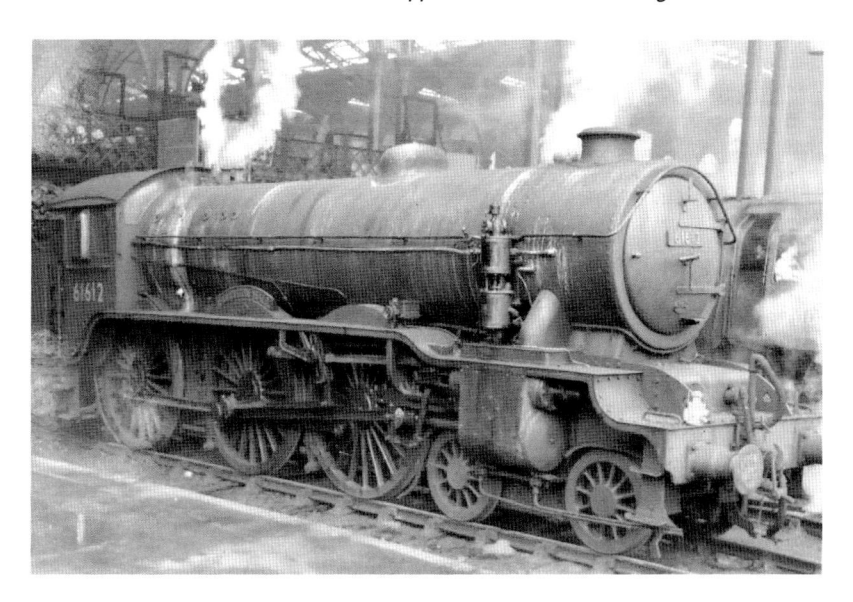

*Class B17, No. 61612, Houghton Hall, was notionally a green express passenger engine. It was seen here, letting the side down, in a filthy state at Liverpool Street.*

175

saddle-tank works engines which, in the ABC, showed them in the 50,000 series, but in reality they bore their pre-nationalisation LMS running numbers. Another surprise was to be shown the stored Lancashire and Yorkshire 2-4-2 tank, 1008, along with 'Coppernob', the ex-Furness Railway 0-4-0, both later to be preserved in restored working condition. We also came across the works narrow gauge locomotive, 'Wren', now resident at the National Railway Museum. There it was, simmering gently, waiting to be useful, and providing another memorable cameo recollection. Locomotives apart, we watched at close quarters, some of the heavy physical work involved in casting rail chairs and making locomotive springs, just examples of dozens of skills on which the railway depended.

Gorton, by contrast, visited in 1959, provided a starker reminder that times were moving on. The name plate 'Valour' was proudly and respectfully displayed on a wall in the works entrance area. This had been retrieved from a former Great Central 4-6-0, withdrawn in 1947. This engine had run as a mobile war memorial to staff who had fallen in the First World War, a similar role to that of 'Remembrance' on the Southern.

When Gorton closed in 1963, this memorial plaque was transferred to a local church, from which it was promptly stolen. I do so hope it was not the deed of an obsessive railway enthusiast. Meanwhile, the inside of the works was full of electric locomotives in various states of undress and maintenance. These served the Woodhead route to Sheffield, whilst out in the yard were forlorn rows of mostly ex-Great Central tank engines, condemned for scrapping. Others were in store, their chimneys covered, but no doubt waiting the same fate.

There was a growing awareness that steam engine numbers were in decline. Obviously, the locomotives of the national system were the ones most sought after before their demise. Nevertheless there were considerable numbers of private industrial engines at work throughout the country, along

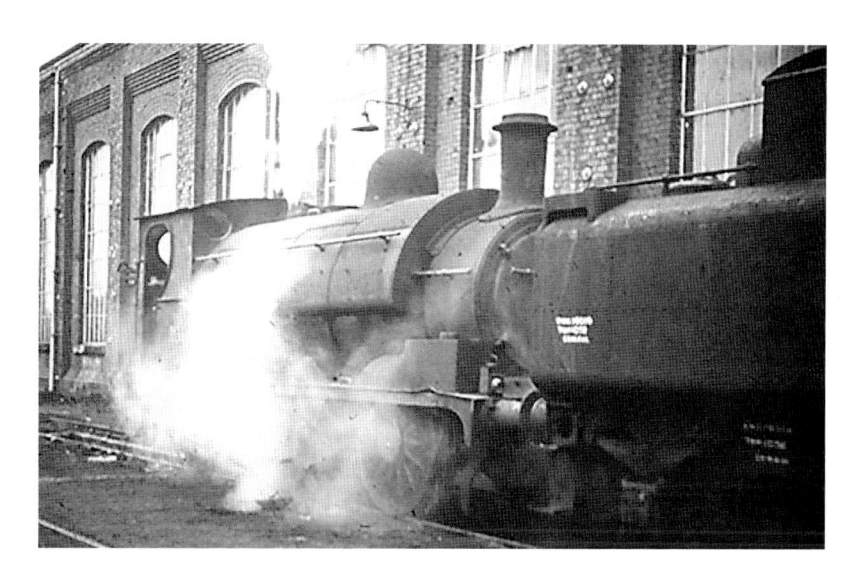

The former Lancashire and Yorkshire Railway saddle tank pictured here in 1960, at Horwich works, was in departmental stock, carrying its old LMS number, 11368. A spot of heavy shunting appears to have bent its buffer beam. L & Y engines generally ended up carrying 50XXX numbers under British Railways.

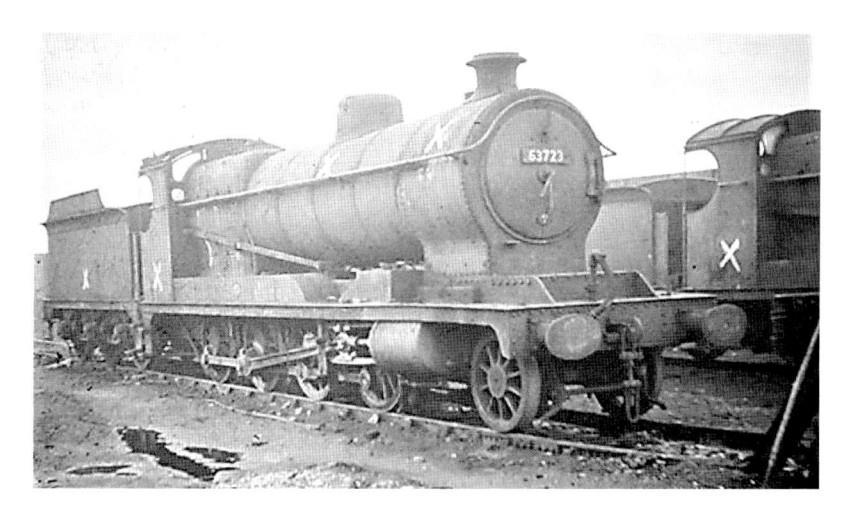

Different yards adopted different markings to confirm an engine was to be cut up. CON or WDN indicated condemned or withdrawn. Often a cross within a circle was adopted or, in this case, 'The Gorton Kiss of Death' for 04/1 class No. 63723, seen in 29 December 1959. The oval buffers were a favourite Robinson design detail for his larger engines for the Great Central Railway.

177

with those of tourist railways, with yet others in store for preservation. Thoughts turned to these occasionally.

Nevertheless, certain factors amongst the loco spotting fraternity mitigated against any real enthusiasm to search out these specimens. Initially, there were no obvious comprehensive published lists of these engines, to draw attention to their existence.

The engines were widely distributed, which could involve awkward travel plans and access issues to private sites. Even finding adjacent public viewing points, could pose problems. After all that, at any particular location, be it mine, quarry, steel works or recreational tourist line, the locomotive fleet would only occasionally exceed half a dozen or so engines.

Perhaps the greatest deterrent to tracking down these specimens was the fact they did not fit easily into the overall sweep of railway history, represented by the pre-grouping companies and their successors. The public, as customers, had always interacted with those. What went on within less publicly exposed private enterprises mostly passed them by.

Loco spotters did like lists. Completing a list where every number had its place gave a certain satisfaction. The challenges resulting from the scattered distribution of industrial locomotives might well have been met by lists of engines of their respective builders – Andrew Barclay, Neilson, Avonside, Peckett and so on – rather than by their company ownership.

Had there been ABCs of industrial and privately owned locomotives, maybe they would have commanded a significant following, at least during those remaining few years after the conclusion of main line steam. As it is, those which have found a home on preserved lengths of former British Rail tracks look quite incongruous to old time spotters, even if they give delight to young families to-day.

There were times when, exceptionally, one did make the effort to search out some of these 'private' specimens. For example, the Romney, Hythe and Dymchurch railway ran like a

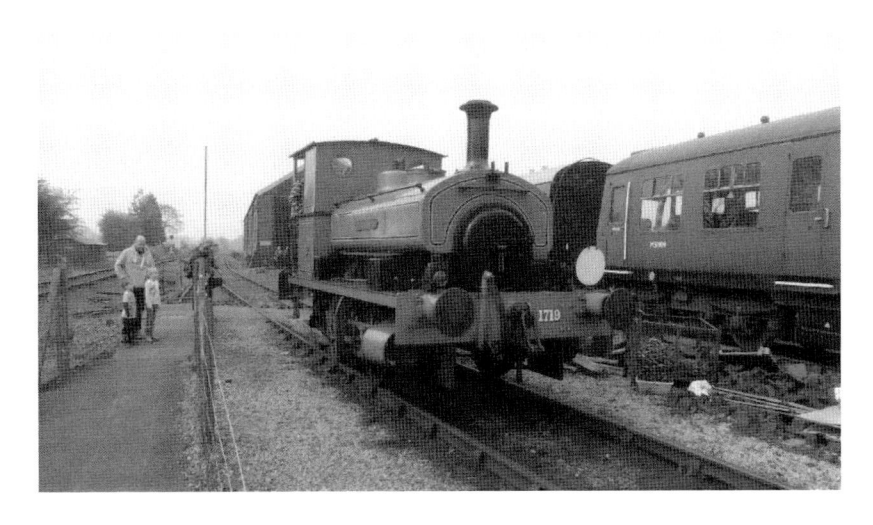

*An Andrew Barclay saddle tank at the East Somerset Railway. Different manufacturers displayed their own design characteristics, in this case their flat sided saddle tanks. As always, the appeal of steam to small boys is evident. They would surely have become to-days' spotters had steam continued.*

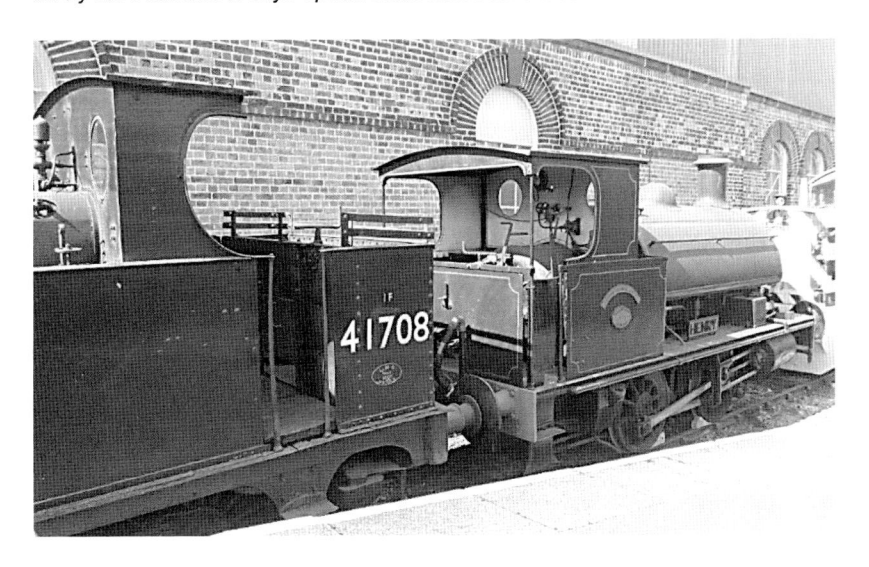

*Faced with this juxtaposition, spotters would have noticed 'Henry', a 1901 Hawthorn Leslie industrial saddle tank, but it would have been the rare ex-Midland Railway half-cab 0-6-0 tank which really caught the attention. These were photographed at Barrow Hill in 2019.*

scaled down full size line, had some impressive engines and served places over its thirteen mile length, capturing some of the feeling of a main line system.

The Vale of Rheidol light railway, with its three locomotives, was another narrow gauge line, from Aberystwyth to Devil's Bridge. It was a curiosity but still a legitimate branch line of British Railways, so there seemed no reason not to visit it, though somehow it was a bit more difficult to take as seriously as the full size equivalents.

Once, having seen V of R No.7, Owain Glyndŵr, awaiting attention on a low loader wagon in 'A' shop at Swindon, it became more pressing to see its sister engines, numbers 8 and 9; even a list of three to complete the class took on a significance. There was no easy explanation for why that should be.

In the case of that other former GWR narrow gauge line, the Welshpool and Llanfair, its two engines were in store and the future of the line remained in doubt. This imparted a mythic existence to the engines.

Whilst in Wales, the Festiniog, like the RH & DR, had some of the attributes of a full scale railway, even if in my spotting days it was still finding its feet. Again though, its entire loco stock was quickly spotted. The Talyllyn railway was similarly re-establishing itself and, once more, whilst fascinating in its own right, it did not present a serious spotting challenge.

On the other hand, there was some real excitement to be had at its Towyn terminus when we visited. Stored in the open air was 'Cecil Raikes'. It has to be explained that this engine was known to very few spotters and certainly did not appear in the ABCs. It was a standard gauge tank, unusually fitted with ungainly condensing apparatus. It was a unique survivor in having an outside frame 0-6-4 wheel arrangement and had been built in 1886 for the Mersey Railway.

Displaced by electrification in 1904, it had passed to a Derbyshire colliery until 1954, and hence escaped inclusion within British Railway's stock. It looked a clumsy brute, its faded dirty blue paintwork contributing to an overall appearance of severe neglect. Happily it was eventually cosmetically restored. Whilst such encounters were incidental to the immediate business of loco spotting, they did add to the stock of peripheral cameo memories which enriched the hobby.

Other than joining an occasional organised excursion, I seemed always to be preoccupied with studies, and therefore disinclined to frequent the large Manchester stations for spotting purposes. I did though, make the most of the choice of routes to London, which then existed. The former London and North Western line from Euston to Manchester Piccadilly was the fastest and the Midland line from St Pancras to Manchester Central was the most scenically attractive.

When there was the time to spare and I was not encumbered with bags and equipment, I rather enjoyed the less direct routes, even when changes of train were involved. Changing not just train, but also station, at Wolverhampton, enabled me to take the Great Western route to Birmingham Snow Hill and onwards to Paddington behind a King class 4-6-0. Equally intriguing was the ex-Great Central possibility from Manchester Piccadilly on the electrified route, via Woodhead, to Sheffield Victoria. Then it was towards Nottingham Victoria, over the girder bridge at Rugby and thus to Marylebone, this time behind a considerably less glamourous B1 4-6-0.

In due course, the Midland route from Manchester Central to St Pancras, became my favoured choice. It was a little longer than the Manchester Piccadilly to Euston option but since I was becoming too old to leap all over the carriage in an effort to spot every loco in range, then I sought alternative compensation. The Midland line always seemed a little more civilized and it was certainly more scenic.

On occasion, I indulged myself by taking afternoon tea in the restaurant car. The comestibles were noteworthy only in their predictability, consisting of modest uniform slabs of fruitcake, apparently mechanically sliced from an infinitely long extrusion, buttered scones and jam in micro pots, calculated to be just enough to cover a scone but never enough for a surplus to spill down one's shirt front, and finally, mahogany red tea to wash it all down.  This elixir was presented, with some ceremony, in silver (plated surely?) tea-pots and hot water jugs, along with their attendant sugar cube bowls and teaspoons. The two uniformed attendants made some show of setting it all out correctly and the fact that this little piece of theatre was always carried out in a first class carriage, added something to the sense of occasion.  There were never many passengers present, and on one occasion, with the formalities over, I noticed the attendants slipped into easy conversation with a lady passenger whom I had noticed before.  I took her to be a business woman of a certain age, as we used to say, no doubt a regular traveller, pleased to relax a while in this cosy escape from the office.

 Having travelled through the Peak District in this fashion left one somewhat vulnerable to feelings of superiority when drawing into Derby.  After all, we had shared a very agreeable time whilst the huddles of passengers now boarding had been waiting below those dreary wind-swept concrete platform canopies, which were part of Derby Midland station at that time. Depending on the time of day, there may well not have been another call for afternoon tea.  In such cases, they had only the nondescript St Pancras station buffet to look forward to. Never mind, they would have found that same fruit cake awaiting them there.  Eventually, on one of these trips we were offered a card to fill in regarding the frequency with which we used the Midland route, our reasons for choosing it, and so on.  There had been whispers about closing this line so I immediately interpreted this as a manifestation of so called passenger consultation, prior to inevitable closure.

 It was going to be a loss, not just scenically, but because it usually still yielded a few cops, perhaps including something in the rarer 50,000 series, even if they did represent mundane classes of engines. That being the case, I resolved to make one last memorable journey on that route when I would travel 1st class. I justified the expense by telling myself that classy comfort would make up for the snowy bleakness of December. It turned out to be a disastrous decision.

There were initially few passengers in that single 1st class carriage in the entire train, and I had a compartment to myself. It was of early 1930s origin, with decidedly firm seats and a heater control which rattled but produced little heat. At least I felt free to crane my head for every potential cop. Unfortunately, it soon became apparent that with so many severe weather cancellations there were few trains to be seen.

All the way to Derby the only interesting moments were a visit from the ticket inspector who looked decidedly downcast when I proffered my white 1st class ticket instead of the $2^{nd}$ class one he was clearly expecting, and the other interest was a sole freight train behind a 2-8-0 8F, looking completely lost in the snow but probably just waiting in a loop for us to pass. Unscheduled stops led to us taking on more and more stranded passengers. Eventually the guard unceremoniously filled the 1st class carriage with 2nd class travellers, including my compartment. My initial indignation duly subsided when I realized they were contributing some body heat to the compartment. As they eyed their surroundings even they did not seem too impressed. I shared their feelings. The entire journey passed under that brooding silence which can accompany heavy snowfalls and leaden skies on a December afternoon.

That valedictory journey really did turn out in the spirit of a sad farewell. At the time, it just served further to extinguish my already waning railway enthusiasm. It was saddening to see groups of condemned steam engines in station yards and the growing number of diesel locomotives, whose novelty value was already wearing off.

These variations of route did usually provide some useful

cops and might have been even more fruitful. As it was, as a young adult, I was conscious of feeling a bit of a twerp, were I to start leaping from one side of the train to the other, and hanging out of carriage windows, in the time-worn pattern of younger spotters.

My final works visit had been to Swindon, in 1960. The presence of 'Warship' class diesel hydraulics under construction, shortly after the completion of 'Evening Star', the last steam locomotive built by British Railways, provided a poignant reminder for the steam enthusiast that there would soon be little of interest left to spot.

It had taken eleven years for the 20,000 or so locomotives inherited at Nationalisation to be reduced by 4,000 by the end of 1958 (implying an average attrition rate of something like one a day.) In the next five years, another 15,500 or so were to disappear (that is at something like 8 or 9 a day), leaving fewer than 400 by the end of 1963. Bearing in mind the number of standard types taken into service, and still under construction until 1960, it was naturally the older types which were in most dramatic decline throughout this latter period.

Just as we had grown progressively into our railway hobby, so we were now being progressively deprived of it. The demise of the steam locomotive took with it the sights, sounds and smells which went with it. So too the built environment, so closely associated with the steam age, was being increasingly modified and eroded out of recognition.

# CHAPTER TWELVE          Somewhat off the Rails

In 1960, I acquired my first car and, because my friend, Blair, shared my interest in exploring rather than just seeking the biggest possible haul of cops, we were able to distract ourselves from the all too evident decline of steam.  Over the next year or so we opted to visit a number of curiosities and forgotten corners.

It started with an unplanned detour to Stanmore Village, where passenger services had ceased eight years previously.  The station was in good fettle with the tracks intact, and still used by the occasional freight train, though not everything had survived so well at future locations we were to visit.

We took a look at the former Kemp Town station at Brighton and made a point of studying the rather unusual 4-way points at the tunnel mouth.  We drove to Verney Junction and explored the environs with some care.  The only train we saw was a diesel multiple unit on the Oxford to Cambridge service but we were easily able to imagine the presence of a Metropolitan engine waiting to depart with a London bound train, as depicted in a well-known HC Casserley photograph.

The empty Metropolitan goods yard enticed us towards the vestige of the line which had once branched away towards Quainton Road and thence to London.  To our delight this continued for a mile or so until it stopped abruptly at the point where it had once crossed East Claydon Road at the site of Winslow Road station.  It turned out that this line was used for carriage storage, offering the unusual spectacle of several full length trains stored end to end in remote countryside.  These represented reserve stock, used solely for extras and excursions during the summer months.

Driving on to Quainton Road, we set out to hunt down the route of the former Brill branch.  It had a tenuous history, with motive power in the form of a modified Aveling and Porter

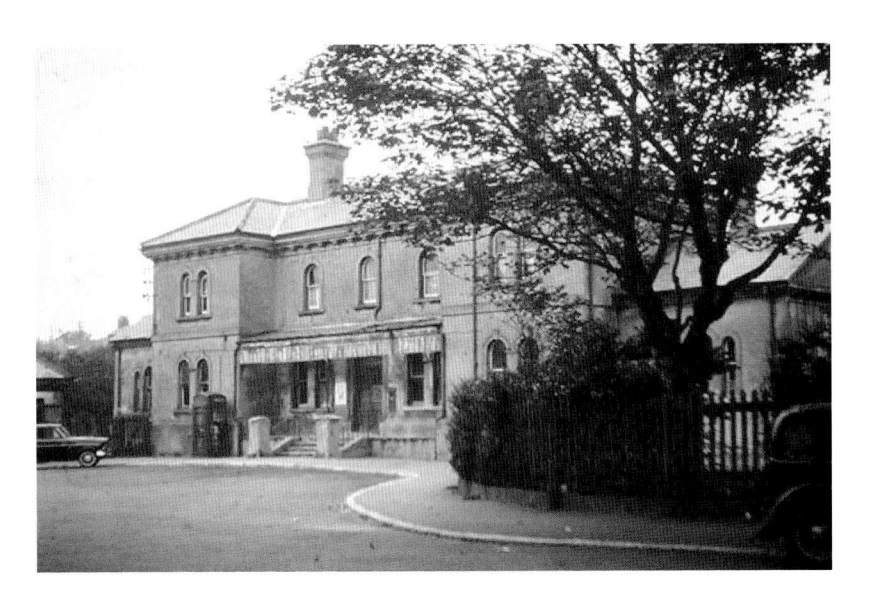

*Kemp Town station, Brighton, closed to passengers in 1933 and to goods iin 1971 seen on 6 August 1960. The telephone box and wall mounted letter box were still in use.*

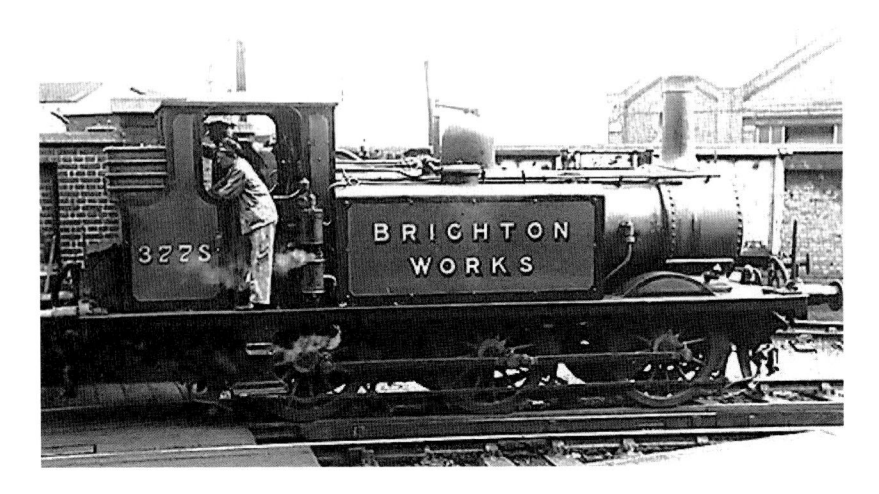

*Since1947, class A1X, 377S, originally LB&SCR No. 35 'Morden', had been the Brighton works shunter, conspicuous in its Stroudley 'Improved Engine Green' livery. Seen here in the shed yard in 1958, it was repainted a slightly darker shade of golden ochre, which it retained when the works closed in 1959, and when it was re-numbered 32635. It was finally withdrawn in 1963. That yard full of yellow engines in LB&SC days must have presented quite a sight.*

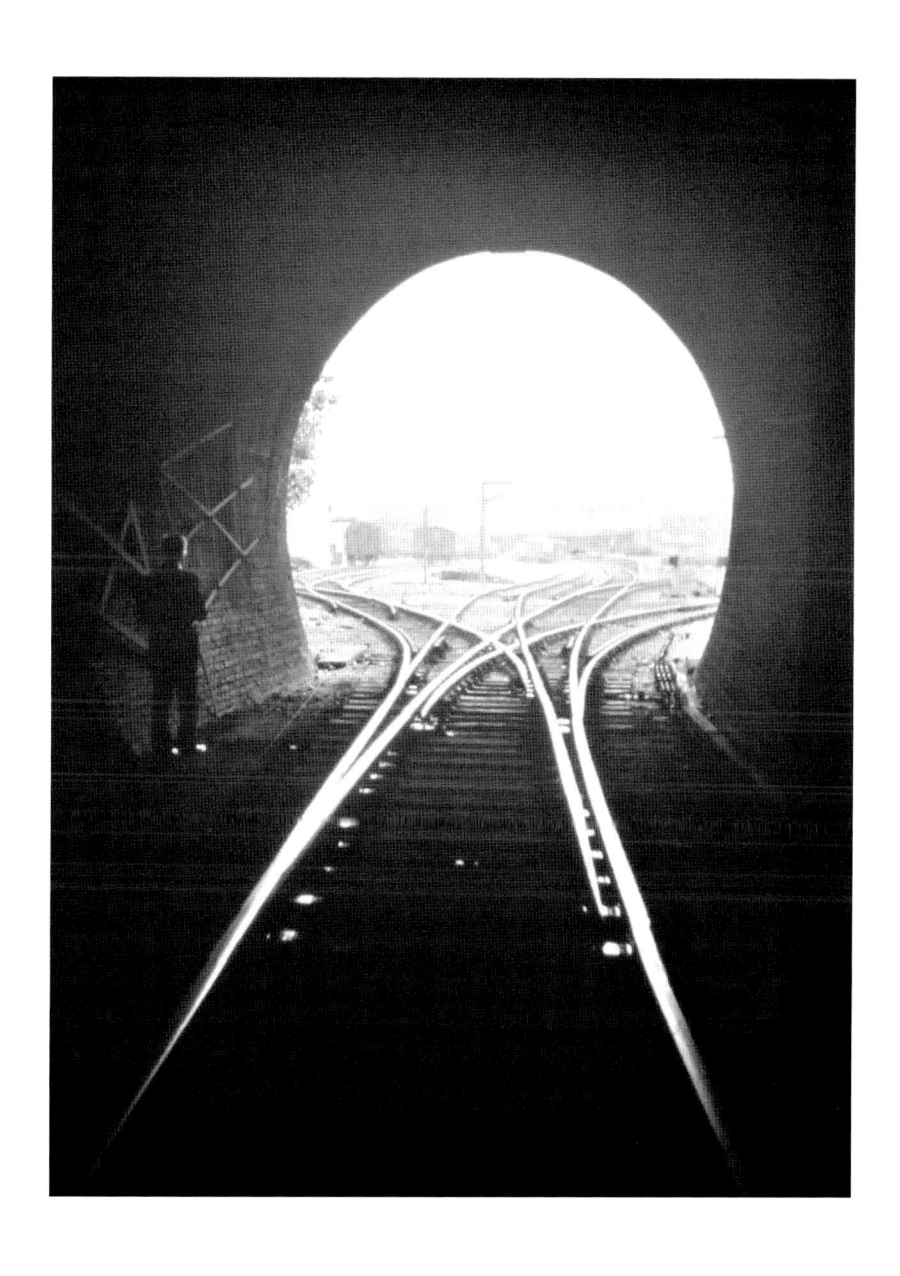

*The 4-way points at the tunnel approach to Kemp Town station. Seeking out such unusual features continued to provide considerable interest as cops became scarcer.*

steam tractor, later to be superseded by Metropolitan Beyer Peacock tank engines. Examples of both are now preserved at the London Transport Museum although, at the time, we knew of them only from photographs. We soon realised we had done insufficient research in advance, bearing in mind there were no quick reference sources like the internet to draw upon, and the range of relevant books was a fraction of what now exists. As clues became fewer, we were eventually confronted by a Ministry of Defence fence blocking our path, from which point we lost the scent.

An enthusiasm for railway locations was understandable enough, but the fascination with locomotives was at the root of it. Consequently we were always inclined to seek out some locomotive interest during our roving explorations.

It was not possible to visit the former outposts of the Metropolitan without being aware of the old Great Central Railway. It was time again to drop in on Marylebone station and Neasden shed. Marylebone had never been a great spotters' venue for the sole reason that not a lot seemed to happen there. Only Broad Street, Charing Cross, Cannon Street and Holborn Viaduct were even less attractive for the steam enthusiast.

In the past an occasional visit to Marylebone would have yielded the odd cop, even if it had been nothing more exciting than a B1 4-6-0 for Sheffield, Nottingham or Leicester. The most glamorous engine we could have hoped for was an A3 on the 'Master Cutler'. We had seen Flying Scotsman itself taking its turn on that service.

To make things more interesting we once made a point of travelling on the single track Wembley Stadium loop. This was possible only on certain occasions, as for example, a national or international sporting event. It had been built to serve the 1924-25 British Empire Exhibition, but there were no excited crowds when we took it. Trains were running at regular intervals and we assumed it was better patronised immediately before or after the event. Whatever the explanation, we enjoyed

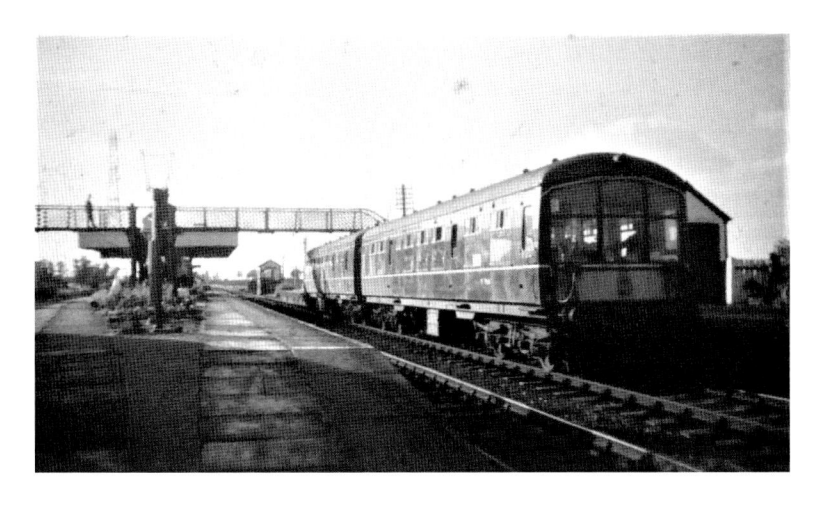

*A Bletchley bound diesel multiple unit pauses at Verney Junction in 1961. Try as one might, it was hard to raise much enthusiasm for diesel multiple units. They would sit there, mumbling to themselves and then lumber off, sounding like buses. Noting down their numbers was not like recording the acquaintance of a machine with personality.*

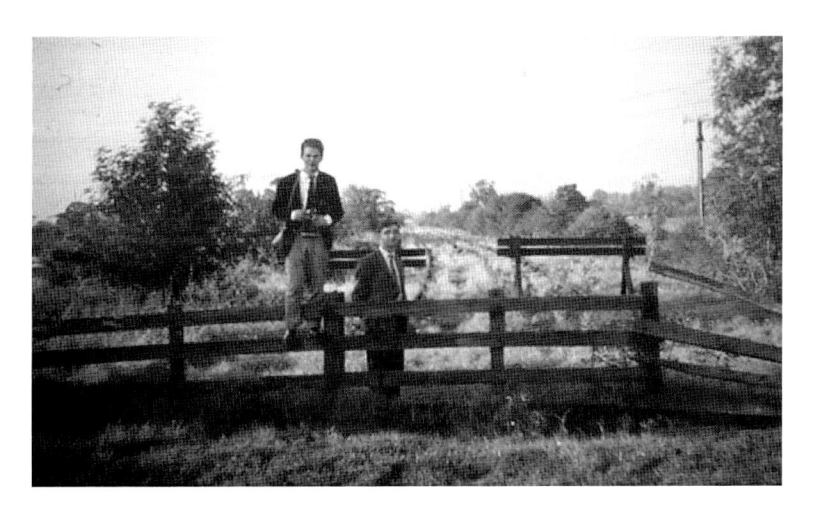

*The end of the line in 1960. The mile long double track stub of the Verney Junction-Quainton Road route finished abruptly just short of the site of Winslow Road station. It was used for carriage storage until 1961. No passenger trains had passed that way since July 1936 and freight traffic had ceased in September 1947. Fellow enthusiasts, Blair Jeary and Ken Mead, are wearing shirts and ties, sports jackets and polished shoes – fairly standard dress for young men at that time.*

a slow plod in a virtually empty train behind an L1 class 2-6-4 tank engine to Wembley Stadium station and then back to Marylebone, without seeing any other engines.

There had been nothing for it but to take the Underground and head for Wembley Park. A few minutes' walk from there brought us to Neasden Motive Power Depot, where we saw a couple of elderly Great Central 4-4-2 tanks, resting between turns of duty on the Chesham branch shuttle, along with some forlorn looking 0-6-2 Great Central tanks, which echoed those seen at Gorton the previous year. A number of L1 2-6-4 tanks, which were used to take Metropolitan trains on the non-electrified section beyond Rickmansworth to Aylesbury, were the other residents.

What was striking on that occasion had been a sprinkling of visiting B1s, Black Fives, and even a Jubilee, which had brought special trains to Wembley Park and were being serviced at Neasden shed in preparation for their return journeys to the Midlands and north of England.

From 1958 the former Great Central route had fallen under the auspices of the London Midland Region. It was no surprise that, by the time of this present visit, most of the Great Central tanks had been replaced by LMS types and the ubiquitous Black Fives dominated the larger engines present.

Interesting cops were becoming harder to find, without embarking on long distance travel. I had been taking photographs for some time and one of the first things my pictures had revealed was just how dark, gloomy and often downright dirty, was so much of the railway environment. So much too was dilapidated, poorly maintained or just worn out, that I started to detect a certain personal despondency towards the entire railway scene.

Many an engine crew too, must have wondered how much longer they could go on cross country jaunts and up and down branch lines, hauling essentially empty trains.

It was a working museum where steam was staggering towards inevitable extinction in the not too distant future. My thoughts turned increasingly to past travels and observations and I enjoyed reading up on railway and locomotive history. That was the trouble though; it was *all* becoming history. Diesel power was increasingly in evidence and station modernisation and rebuilding were beginning to get under way. The railways, as we had known them, were so much ingrained in my consciousness that it was hard to grasp just how dramatic forthcoming changes were to be.

I think it was this awareness of change, even when not conscious, which led us to poking around in obscure corners of the system, in an attempt to conjure up the past, even when the locomotives and trains had long since vanished. We could not have been alone in this, since from about that time, there started to appear on the market a seemingly endless flow of locomotive and associated railway publications.

Turning to South London, we were to visit Crystal Palace High Level station. This had been abandoned after the withdrawal of services in 1954. Whilst not an obvious victim of vandalism, it was fast decaying and notices warned of the unsafe structure. The modest entrance and ticket office lobby gave onto a wide gallery with steps down to the platforms. With missing floor boards and rotting timbers, rumours of rats, the tracks all lifted and much of the roof glazing missing, there was little inducement to explore the interior in detail. Instead, we looked around the outside, and traced where the sidings had been, along with the former turntable pit, just beyond the south end of the station which had, of course, been a terminus.

Designed for the anticipated crowds visiting the re-located version of the 1851 Great Exhibition, the platforms were arranged so passengers could alight quickly from both sides of their train. The main entrance to the building seemed rather poky until we discovered the remains of the broad flights of steps at the London end of the platforms. These led to the pedestrian passageway, under Crystal Palace Parade, which had been provided for direct access into the Exhibition site, on the opposite side of that road. Access was blocked but the view into the subway was breathtaking. It was (and remains) a wide vaulted concourse, exquisitely built with precision brick work and reminiscent of a medieval undercroft. Here, at least we could imagine the visiting crowds. Continuing up the steps, a scramble over a low wall saw us on the pavement opposite the former Exhibition site. At this point we were walking at the eaves level of the station building, rather oddly passing next to the large stone ball finials which topped the flanking wall of the building, like giant cannon balls.

Again, in the London area, we explored the still substantially intact station buildings of Cranley Gardens which, like Crystal Palace High Level, had also lost its passenger service in 1954. The former Alexandra Palace branch on which they stood, represented a sort of northern counterpart to the Crystal Palace branch. Ghost stations like that had a strong presence, as if waiting for a train which was never to come. On another occasion, we made our way to Kensington Olympia to catch one of the unadvertised services over the West London Extension line, to Clapham Junction. The engine at the head of the train was just a familiar Nine Elms Standard tank but we were pleased to have made the effort. At the time, joining one of those crowded evening steam hauled trains, full of postal workers, was the only way to traverse this route, which was such an anomaly amongst the otherwise all electric Southern suburban lines. It was a line which displayed vestiges of war damaged or abandoned stations, just as we had previously encountered on the route from Broad Street. They all exuded a forlorn nostalgic presence, compared with the then still reasonably presentable Cranley Gardens station buildings.

Our train stopped at the most southerly platform at Clapham Junction whereas, in the reverse direction, it would depart from the most northerly platform. There, below the tracks, a pedestrian passageway revealed a row of destination names above firmly shuttered booking office windows. The last one read 'Kensington Addison Road', a name which had been officially superseded by 'Kensington Olympia', as long ago as 1946. Exploring still brought its little rewards.

It was also at this time, we became more aware of the embryonic preservation movement, with visits to the Bluebell railway and the Kent and East Sussex. We had no idea of just how dependant we would become on them, for our occasional dose of steam in the future.

I had spent seven years as a spotter, patiently awaiting the next fluster of activity from my lineside position, feeling comfortably at ease taking in the overall scene. It was true there had been moments, if the wait became too long, when the reality would dawn on me. Within the next few years, all this would be replaced by electric and diesel power, engine sheds and works as we knew them would disappear, stations would vanish, and so on. The straws were already in the wind and these thoughts were occurring with greater frequency. Before long, that next steam-hauled train I was waiting for, was not going to arrive – ever again.

So it was, on this rather downbeat note that my spotting days dwindled to their close. There were already fewer spotters at the old haunts and they were younger and apparently quite excited by the new diesels. Richard Beeching's 1963 report, 'The Reshaping of British Railways', unleashed a public outcry which has not entirely subsided to this day. It was a reaction, much inflamed by resistance to change, degrees of potential inconvenience and one might suggest, not least by a deeply ingrained subconscious attachment to the steam train in the British psyche – reminders of bucket and spade holidays, long distance trips to visit family, the moving plume of steam in the landscape, and so on.

None of this confronted the hard economic realities at a time when one third of the route miles carried 1 % of total passenger miles and in a period when road transport and package holidays abroad were fast displacing traditional travel patterns. With the benefit of hindsight, some of Beeching's judgements may have proved inappropriate. So too, some of his methodology might be questioned, but change there had to be.

There were no grounds for loco spotters to draw a long face at the mention of Beeching's name, as far as locomotives were concerned. By the end of 1963, the year his report was published, fewer than 400 steam locomotives remained in service in any case.

As early as 1955 I had seen a poster at Doncaster station which announced the forthcoming withdrawal of services from Park Drain station. That unglamorous name was not enough to let the matter pass unnoticed. Although I already knew about numerous historical line closures, there was a certain shock in being faced with the immediacy of this announcement. How often was this going to happen? Soon enough, we were to find out.

In reality the Beeching report of 1963 simply accelerated this process which had been underway for some years. It was only at this point that the frequency of closure notices shocked us into awareness as to just how much the spotting scene was about to change. From the enthusiasts' standpoint, the attendant outcry, had they stopped to consider it, was more against the destruction of the spotter's 'habitat', rather than the demise of the steam locomotive, which was well on the way to its conclusion by the time of Beeching.

As if this was not enough, from September 1964 numerous engines started to appear with a diagonal yellow stripe painted across their cab sides. This was a prohibition sign against locomotives with insufficient clearance to run below the overhead wires on the newly electrified West Coast Mainline south of Crewe. Seeing these markings was a constant reminder that steam was very much in final retreat. Those steam locomotives which had survived to that point started to receive less cosmetic attention, presumably given the difficulty of recruiting young cleaners who, in the past, would have progressed towards work on the footplate. Missing nameplates did nothing to maintain morale, when cleaning might consist of nothing more than a wipe over the cab-side number.

My only regret was my absence abroad during the last two years of steam. I gather there had been some scintillating last fling performances with the Bullied Pacifics on the South Western main line out of Waterloo – the very line where my steam enthusiasm had been kindled as a young lad. On the other hand, I suppose if I had witnessed the Farewell to Steam specials in those final days, along with inevitable visits to breakers' yards and almost empty engine sheds, then the sense of loss would have been even worse. As it was, we all had to come to terms with changed times. For many of us it meant entering a period not unlike mourning and which, for some, took decades to overcome.

When mainline steam finally drew towards its conclusion, there was still a sense of shock and incredulity, in spite of the fact we had been watching it coming for the previous five or six years. Some spotters expressed indignation that so many sound and far from worn out engines were being condemned, pointing particularly at the London and South Western main line, which was apparently still functioning perfectly well under an essentially steam regime.

There followed a period of reflection, obviously involving regret but also coming to terms with the realities of the time. However youthful were quite a large number of locomotives, they represented old and uneconomic technology. They were victims of the wider struggle to make the railways pay and their loss had to be seen in that context. No amount of criticism of the shortcomings of marketing, political policy or financial investment, would have changed things very much. At best, it might have delayed the demise of steam for a few years. There was evidence of that in Germany where steam was phased out, rather than the all or nothing approach we adopted in Britain.

For the long-standing loco spotter, the replacement diesel locomotives were fairly soulless. Consequently, the excessive reliability issues they displayed at that time seemed to vindicate the steam die-hard. What is more, diesel and electric multiple units seemed even less appealing. There was still a number of private owner industrial steam locomotives at work, but they too were heading for extinction. In any case, they were an unknown quantity and industrial shunters had none of the glamour of the mainline.

Thus it was, those steam spotters of several years experience were left high and dry. Some must have closed their ABCs for the last time, and that was it. For those with more steam in the blood, there were withdrawal symptoms to endure. The growing achievements of the standard gauge preservation movement were apparent and so too was the increasing availability of railway publications. The sixties had seen a steady output of books, dealing as much with the railway environment as with locomotives and trains alone. Then, that relative trickle turned into a deluge of publications, spanning architecture, historical geography, railway engineering and, of course, locomotives and rolling stock, sometimes in the most intense detail.

Most of this output fed not just academic interest but went some way to satisfy the widespread nostalgia for all things to do with the steam era. Whilst this helped to some extent, the most effective way to nurture that nostalgia was to revisit old haunts, accompanied by one's memories. For the first decade or so after the end of steam there was much of the old infrastructure still in place. Certainly, in my case, I would find myself making detours during a road journey in order to visit a closed station or sometimes an empty former engine shed. What could have been more poignant than a still dripping water crane, an abandoned coal wagon bearing the marking 'Loco Coal' or sometimes a former loco tender without its engine, reduced to serving as a water tank?

When the occasion arose, it had always been fascinating to explore closed stations or railway lines, but then that was an extension of the spotting hobby and all that it entailed. Once steam had gone, there remained *only* such explorations and it was hard to accept that reality. The transition years of diesel haulage kept alive some of the old feeling of steam days, but it was no substitute.

The range of newly published material showed just how much pent up knowledge and railway experience was on offer. Whilst it would be foolish to suggest all that had been a product of train spotting, one can be confident that the bulk of the writers had been spotters at some time, even if only briefly. What was loco spotting, anyway? There were no rules. One did not *have* to collect numbers to be a spotter. An interest in trains inevitably drew locomotives to one's attention and that done, interest could intensify or evolve in many a direction.

So it was, one could simply accept times had changed, putting up with a feeling of bereavement and plunging oneself into books and visiting old haunts or, to be more actively engaged, one could still bring alive much of the material one studied by simply visiting railway locations. It was still very possible, armed with some knowledge, to derive enormous pleasure from exploration. For those whose interests had not remained dependant on the steam engine alone, it was perhaps easier to maintain those interests through further exploration.

More and more as time went on, the physical vestiges were eroded, so that some of those explorations would incline increasingly towards industrial archaeology. For example, at the peak of my loco spotting activity I was always aware of how few inroads I had made into Scottish loco classes. The situation was never remedied and then, as much as thirty years after the end of steam, even those locations previously visited, or sometimes known only from photographs, would be sufficient to evoke many a locomotive memory. It may not have been loco spotting, but nostalgia and the mind's eye are powerful companions.

In the spirit of attending to unfinished business, I set out from Leeds over the Settle and Carlisle line, which needs good weather to fully appreciate it. Most of the way it was wet and misty, so the grandeur of the scenery was lost. Nevertheless, even under diesel power one could imagine the challenge that route presented in steam days and the enormity of the engineering. Approaching Carlisle, I was taken aback by the unexpected sight of a red 'Duchess', simmering away on the adjacent track and presumably there in connection with a rail-tour special, though no carriages were in evidence.

If that was a nice little surprise, yet another was to follow. Connecting with a Glasgow bound train, it was announced that because of engineering works it was to be diverted by the former Glasgow and South Western route via Kilmarnock, a route I would not otherwise have ever expected to take. Next day, bound for Fort William, we started off with little fuss up the once notorious Cowlairs bank, this time by diesel multiple unit from Queen Street High Level. Consequently, not before reaching Dalmuir did I re-join the route from Queen Street Low Level and hence onward towards Arrochar and Tarbet, recalling that holiday of youth hostelling and push-and-pull footplate travel.

At Crianlarich, the now empty track bed of the former line from Dunblane was clear to see, as later were the earthworks where the Fort Augustus branch had left Spean Bridge, until it was finally closed to freight in 1947, just over thirteen years since the last passenger train had run. Then, running into Fort William, was another flurry of interest with the sight of a Black Five, no doubt serving the tourist train to Mallaig. That was all it took to stir memories of that train behind its Black Five, arriving at Dalmally from Dunblane, some forty years previously. Fort William was where the diesel multiple unit train reversed on its way to Mallaig, before taking in the Glenfinnan viaduct and the various remote stations on that line. It was noticeable how hardy-looking hikers would descend at these points, swing their rucksacks over their backs and promptly disappear into the landscape. There seemed to be scarcely a path or significant roadway in sight. It was not a landscape I would want to be out in at night or during a storm.

Mallaig station was something of an anti-climax and here it was a short walk to the bed and breakfast I had arranged. In fact, everything was a short distance from the station, which had been built to serve this fishing community. The next morning, chatting over breakfast with the proprietor, he asked what had brought me to Mallaig at the very end of the tourist season, so I mentioned my interest in the railway, expressing my admiration for the navvies who had worked in such bleak conditions. There was a moment's pause and then he spoke. "Yer know, 'twas all built on death." There was a touch of, "We are all doomed", in his voice, and I wondered what was coming next. "Ay", he continued, "it was built so the Lords and Ladies from down South could reach their estates for shooting the grouse." I thought that was enough of an explanation but he went on, "and then there were the fish trains to England." England sounded like a far off country and in any case the fish at least died in a good cause. I took another bite of toast and chose not to pursue the subject. Taking the ferry across to Skye in the crisp morning air was a good antidote to this gloom. Unsurprisingly the waiting bus driver confirmed that his was the very last connection with the boat until the next season. Travelling via Skye may have been somewhat roundabout but that was the simplest, perhaps the only way, to reach Kyle of Lochalsh, and hence the old Highland Railway route to Inverness and on to Perth.

Kyle of Lochalsh station was immediately recognisable, almost unchanged from the early photographs of it which I had studied, except for the absence of the Skye Bogie 4-4-0s. Those nine engines, introduced by the Highland Railway in 1882, were synonymous with the line and the last two had remained in service until 1930. So often, loco spotting could induce a feeling of, 'If only I had been there at the time of the grouping'. Sometimes, it could even be aggravating to think one had missed seeing a particular type of engine by as little as only a few months. There is still a fine steam railway legacy in Scotland, now mostly focussed on stations and civil engineering works. Many of the bridges and viaducts are remotely situated and easily overlooked. My circuit continued to Inverness and onwards to Perth, both of which had made important contributions to railway history, before continuing to Dundee. The plan was to return to Edinburgh by way of the two most famous railway bridges, the Tay Bridge and the Forth Bridge.

From Dundee, the diesel multiple unit to Edinburgh was full of passengers, sitting morosely or engrossed in magazines and newspapers. At that point the burden of history started to tell on me as I recalled the details of the Tay Bridge disaster of 1879. On that occasion 75 people were killed when a section of the bridge collapsed in a storm, when the train was half-way across. Although we were crossing on a replacement structure, much of it incorporated many of the original spans. I had to tell myself there was no cause for panic, but it did not help when the thought crossed my mind that maybe that was the reason why so many passengers chose to distract themselves with their newspapers. Certainly, nobody was admiring the view.

I felt none of that anxiety in crossing the Forth Bridge, just huge admiration for its engineering and a sense of disappointment that I had to be back home the next day. So, there was still unfinished business in Scotland, preserved locomotives to be seen and more railway exploration to be undertaken. Twenty years on, much fascinating infrastructure still remains to be seen throughout the country and surprising numbers of locomotives, albeit in a new context, remain to be spotted, perhaps still to be copped!

# CHAPTER THIRTEEN　　　　　　　　　　　Legacy

The nationalisation of Britain's railways in 1948 marked the beginning of an attempt to restore the national system to health after the ravages of World War II.

The first move was to get some order into the numbers of locomotives and carriage types inherited by British Railways. In the normal scheme of things much of that stock would have been withdrawn by the start of the Second World War. Consequently, the tired remnants of formerly more numerous classes were cut up, often before they acquired their newly allocated BR number.

The rest was a prolonged process, afflicted as it was by political interference and inadequate investment. Arguably, a lack of direction and systematic objectives did nothing to expedite the regeneration process. One significant consequence was the reprieve of the steam locomotive, which was something the enthusiast could be grateful for.

More than half a century since British Rail abandoned it, steam still has a huge following and it is little short of miraculous that several hundred steam locomotives have survived, a good percentage of them in working order. The nature of that following is bound to be different between those who knew the steam railway and younger devotees who have come to learn about it. Those who were there, experienced an environment and atmosphere which has all but totally disappeared, but which provided the backdrop for our activities.

The heritage and preservation groups do a tremendous job but it is inevitable that they can hardly hope to reproduce more than an echo of steam days. For example, a beautifully restored train and country station, its platform occupied by several dozen visitors, cannot be compared to the same scene fifty or sixty years earlier. In those days perhaps only one or two people left or boarded a train, itself less than spotless, and often hauled by a grubby locomotive. As often as not the station too could have done with a coat of paint. How could a heritage line attract visitors if it did not spruce up both trains and stations?

Headboards bearing the names of famous trains but with inappropriate locomotives or rolling stock, and even worse, cheeky faces applied to smokebox doors, take us further from authenticity. That said, one understands the commercial necessity of the situation. Much as we might regret it, it is probably inescapable that most heritage groups become increasingly part of the entertainment industry. Complete authenticity is indeed very difficult to reproduce and perpetuate, and even then it is vulnerable to rose-tinted interpretations of the past. Nevertheless, misplaced enthusiasm, like an overcrowded display of enamelled advertising signs or the questionable placing of picnic tables, are easily avoidable examples which detract from authenticity.

An interesting aspect of the heritage world can be seen in its in-train catering. I have seen examples of magnificent buffet cars with neither a rock cake nor a limp sandwich in sight. Sadly, nor were there any other refreshments on offer. Either of those alternatives could have been seen as authentic but they would have done little to increase revenues. When it comes to restaurant car services, that is another story. Many a heritage line makes great efforts with its dining car operations and some really do manage to recreate much of the historic experience. However, increased foreign travel since steam days has exposed travellers to rather more sophisticated menus than are generally offered at the prices charged, in spite of the grand language of some menu cards. Still, it would be churlish to be critical in that regard since some restaurant car catering loses period authenticity only by exceeding expectations. It is another illustration of the constant struggle between authenticity and commercial viability.

The more formal, and essentially static preservation scene, as represented in specialist museums, again does an excellent job, especially for the more informed student of railways, and locomotives in particular. One thinks for example of 'Head of Steam' at Darlington North Road, the National Railway Museum at York and its locomotive reserve collection at Shildon, and 'Steam' at Swindon. The latter, for example, does a splendid job of encapsulating the whole of the Swindon Works story and yet one can read complaints from visitors that there is not enough for children to do, not enough steam engines to climb on, and so on. There are huge expectations of both constant novelty and passive entertainment. Consequently the difficult balance between casual family leisure and the bringing to life of history, is a huge and possibly insoluble challenge. In addition, one should not overlook the outstanding achievements in the field of rolling stock restoration. The Midland Railway Trust at Butterley, for example, along with others, have fine collections. Even so, there remains for some the difficulty of reproducing authenticity, by way of at least half a dozen compatible vehicles to create a convincing period train.

Given the large numbers of preserved steam engines, along with their electric and diesel successors, one might have expected a new generation of spotters, keen to seek them out, but that has not materialised in anything like the previous numbers. Old time copping and bunking cannot be reproduced. We have more opportunities to read up and study photographs. We know, for the most part, where to pin point our quarries and the whole process is reduced to collecting predictable numbers.

That modest level of engagement is, I am sure, a major reason why many spotters in the past pursued the hobby for no more than a year or two having, in the process, failed to look beyond simple lists of numbers. Others might not have had access to many locos or the opportunities to seek them out and hence experience the appeal of the wider railway scene.

Certainly up to the 1950s, country stations, well patronised or not, were still characterised by all manner of furnishings and equipment, which could impart a misleading

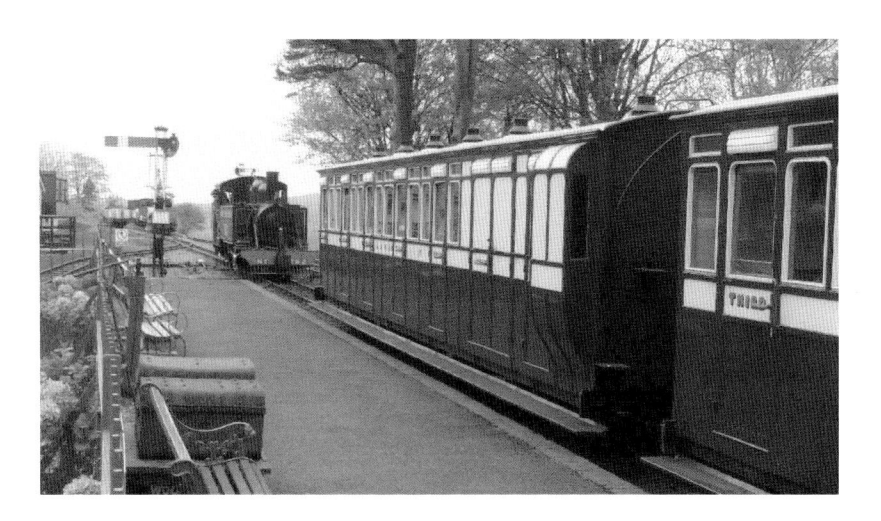

*These splendidly restored carriages are seen at Woody Bay station on the revived section of the Lynton and Barnstable railway. It is questionable whether, given the passenger numbers, the generous provision of platform benches was ever justified.*

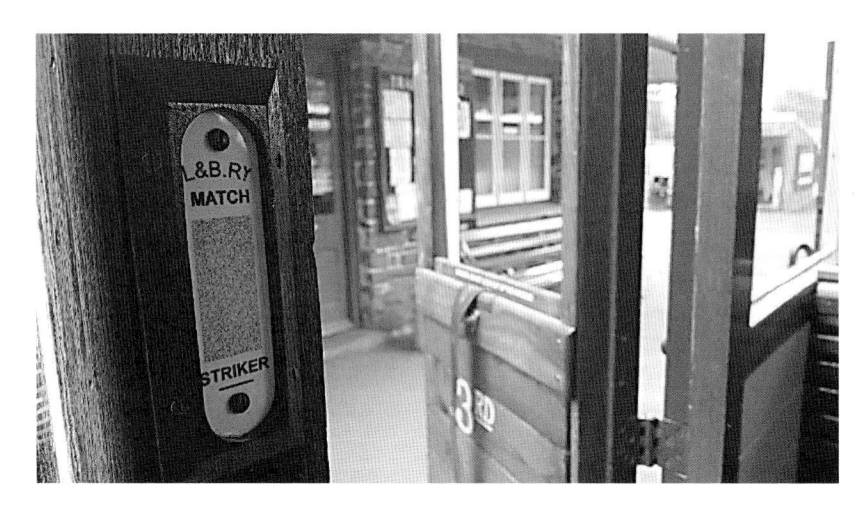

*This match striker is a nice detail, along with the door with its 3rd Class marking. Second class had generally been abandoned in 1918 but it was still felt necessary, even in the face of bare wooden seats, to remind passengers of the class distinction. No anonymous Standard Class in those days! Notice the leather strap, which was a familiar way to raise and lower carriage windows well into the 1950s.*

impression of a station's importance, or busyness. Most of this was the legacy of pre-nationalisation practice.

Platform advertising, now promoting British Railways' services and the destinations served, remained commonplace. There would be a parcels scale to weigh packages destined to be forwarded by train and these would be left to wait on a platform trolley, conveniently near where the guard's van of the awaited train would stop. There would be porters' barrows and certainly platform benches for waiting passengers. Many such benches still displayed the arms or initials of their originating pre-grouping company, in their cast iron frames. Then there were the rows of red-painted fire buckets, filled with sand or water, but it was never self-evident what particular fire hazard they might be guarding against. There would be signs indicating ladies' and gentlemen's toilets and the platform exits, along with instructions to cross the line by the foot bridge, to buy a platform ticket or to show all tickets. Those instructions seemed to belong to a more innocent age. The occasional slightly startling encounter with a drinking fountain or 'Do Not Spit' order, took one back yet another generation. There might well have been a station cat too, and certainly platform brooms and galvanised buckets or watering cans were commonplace.

Loco spotters would generally be attracted to rather more important stations unless there was plenty of through-train activity to observe. There, they might find, in addition to all this, train and platform indicator boards, chocolate vending machines, weighing machines and perhaps a metallic strip name plate printer and even, in some rare cases, a discreetly parked coffin trolley. Equally rare, but more conspicuously displayed at busy stations, was the odd stuffed dog, long since dead but still collecting coins for a railway charity from within its display case.

On the operating side there would be semaphore signals, water cranes, signal boxes, sidings and perhaps level crossing gates and a coal office, together with a one and a half ton crane and a goods shed.

All this paraphernalia applied, in varying degrees, to both suburban and country stations. Just its recollection conjures up the richness and complexity of the typical spotter's habitat. No wonder it created an ambiance in which a spotter would be happily distracted until the next train approached. There was no escaping from it all, even if spotters were famously identified solely with platform ends.

The void produced by the extinction of steam and its historical environment turned out to be the worst possible legacy for spotters. Without the infrastructure – the engine sheds, the big city stations, the goods yards, the loco works, the sounds, the smells and the motion of the steam locomotive, we old diehards are bound to find it hard to grasp why there are still occasionally spotters to be seen taking down details of anonymous looking sets of carriages or locomotives, for us, low on glamour or personality.

So, when the train did come, did it really used to be worth the wait? At a quiet location the sound of dinging bell codes in a nearby signal box would draw attention to pending activity. Perhaps a glimpse of the signalman reaching for a lever would correspond with the clunk of points being set, followed by a twitching of signal cables, carried on rattling pulleys affixed to the wall of the platform opposite. There followed a period of two or three minutes of silent but growing anticipation. Would it be a freight, an express or a local stopper? Would it be a cop?

That flash in the distance – was it the sun catching a car's windscreen? Was anything happening on that hazy horizon? Then, there it was, a wisp of white, unmistakably moving and perhaps still a mile away. The tiny dark patch started to take on form as it grew slightly larger. We strained our ears for a sound and were rewarded with silence. Now a shape was visible, unidentifiable but approaching fast with a plume of steam and an exhaust beat which came and went with the wind. There was just time to notice a fleeting rumble, a vibration in the nearby rails and there it was surging towards us, exhaust beat strong, looming up upon us with a screeching whistle to focus the moment to glimpse the number. How could it all have taken so long, when it was with us for a split second right in front of us, next to us, gone – trailed by flashing carriage windows, clicking bogies and a flurry of platform dust and summer pollen?

Only the faintest hint of sulphurous air remained to confirm what we had just witnessed, as the clang of a semaphore signal fell to 'danger' and invited us to wait for a re-run of the entire sequence.

Is that fact or the product of nostalgia? Happily it could well be both.

What is interesting is just why so many of those recollections of steam spotting, should remain so indelibly vivid in the memory. They could have been last week. Even now, a distant plume of steam in the landscape can spontaneously evoke an initial curiosity as to the engine producing it, quickly deflated by the realisation it is fifty odd years too late … or is that always the case?

Along with the still slowly growing numbers of restored engines, is a tiny trickle of new-builds. The expensive recreation of long since vanished loco types, may be criticised as unauthentic, wasteful, backward-looking, romantic, nostalgic, and so it goes on. It is possibly all these things. Who is to judge? These projects give enormous satisfaction to their participants at all levels. They preserve skills, increase knowledge, provide jobs, bring people together and all that before providing pleasure for people of all ages.

Maybe there is just one valid reservation. The reproduction of a truly unique loco might leave one uneasy. There was only one 0-10-0 Lickey incline banker, only one 4-6-4 LNER 'Hush-hush', and so on. They were one-offs with their very own personalities and histories. A historically late addition to a previous class does feel more comfortable since there is no pretence at it being something it is not. Interesting as it is, a working replica of the 'Rocket' is still not **the** Rocket.

Amongst the former natural haunts of loco spotters, it is hardly surprising there has been tremendous change. Plenty of stations, for example, do remain recognisable. However, bereft of their goods yards, water cranes, semaphore signals, oil lamps, period signage and publicity material, they are sanitised versions of the places we knew and certainly free of the attendant sounds and smells which are so evocative of the past.

This extends to even the most monumental locations. There is hardly a London terminus which has not undergone major updating or indeed, in the case of Broad Street and Holborn Viaduct, simply disappeared. Similar observations apply to the major provincial centres. Today's Birmingham Snow Hill is no more than a reference to its namesake. Only a clock tower remains of Nottingham Victoria, Manchester Central is now an exhibition hall and Glasgow St Enoch has vanished, and so it goes on.

Comparison between past and present may engender fond memories but too much nostalgia lays us open to maudlin discomfort. Nostalgia apart, we old hands are privileged to have witnessed, at close quarters, the operation and environment of the last years of main line steam in Britain. If something of it can be preserved, it will at least resonate with that streak in our national psyche which will always delight in Edward Thomas' 'Adlestrop', WH Auden's 'Night Mail', or railway references by Charles Dickens, Conon Doyle or Agatha Christie.

The train spotting fraternity has essentially disappeared from public consciousness but not so the steam railway. In the summer of 2016, Flying Scotsman returned to main line excursions after a long overhaul. During a lengthy signal check at Reading West, I observed a woman waving to it continually for a good ten minutes, from her bedroom window. I am sure she expressed the feelings of thousands of people, welcoming back an old friend and what it symbolised.

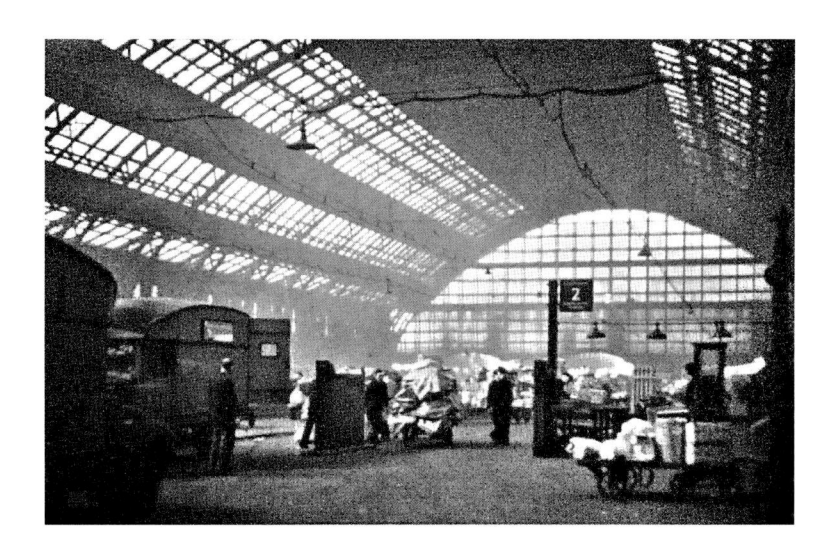

Manchester Central in 1962. There is plenty of mail and parcels traffic but unusually, not a train to be seen. The roof was somewhat more modest than its counterpart at the London end of the Midland Railway route. Unlike at St Pancras, it was elliptical rather than slightly pointed and in addition a glazed end screen reached down to train roof height.

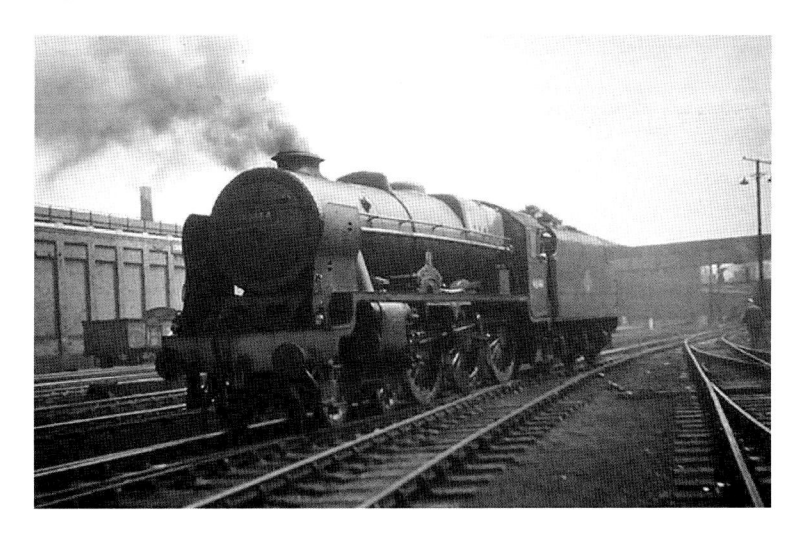

Rebuilt Royal Scot 46144, Honourable Artillery Company, leaving Camden motive power depot on 12 April 1959, its tender well filled and preparing to back down to its train at Euston. The Scots were stalwarts of Euston to Liverpool and Manchester expresses and equally from St Pancras to Manchester by the Midland route.

Globally the changes are for the better and it is meaningless to pretend the railways, as a public service, are not much improved on those of half a century ago. We live in different times. For that reason alone, loco spotting as the social phenomenon it was, belongs to the past ... good fun while it lasted.

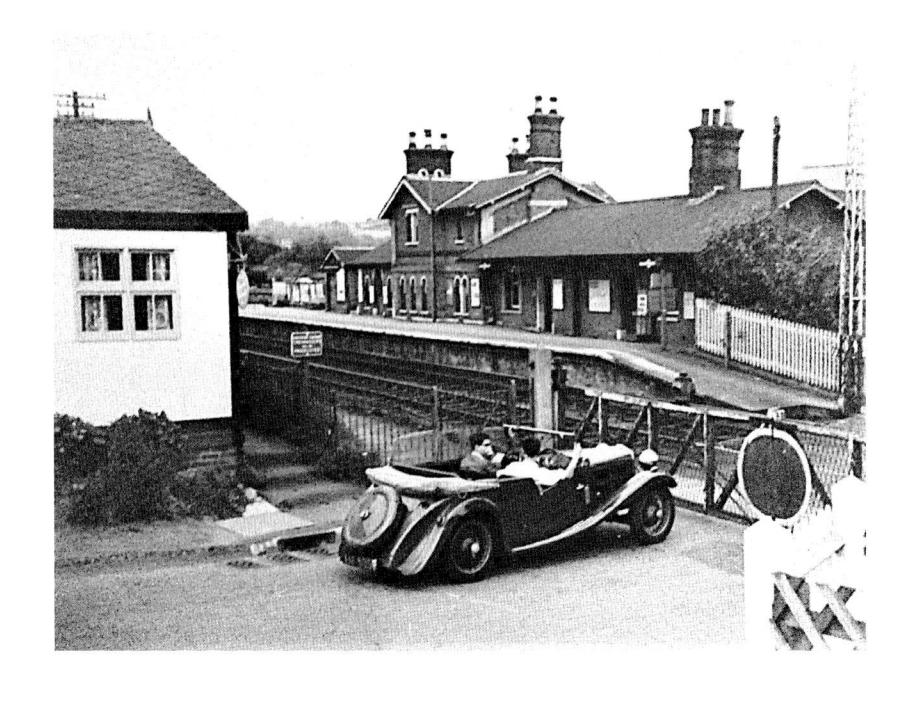

*The author with friend, Ken Mead, at Robertsbridge in August 1962 off to explore the Kent and East Sussex line and the remains of the Hawkhurst branch. The car, incidentally, was a 1934 Triumph Gloria.*

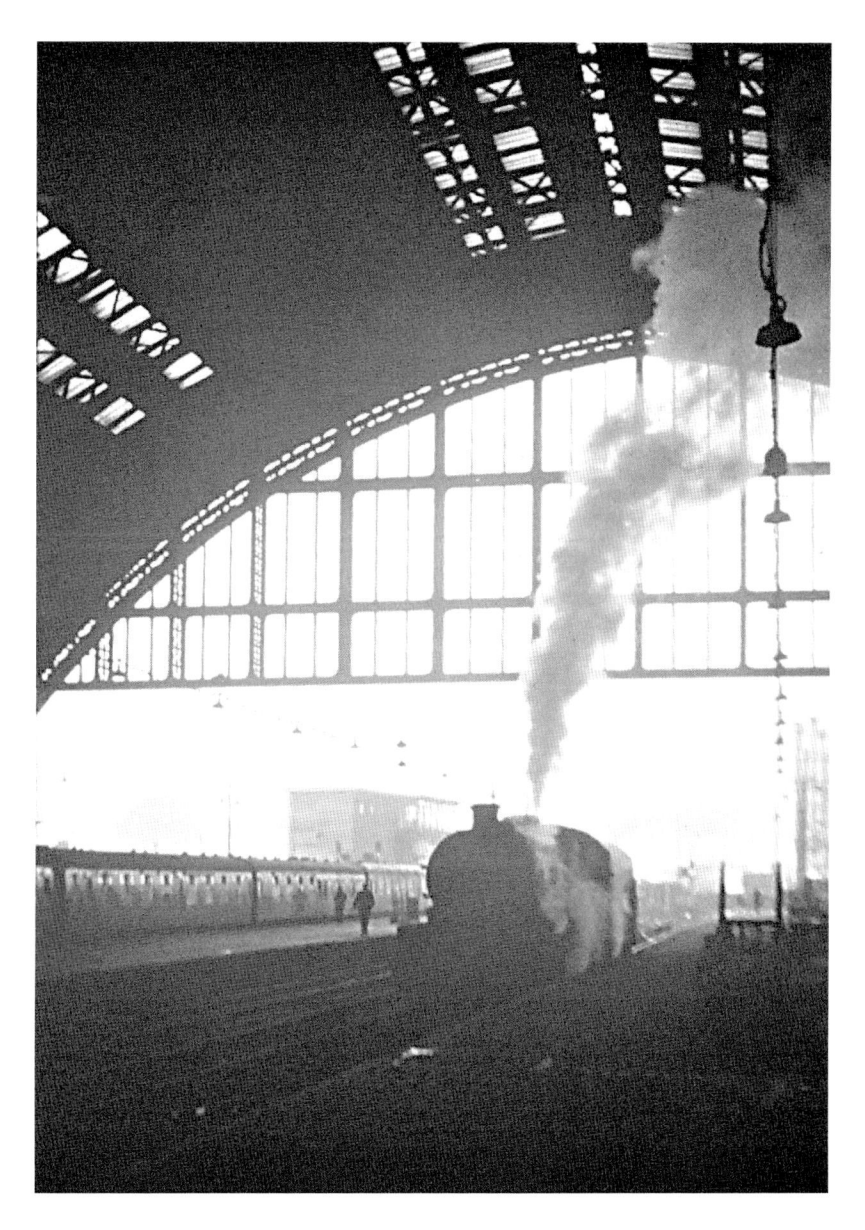

*All but silence reigned under the 243ft roof span of St Pancras, in this late 1950s view. There was never enough activity to sustain the interests of spotters who were better served by visits to Kentish Town and Cricklewood sheds. It provides stark contrast with the international terminal now occupying these platforms.*

# POSTSCRIPT

At the height of the loco spotting phenomenon, few casual observers would have had the slightest idea why people collected engine numbers. Put that bluntly, it was unlikely spotters themselves could have explained why they did it. Why people collect things at all is the wider question. Perhaps psychologists can offer meaningful explanations.

It might be coins, postage stamps, bus tickets or cookery books. The list is endless but there is usually a diversity within the chosen subject. At first sight one might as well collect car registration numbers from the infinite lists available. In such a case there is little inherent information in the numbers and any incidentally acquired knowledge about the vehicles themselves has no connection with the activity of number taking.

Some people collect glass marbles because they like the colours, or even novelty rubber erasers because that makes them smile, but it is hard to imagine that sort of collecting could inspire wider interests or sensibilities. The aesthetics of the steam railway, however, were very special. Some heritage lines have preserved some of the atmosphere, albeit often in a sanitized tourist orientated form. Model railway enthusiasts are a related group whose skills recreate that atmosphere in model form, representing another example of a spin-off interest.

Some youngsters did go no further than collecting numbers for their own sake and, indeed, the appeal waned after a year or two. For those who persisted, one suspects there was an element of camaraderie at play. Instead of hanging out on street corners, or kicking a ball around, the railway environment provided the venue whilst the visual activity substituted for the background chit chat. It also suited the more introverted, or at least the less expansive personalities, along with the *non sportifs*.

The fact that steam locos fell into distinct types or classes meant the numbers were identifiers. Specific engines were easily pin-pointed too. It did not much matter if numbers were in neat blocks or if a class was apparently numbered randomly. The existence of quantities, measurable against specific numbers, allowed the class size to be determined and hence the rarity of certain locomotive types. Rarity stimulated curiosity. Was an engine a one-off prototype or a survivor from a previously numerous class? Why did a prototype not proliferate? What caused the decline of a once larger class? Where did a particular locomotive fit in the evolutionary chain?

Then again, who were the designers and how did their personal talents affect innovation and developments? Was this evident when observing particular locomotives? Many of these answers hung on personal research, whereby the single minded pursuit of spotting engines led to more lines of enquiry. It could be not unlike any pastime when followed intensely.

Curiosity led to questions of location; where the quarry might be found – the hunting instinct. That in turn imparted a degree of geographical knowledge. It also exposed us to industrial and engineering environments we might otherwise not have encountered, such as railway works, locomotive sheds, freight handling yards, busy stations and so on. What engines were designed to haul led to interests in rolling stock, both passenger and freight. Locations themselves could raise interest, whether it was the complexity of a dock yard and what made certain locomotives suitable to work there, or perhaps a sharp eye which spotted a coherent order in the station architecture along a particular route.

The point is that the initial pastime of loco number collecting could readily lead to an explosion of curiosity or interest in multiple inter-related subjects. Other collecting hobbies too have the potential to expand curiosity and knowledge beyond the immediate subject matter. In a way one might see parallels between railway enthusiasm and learning a language. There was a sort of osmosis which occurred through constant and repetitive exposure, in the case of railways, to particular routes or locations. One could choose to be very knowledgeable about certain aspects of locomotives and the wider railway scene or to be content with a more diffuse appreciation, but either way, a lot of knowledge seemed to be unconsciously absorbed.

Wherever one fell on that spectrum, there was an aesthetic element at play. With the initial motivation of loco spotting it has already been described how protracted waits between trains and loco activity could lead to a more studied examination of the static surroundings. Similarly, between outings, there was the drip feed input stemming from magazine articles, books and imagery. Things started to link up in a way where even aspects of school history and geography lessons could make more sense.

To-day, people spend significant sums of money on railway models, way beyond the means of most teenage boys. Others, of the older generation in particular, will pay high fares for the pleasure of a steam-hauled excursion behind an engine type familiar in their youth.

Nostalgia and evocation of times past, whether in model form or memory, is a powerful force which can perpetuate the rail related interests of lost youth. If subsequent generations have discovered train watching, their activities presumably hold some parallels to those of steam spotters of old. Nevertheless, the publications covering modern topics and the occasional lonely figures on platform ends suggest that spotting without steam has lost most of its appeal, which leads us to the question of what was so special about steam?

There is an elemental quality about the inter-relationship of earth, air, fire and water, to produce movement. The rhythmic motion of coupling rods and valve gear implies life. By some psychological path one can start to make the connection between machine and person. Again, in steam days one could see the footplate crew at work. Their locomotive had to be coaxed and handled as was the case of their predecessors, the stage coach drivers and their horses. It was a rapport between living things. There was good reason for a steam locomotive out of steam being described as 'dead'.

Locomotives and trains, like stage coaches, were regularly given names. Although these would often celebrate places e.g. City of Chester, or abstractions e.g. Renown, considerable numbers of others represented living creatures, be they birds, race horses, mythical or fictional personalities or people.

All this enhanced the temptation to anthropomorphise the steam locomotive, narrowing the gap between watching people and watching locomotives in steam. More than one children's writer has developed that theme. There existed a distinction between engines in steam, where the merest whiff of steam could be equated with a breathing creature at rest, and a dead engine, which immediately became no more than an artefact.

The interest in loco spotting came predominantly from teenage boys. Is it therefore so fanciful to suggest the steam locomotive played a role, useful for some, in the passage of adolescence? At a time of discovering new horizons, one's place in the world, perhaps a time of emotional adjustment and learning appropriate communication skills with adults, could not loco spotting have been a way to sublimate or detract from these concerns?

The recollection of meaningful numbers encouraged an orderly way of recording information and using points of reference. Travel broadened awareness and demonstrated personal independence, whilst travel time-tables imposed an order on the activities of the day. Be that as it may, many a young man must have acquired lifelong habits, interests and awareness via their hobby, be it through history, geography or engineering. Indeed, when steam declined and eventually disappeared, it was the residual 'steam in the blood' which kept the interest alive. It is a thought that to-day's passionate car enthusiasts happily embrace the term 'petrol head'. In our day, nobody was called a 'steam head'. We had to be a little cautious with whom we discussed our interest, especially as we got older, if we were not to be mocked as 'puff-puff watchers' or worse. Those not in the know will never understand what a privilege it was to have witnessed at close hand, the final decades of the steam railway in action, and all that went with it.

Ultimately, it remains difficult to describe the appeal of locomotive and rail enthusiasm during those years. The experience was unique to each one of us and yet we all knew we shared so much in common.

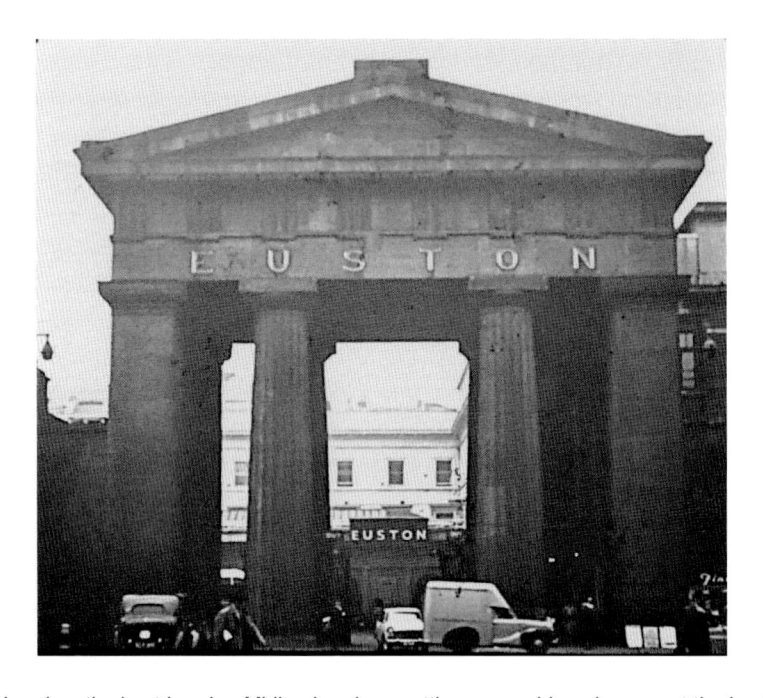

*In London, the best London Midland region spotting was achieved amongst the jumble of the old Euston. The Euston 'Arch' was built in 1837 as the gateway to the very first trunk railway, the London and Birmingham. Demolished in 1963, it all but lasted the entire steam age. Much of the masonry has since be located in the noble hope that reconstruction may yet one day be possible*

Dear Reader

It has been suggested that as many as 250,000 spotters were once active. They surely represented a slice of social history, worth further recording.

With this in mind, I am hoping to publish a collection of memories, reflections and anecdotes which would embrace a much wider geographical area than I was able to cover in this book.

If you have any fond recollections from steam spotting days, which you would like to share and contribute, I'd be delighted to hear from you.

Let's keep enjoying steam!

Maxwell Jackson
jacksonhms@googlemail.com

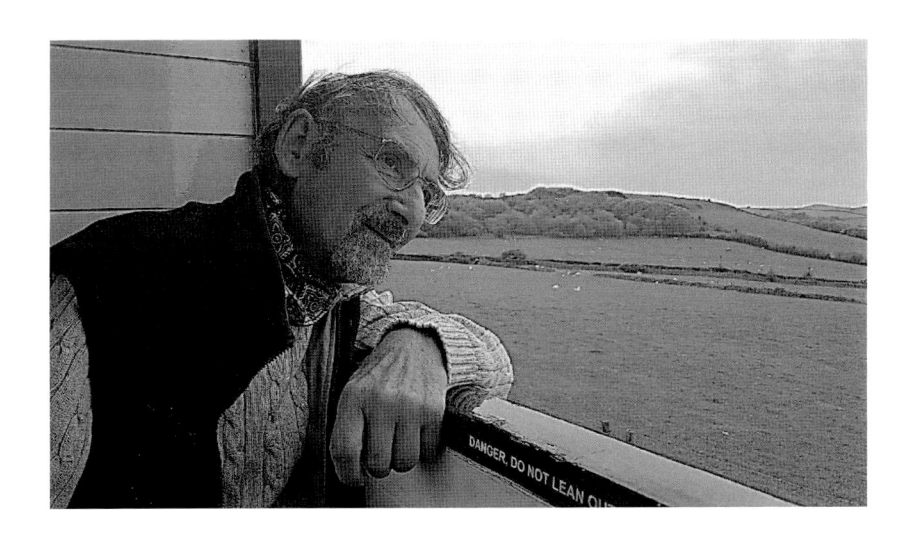